HARLAN LANE

The Mask of Benevolence

A specialist in the psychology of language and linguistics, Harlan Lane is Distinguished University Professor at Northeastern University. In addition to his work on deaf language, education, and history, he conducts research on cochlear implants in deafened adults at the Massachusetts Institute of Technology.

Besides his pioneering history of the deaf, *When the Mind Hears*, Dr. Lane is the author of *The Wild Boy of Aveyron*, a highly acclaimed study of the life of a feral child and the foundations of special education, and co-author (with Richard Pillard) of *The Wild Boy of Burundi*, on the psychological catastrophes of childhood. He is editor of *The Deaf Experience*, readings in translation on the history of the deaf, and co-editor (with François Grosjean) of *Recent Perspectives on American Sign Language*, a survey of contemporary scholarship concerning the language of the American deaf community.

Dr. Lane is the recipient of numerous awards, including the Distinguished Service Award from the National Association of the Deaf and, in 1991, a MacArthur Fellowship. Although he is not deaf, he speaks ASL and is well known to deaf communities in America and abroad. He lives in Boston, Massachusetts.

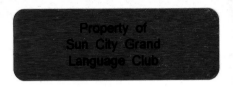
The Mask of Benevolence

The Mask
of Benevolence

DISABLING THE DEAF COMMUNITY

Harlan Lane

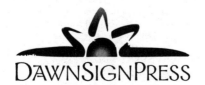

DAWNSIGNPRESS

Manufactured in the United States of America.
Published by DawnSignPress.

Library of Congress Cataloging-in-Publication Data

Lane, Harlan L.
    The mask of benevolence: disabling the deaf community / Harlan Lane.
        p.   cm.
    Originally published: 1st ed. New York: Knopf, 1992.
    Includes bibliographical references (p.) and index.
    ISBN 1-58121-009-4 (paperback)
    1. Deaf—United States. 2. United States—Social policy.
3. Social control. 4. Deaf—Education—United States. 5. Deafness—Treatment—
United States. I. Title.
[HV2537.L36 1999]
305.9'08162'0973—dc21   99-13183
                                                              CIP

10   9   8   7   6   5   4   3   2   1

I am indebted to a great many deaf people for their instruction, their patience, and their friendship. This book is dedicated to them.

The real political task . . . is to criticize the working of institutions that appear to be both neutral and independent; to criticize them in such a manner that the political violence which has always exercised itself obscurely through them will be unmasked so that one can fight them.

MICHEL FOUCAULT, 1974

Contents

PART ONE
Representations of Deaf People: The Infirmity and Cultural Models

PART TWO
*Representations of Deaf People: Colonialism, "Audism," and the
"Pyschology of the Deaf"*

PART THREE
*Representations of Deaf People: Power, Politics, and the
Dependency Duet*

Preface to the Second Edition
(revision January 20, 1999)

"The moving finger writes," Omar Khayyam warns us, "and having writ moves on," but writers *do* get to amend their works when there is a second edition—the case here with *The Mask of Benevolence*. In the eight years since the manuscript for the first edition was prepared, there has clearly been an escalation of the fundamental struggle concerning culturally Deaf* people. On the one side of the struggle, there are Deaf people themselves and their hearing allies; on the other, the technologies of normalization. Thus, paradoxically, both an additive understanding and a deficit understanding of culturally Deaf people have become further entrenched. On the additive side of the ledger, Deaf culture and language are surely better understood and documented and more widely appreciated. There is growing formal recognition of ASL in the United States. Many state legislatures have adopted resolutions recognizing the language and numerous high schools and universities accept ASL in fulfillment of the requirement to study a language other than English. Signed languages elsewhere in the world are likewise gaining recognition—for example, the European Commission has urged its member states to protect and encourage their national signed languages.

There are many more studies of the history of Deaf cultures here and abroad than there were just a decade ago. More political analyses of the struggle of Deaf cultures for autonomy. More about minorities in the Deaf-World. Numerous books about the experiences of Codas (hearing children of Deaf adults). More about ministry to Deaf people and more on culturally informed counseling and mental health services. More about Deaf peoples' gifts in perception and cognition and more about how their brains

---

*Since the first edition of *Mask*, the practice has become more widespread to capitalize *Deaf* when writing about the culture and the children and adults who are its members. The term *Deaf-World* is a gloss on the signs in ASL with which members of that culture refer to it.

process information. More linguistic and sociolinguistic studies of ASL and other signed languages. More on the acquisition of ASL as a native language. More dictionaries of signed languages and more textbooks and videotapes for learning those languages. More about the profession of interpreting and the ethics, skills, and knowledge involved. More biographies of great Deaf people. More publications about—and schools implementing—bilingual-bicultural education of Deaf children. More works of ASL poetry and narrative. More books of Deaf culture art. Our society is, further, witnessing the development of Deaf Studies programs in schools and colleges and the growth of the field as a professional specialization. There is more attention to winning fundamental human rights for Deaf people around the world. More Deaf leadership in programs for Deaf people. And the first comprehensive textbook about the Deaf-World has appeared (my book with Robert Hoffmeister and Ben Bahan, *A Journey into the Deaf-World,* DawnSignPress, 1996).

Yet, at the same time, the opposing forces that promote a disability model of Deaf children and adults have won two stunning victories, both in 1990—the inclusion of Deaf people under the Americans with Disabilities Act, and *carte blanche* for cochlear implant surgery on Deaf children. The much heralded Americans with Disabilities Act (ADA) is the fruit of one of the greatest, and saddest, ironies in the annals of minority oppression. The 1988 Gallaudet Revolution was fought and won on behalf of a cultural model of culturally Deaf people. As one of the students who led the Deaf President Now movement explained to the press, "There's more of an ethnic difference than a handicap difference between us and hearing people."[1] At that time, the ADA was "dead in committee" in the U.S. Congress.[2]   However, when the Congress witnessed the great outpouring of support nationwide for the Revolution, they were moved to pass—not legislation promoting what the revolutionaries sought—acceptance of their language and culture and, on the model of African-Americans whose banner they carried, self-determination—but rather legislation protecting the rights of quite a different group, with whom they felt no particular affiliation at all, people with disabilities.

All Americans, Deaf, hearing-impaired, and hearing alike, can support the ADA's provisions to guarantee rights to our fellow citizens with disabilities. But the Deaf-World faces a dilemma with regard to the provisions in disability law that concern Deaf people. On the one hand, disability legislation aims to provide Deaf children and adults with an education, access to information, and protection of their civil rights; they must have these provisions if they are to live fulfilling lives and be participating citizens in our democracy. Therefore, the Deaf-World supports such legislation. On the other hand, the Deaf-World is a linguistic and cultural minority quite unlike disability groups and with a distinctly different agenda. Moreover, to be Deaf is not a disability in Deaf culture, and most members of the Deaf-World see no disability in their way of being. To give up their legal rights would be self-defeating; to demand them under disability law seems like hypocrisy.

Worse yet, subscribing to the disability construction of culturally Deaf people undermines the Deaf agenda, which aims for acceptance of ASL and Deaf culture. It is because disability advocates think of Deaf children as disabled that they have sought, at times successfully, to close special schools and absurdly plunge Deaf children into hearing classrooms in a totally exclusionary program called inclusion. It is because government is allowed to proceed with a disability construction of culturally Deaf people that the U.S. Office of Bilingual Education has refused for decades to provide special resources for schools with large numbers of ASL-using children, although the law requires it to do so for children using any other non-English language. It is because of the disability construction that laws requiring schools to use their pupils' best language do not apply to children whose best language is a signed language; so Deaf children are mostly in classrooms with teachers who cannot communicate fluently with them. It is because of the disability construction that the teachers most able to communicate with Deaf children—Deaf teachers—are excluded from the profession on the pretext that they have a disqualifying disability or limited language fluency. It is because of the disability construction of culturally Deaf people that the U.S. Congress passed a further law in the wake of the Gallaudet Revolution establishing another institute of health, The National Institute on Deafness and Other Communication Disorders. That institute is operated by the deafness-as-disability industry, and it sponsors research mostly of interest to hearing people, not Deaf people. The institute even seeks to gravely diminish the ranks of the Deaf-World by research on the causes of hereditary deafness, and it pays for the cochlear implant surgery on Deaf children that is carried out by research teams around the nation.

Cochlear implant surgery has burgeoned in the United States and Europe since the first edition of *Mask*. The client base for the surgery has been expanded: Deaf children are implanted earlier; the trial of hearing aids originally required is often dispensed with; and children with residual hearing are being implanted. More manufacturers are involved in these programs and research in the field is more intimately connected with manufacturing.

Several new research studies of implanted children have been published. The poor initial results in speech perception with those born Deaf, reported in the first edition of *Mask*, were excused at the time by implant advocates with the contention that earlier implantation, longer use, and more rigorous oralism would deliver the desired results. Now there is some evidence on those claims: for most implanted children, the desired results are still far out of reach. There remains no research on the potentially negative consequences for implanted children's social and psychological development and delayed acquisition of fluent manual language. There is still no research on the comprehensive outcomes that are important to the patient and family—although the first children to receive multichannel implants did so thirteen years ago. There is still no published case history of one single child acquiring spoken language thanks to an implant.

The ethics of childhood cochlear implantation has been challenged recurrently in the bioethics literature of the past few years and defended by surgeons in the surgical literature. Deaf organizations around the world have studied the issues surrounding childhood implant surgery and have condemned it.

So much has happened with regard to both the science and the ethics of cochlear implant surgery on Deaf children and so many people are looking for a culturally aware account of those developments that this second edition of *Mask* has an entirely new chapter (written in collaboration with Gallaudet University Deaf Studies professor, Ben Bahan). Also, in the numerous reviews of *Mask*, some suggestions were made concerning wording and citations and these have been taken into account in the second edition.

Nevertheless, the fundamental terms of the struggle between a cultural understanding of culturally Deaf people and a disability understanding have not changed. Deaf children and adults still struggle for the right to be different, and the technologies of normalization still struggle to own the perceived social problem. What *Mask* has to say about misrepresentations of Deaf people, bigotry, the failure of Deaf education, and the abuse of bio-power is as true today as it was eight years ago. Increasing numbers of lay people, however, are hearing the message. A revolution in thought concerning Deaf people is taking place, a change in construction as sweeping as the change that put African-American citizen in place of slave property; that put gay minority in place of homosexual sufferer; that put equal partnership for women in place of narrowly stereotyped roles such as nurse and housewife. In this revolution of thought, deafness-as-disability is increasingly replaced by Deaf as linguistic minority. To quote the former secretary-general of the United Nations: "For me and my colleagues, Deaf people are not a disability group [but] a linguistic minority. And I understand that recognizing Deaf people as a linguistic minority goes hand in hand with respect for the Deaf community."[3]

Notes for The Preface of the Second Edition

1. G. Hlibok quoted in *USA Today*, March 15, 1988, p. 11a.
2. I. K. Jordan, The roots of equal opportunity in education. *Deaf Worlds*, 1997, 13, 27–32.
3. A. Mäkipää, Focus on the human rights dimension of deafness. *World Federation of the Deaf News*, February 1993, pp. 13–14.

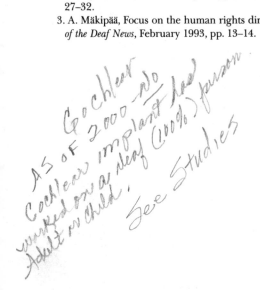

Preface

Our current views of deaf people, our ways of talking about them, are a product of history. In my book *When the Mind Hears,* I undertook to trace that history. In this book, I present the case that these views ill serve deaf and hearing people. I argue for a way of thinking about, and relating to, the members of the deaf community that is different from the one largely practiced now, an approach inspired primarily by the views of the deaf community itself, and by linguistic discoveries concerning signed languages.

Most Americans who have impaired hearing are not members of the American deaf community. They were acculturated to hearing society, their first language was a spoken one, and they became hard of hearing or deaf in the course of their lives, often late in life. This book is not about them; it is about people who grow up deaf, acculturated to the manual language and society of the deaf community. More exactly, I am concerned here with the relations between hearing people, especially those who claim to serve deaf people, and members of the deaf community themselves. The present hearing views of how best to describe, educate, and rehabilitate deaf children and adults are closely interrelated, as are the numerous professions that, proceeding on these views, shape and even regulate the lives of deaf people. Those views reveal a common premise: deaf people are disabled. The deaf community has quite a different premise, one that guides this book: the deaf community is a linguistic minority. Having recorded our changing ways of conceptualizing culturally deaf people across several centuries, I can hardly maintain that the conception I advance here is the "true" and final one. Nor can I peer into the future, a future in any case that I hope this book will contribute to shaping. The best I can do is to juxtapose my view of deaf people as a linguistic and cultural minority with the contrasting view, dominant in our society, that deafness is a tragic infirmity, and let the reader judge which conceptualization is more coherent and compassionate.

Although I am here engaging the issue of how best to conceptualize and relate to members of the deaf community, reflections on this matter rapidly lead to the broader and more fundamental question of the place we want to make in our society for the many distinct communities that constitute it. For those who think we'd best get on with making the *pluribus unum,* measures that seem to acknowledge and even reinforce our differences, such as bilingual and bicultural education, appear dangerously divisive. For those who think, as I do, that the heterogeneity of our society is its most valuable resource, the growing use of technology from the biological and social sciences to minimize and even obliterate our differences is alarming indeed. This book probes our commitment to tolerance by exploring how far we are ready to go in respecting the legitimacy of a linguistic and cultural minority that arises from a physical organization different from our own.

I am making public a private process. As a psychologist, I am concerned with the ways in which conceptions of mankind shape the measurement of man so that it seems to validate those prior conceptions. As an educator, I want to formulate wisely the unique challenge of educating deaf children, of making them literate and enhancing their ability to lead fulfilling lives in work, love, and play— as distinct from the broader challenge of educating young people in general. As a scientist conducting research concerning auditory prostheses, I mean to grasp some of the ways in which science and human values conflict or, at other times, harmonize. I am making the process public for two reasons. First, I hope to foster a bolder and more critical reexamination of current practices with deaf children and adults than has taken place heretofore. Second, I am aware that many of my deaf friends around the world, and deaf people who are dear to them, suffer needlessly from the practices of hearing people; indeed, so do the hearing people engaged in those practices. I do not presume to tell deaf people what to do. I offer here my understanding of how conflict has arisen between deaf communities and hearing societies. I hope it will be a tool in the hands of deaf people and their hearing allies who choose to use it.

Hearing people in the professions serving deaf children and adults have come to remain silent about the fundamental divergence between their view of deafness and that of the deaf people they profess to serve. They rarely discuss these disagreements with one another or with deaf leaders; life is more pleasant that way. This silence of hearing professional people is an adaptive response to an age-old feud, a wearying struggle that seems never to end, no matter how outlandish the steps taken to end it, because it is the inexhaustible struggle of a linguistic and cultural minority for self-determination. Many leaders in the deaf community, moreover, join in the conspiracy of silence, believing that the greatest progress is made when those in power are not offended but treated with discretion. Other deaf people fail to protest and to seek their rights aggressively, for they long ago abandoned the hope that hearing people would respect their culture and language and their ability to manage the affairs of deaf people. At the risk of offending many, out of my love for most, deeply convinced that hearing and deaf people can live better together by examining our differences in the light of day, I have chosen to break the silence.

The president of the World Federation of the Deaf, Dr. Yerker Andersson, has deplored the limited knowledge of deaf people possessed by hearing authors who write on deaf issues, and he proposes that we "come clean" and describe our own communication skills and knowledge of deaf people in our reports. I am happy to comply with that request. I was introduced to American Sign Language (ASL) and to members of the American deaf community in 1973 by Dr. Ursula Bellugi, who, with Dr. Edward Klima and deaf collaborators at the Salk Institute, was conducting pioneering research on the grammar and use of ASL. When I established a laboratory for research on ASL at Northeastern University a year later, my collaborators and ASL teachers were two young deaf women who have since achieved international distinction in education and the arts: Marie Philip and Ella Mae Lentz. In the ensuing years, I have been learning ASL and learning about ASL and its community of users. I have sought the answers to questions in my laboratory, in books and journals, in deaf clubs and the homes of deaf friends, and in schools for deaf children around the world. It has been my good fortune to come to know many deaf leaders in many countries. In general, I have found deaf people extraordinarily candid, patient, and generous in befriending me and helping me. I think this may be because hearing people are so rarely willing to really listen with an open mind to what they have to say; but I may be wrong. I sometimes find it taxing to understand what my American deaf interlocutors have to say in ASL, but I generally understand them and they always understand me. (I might say as much of my French interlocutors.) This reflects partly the skill of my ASL teachers, to whom I acknowledge my great debt, but mostly the competence of many deaf people in circumventing communication barriers. In deaf communities outside North America, I was necessarily served by interpreters, as I have often been here.

I recognize that my pursuit of knowledge about deaf people, however intense and prolonged, will never give me the knowledge of a deaf person. In response to an editorial of mine published in the *New York Times*, which urged a role for reinvented residential schools for deaf children, one deaf young man wrote me to ask by what right I, a hearing person, made pronouncements on deaf issues. I answered that he had a point: I could only know what it means to be a deaf person from the outside in, by means of mental constructions and empathic leaps; I could not know it from the inside out. Yet both kinds of knowledge are illuminating for both parties, the outsider and the insider. When hearing linguists, collaborating with deaf people, presented their first studies of ASL, many deaf people responded with interest and excitement. In the end, that research proved empowering for deaf people. Conversely, deaf people have a privileged access to what are the crucial issues and where the natural fault lines lie; they can guide the outsider to the richest vein. So there are two different ways of knowing a culture. The two modes tend to have different kinds of discourse. In the first, I, a hearing psychologist, might say, for example, that the average deaf high school student scores seven grades behind his hearing counterpart on standardized tests of reading English. In the second, a deaf adult might say: I don't often pick up a book; they never really taught us English in my high school; the teacher couldn't get his ideas across to the class.

As a hearing person and a member of the society that engulfs the American deaf community, I can take the double perspective on hearing culture that is required for this particular story of the relations between our two communities. When it comes to the deaf side of the story, I can look from the outside in and I can listen to the voices that speak from within—I mean deaf scholars, deaf leaders, and deaf friends. The deaf community will judge for itself whether I have been an attentive listener. I hope it is clear, then, that I cannot and do not speak *for* the deaf community. Deaf people speak for themselves in many books, magazines, newspapers, videotapes, and public lectures. I mention several in the pages of this book.

The deaf community is not, however, of one mind—any more than is, say, the Hispanic-American community. It may even be peculiarly diverse, as some deaf people come from deaf homes, others from hearing homes. And within the deaf community there are deaf people who are at the same time, if secondarily, Hispanic-American, African-American, Native American, Asian-American, gay or lesbian, and deaf people with physical or mental disabilities.

Hearing professional people who work with deaf people are also far from being of one mind. When I condemn the practices of hearing professional people in these pages, some of those people are unjustly accused—they are doing all they can to empower deaf people. And then there are, culturally speaking, hearing people who have lost some or all of their hearing, and these people may well say, "A pox on both your houses!" Another deeply concerned group, with its own variegated points of view, comprises the parents of deaf children; they, too, wish their voices to be heard and considered authoritative. It is difficult to urge reforms, as I do here, and still respect so many diverse, even conflicting, points of view. There is, at least, this much consensus, which can serve as a starting point: The relations between hearing people and deaf people in America, as elsewhere around the globe, are unsatisfactory. We urgently need to reexamine the principles that underlie those relations and where they are leading us. This book is devoted to that end.

Any writer in America today, and especially one who advocates a change in vocabulary for discussing the concerns of a minority, must tangle with the issue of pronouns and gender in English. I find none of the alternatives appealing—neologisms; doubling of pronouns; using the passive or the plural when the active or singular is clearer; using "she" when neither gender is intended in particular; or simply staying with the old practice of using "he" as the unmarked form, as if the matter had not been hotly debated. I have chosen to follow the dictates of clarity, at the risk of losing some valuable allies.

Acknowledgments

I am indebted to Northeastern University for appointing me University Distinguished Professor and releasing me from other duties so that I could conduct the research reported in this book. Some of that research was also conducted while I held the Powrie V. Doctor Chair of Deaf Studies at Gallaudet University, to which I want to express my deep appreciation. This book grew out of a suggestion by Arthur Rosenthal, vice-president and publisher, Hill and Wang; it is a pleasure to record my thankfulness. I gratefully acknowledge the instructive discussions and comments on sections of this book contributed by colleagues; I did not always agree with their remarks, but I invariably benefited from them. Warm thanks to: Mr. Ben Bahan, Graduate School of Education, Boston University; Dr. Michael Karchmer and Dr. Kathryn Meadow-Orlans of Gallaudet University; Dr. L. Peterson, Department of Social Medicine, Harvard University Medical School; Dr. Donald Eddington, Massachusetts Eye and Ear Infirmary; Dr. Mario Svirsky and Dr. William Rabinowitz, Research Laboratory of Electronics, Massachusetts Institute of Technology; Dr. Donald Sims of the National Technical Institute for the Deaf; Dr. James Gee, University of Southern California; Dr. Robbin Battison, of the International Business Machines Corporation, Stockholm; and Dr. Tony Smith, Tufts University.

I received many valuable suggestions concerning the manuscript from: Mr. Franklin Philip, of Boston; Dr. Richard Pillard and Dr. Robert Hoffmeister, Boston University; Ms. Marcella Meyer, Greater Los Angeles Council on Deafness; Dr. Vicki Hanson, International Business Machines Corporation; Dr. Moise Goldstein, Johns Hopkins University; Dr. William Isham, Northeastern University; and Dr. Carol Padden, University of California, San Diego. My editor, Corona Machemer, has helped me to conceive and craft this book, to be clearer and more graceful; moreover, she is one of those hearing people who, when presented with the facts, develops great empathy for the cause of deaf people.

The notes, including references, are arranged at the back of the book, keyed to the text by significant words and page number. References for every quotation, as well as for books and investigations, appear in the notes. When a note gives more than a reference—for example, supplementary remarks or a list of relevant works—this is signaled in the text by an asterisk.

PART ONE

Representations of Deaf People: The Infirmity and Cultural Models

A Different Center

On June 27, 1990, the United States Food and Drug Administration approved a proposal by the Cochlear Corporation to market a "bionic ear" for surgical insertion in deaf children over the age of two. More properly called a cochlear prosthesis, this device converts sound waves into electrical currents that are delivered to a wire implanted in the child's inner ear. With the headline "New Hope for Deaf Children: Implant Gives Them Hearing and Speech," *American Health* enthused: "Results promise to be even more dramatic for very young children [than they have been for adults]. The implants will actually allow them to speak." The modern miracle of biotechnology, you say, as do the media, and yet the National Association of the Deaf has called the FDA approval "unsound scientifically, procedurally, and ethically." Audiologists and otologists—those who measure hearing and those who treat it medically, experts who "have only the best interests of deaf children at heart"—proclaim a dramatic advance; yet the American deaf community, whose members could not love deaf children more, proclaim a dangerous setback to their interests.

Cochlear implantation is a surgical procedure, lasting about three and a half hours under general anesthesia, and it requires hospitalization for two to four days. A broad crescent-shaped incision is made behind the operated ear, and the skin flap is elevated. A piece of temporalis muscle is removed. A depression is drilled in the skull and reamed to make a seat for the internal electrical coil of the cochlear implant. A section of the mastoid bone is removed to expose the middle ear cavity. Further drilling exposes the membrane of the round window on the inner ear. Observing the procedure under a microscope, the surgeon pierces the membrane. A wire about 25 millimeters long is pushed through the opening. Sometimes the way is blocked by abnormal bone growth in the inner ear; the surgeon will generally drill through this but may have to settle in the end for only partial insertion of the wire. The wire seeks its own path as it moves around and up the coiled inner ear, shaped like a snail and called the cochlea, from the Latin for "snail." The exquisitely detailed microstructure of the inner ear is often ripped apart as the electrode weaves its way, crushing cells and perforating membranes; if there was any residual hearing in the ear, it is almost certainly destroyed. The auditory nerve itself is unlikely to be damaged, however, and the implant stimulates the auditory nerve directly. The internal coil is then sutured into place. Finally, the skin is sewn back over the coil.

Not long after the FDA gave the green light to surgeons to implant the Cochlear Corporation prosthesis in children, the manufacturer announced a promotional meeting in Boston and I attended. Two sets of satisfied parents and their implanted children were flown in for the occasion and seated center stage. "Barry," nine, had become deaf when he was six and a half; "June" was four and a half and born deaf. Both children had been using their implants for about a year, and both attended special programs for deaf children housed in ordinary public schools. Barry could understand much of what his teachers said, but June required a sign language interpreter. Both children spent several hours every day practicing listening and speaking, under their mothers' tutelage or that of therapists.

During the presentation, researchers from the Cochlear Corporation reported on their investigations with several hundred implanted children, and then the members of an implant team spoke in turn: first the surgeon, then an audiologist and a speech therapist, and finally a special educator. While the scholars held forth and the parents beside them listened attentively, I noticed the two children, half-screened from the audience behind their parents' backs, signing furiously to each other across the stage.

Will the typical deaf child, who was born deaf, like June, or who became so early in life, be able to understand ordinary conversation after undergoing the surgery and a lot of training? Probably not. Will he or she be able to speak intelligibly? Probably not. Will he learn English better than he would have without the implant? Probably not, but we do not know. Will he be able to succeed in an ordinary school with hearing children? Probably not. Will he then generally rely on vision rather than hearing? Yes.

Although the implanted deaf child will not move easily in the hearing world, it is unlikely that he will move easily in the deaf community either, unlikely that he will learn American Sign Language (ASL) fluently and make his own the fundamental values of that community. So there is a real danger that he will grow up without

Studies now complete w/ dire results.

any substantive communication, spoken or signed. He may develop problems of personal identity, of emotional adjustment, even of mental health—this has not been studied. You may well ask: If the benefits are so small and the psychological and social risks so great, why did the FDA approve general marketing of the device and why do surgeons implant it?

Why indeed? Why would such heroic medicine be practiced on young deaf children? For this to be justified, the plight of the deaf child must be seen as truly desperate. But surely, you say, the plight of the deaf child *is* desperate. The child is unable to communicate with his mother and father—nine out of ten deaf children have hearing parents. He will receive a "special" education —in fact an especially unsuccessful education that commonly leads to underemployment. He will take a deaf spouse and be shut off from the world of his hearing parents and the mainstream of American society.

No longer true

Most people who were born deaf or became so early in life, like the child we are discussing, and who grew up deaf as part of the deaf community have a different point of view. They see themselves as fundamentally visual people, with their own visual language, social organization, history, and mores—in short, with their own way of being, their own language and culture. Scholarly research since the 1970s in such fields as linguistics, anthropology, sociology, and history supports them in this claim. Yes, the deaf child faces many obstacles in life, but the lack of communication at home, inferior education in school, discrimination in employment, are obstacles placed in his way by hearing people who, if only they came to know the deaf community, could readily remove them.

In their book on American deaf culture, deaf authors Carol Padden and Tom Humphries say that hearing professionals who work with deaf people have a different "center" than their clients, which they illustrate with this observation: From a hearing point of view, it is better to be hard of hearing than deaf; someone who is "a little hard of hearing" is much less deaf than someone who is "very hard of hearing." Deaf people see things the other way around. When they sign that an acquaintance is A-LITTLE HARD-OF-HEARING† they mean

---

†English glosses for the signs in American Sign language (ASL) are conventionally written in capital letters. Hyphens connect glosses that are one word in ASL. It is important to note that glosses omit most of the grammar of ASL. They are *not* translations.

that the person has some of the ways of hearing people but basically is quite deaf. When they sign that someone is VERY HARD-OF-HEAR-ING, they mean that the person is very much like hearing people, scarcely like deaf people at all. The same opposing points of view of the hearing benefactor and the deaf beneficiary are revealed in this observation: Members of the deaf community commonly condemn a deaf acquaintance who is ORAL —that is, who does not fully acknowledge that he is deaf. They say disparagingly that that person ALWAYS-PLANS actions for every situation, in order to pass acceptably in a hearing world. Hearing experts, however, do not understand why some deaf people condemn others who are oral and trying to pass; they use terms like "afflicted" for the first group, deaf people who do not speak, and applaud the efforts of those who try to.

Two cultures, two points of view, two different "centers." This book is an exploration of the gulf that separates these two vantage points.

Hearing Representations of Deaf People

What are deaf people like? There are at least three approaches to answering the question. You may, first, reflect on the social identity of deaf people; they belong to a category, and the category has attributes that are part of our popular culture, as a result of the treatment of deaf people in literature and in the media. Second, you may make an extrapolative leap and try to imagine what your world would be like if you were deaf. Most hearing people, if they are led to think about deaf people, soon make this extrapolative leap, for they have little else to guide them; they have not read about deaf language and culture, and extrapolation must stand in for real knowledge. If it happens that you know someone who is deaf, a third way of apprehending deafness is open; it takes on the characteristics of that particular deaf person, as in: "John understands me when I talk to him directly; therefore, deaf people can lip-read."

All of these approaches commonly lead hearing people to the same point of departure in their representations of deaf people: Deafness is a bad thing. In hearing society, deafness is stigmatized.

The sociologist Erving Goffman distinguishes three kinds of

stigma: physical, characterological, and tribal. "There is only one complete, unblushing male in America," he explains. "[He is] a young, married, white, urban northern heterosexual Protestant father of college education, fully employed, of good complexion, weight, and height, and a recent record in sports." Any deviation is likely to entail a stigma, and we tend to impute many stigmas when we find a single one. All three categories of stigma are ascribed to deaf people. Physically they are judged defective; this is commonly taken to give rise to undesirable character traits, such as concreteness of thought and impulsive behavior. Hearing people may also view deaf people as clannish—even, indeed, an undesirable world apart, social deviants like those Goffman lists: prostitutes, drug addicts, delinquents, criminals, jazz musicians, bohemians, gypsies, carnival workers, hoboes, winos, show people, full-time gamblers, beach dwellers, gays, and the urban unrepentant poor. But even if the American deaf community were known for what it is, a linguistic and cultural minority with a rich and unique heritage, it would still be subject to a tribal stigma, as is, for example, the Hispanic-American community.

Stigma is relational. In the deaf community, to be called ORAL, we have seen, is unacceptable. ORAL means you have made the wrong life choices, you have uncritically embraced alien values that place a premium on speech. Hearing people fail to see what is wrong with deaf people's being ORAL; articulateness is prized in American society; gesturing is not.

In the hearing stereotype, deafness is the lack of something, not the presence of anything. Silence is emptiness. The deaf community, say Padden and Humphries, recognizes that "silent" "is part of a way of viewing deaf people that is pervasive in hearing society; they accept it and use it as an easy way for others to recognize them." Thus the magazine published by the National Association of the Deaf (NAD) was long called *The Silent Worker*. But for hearing people, "silent" represents the dark side of deaf people. They must not have the orientation and security in their environment that we have; of course, they can't appreciate music, we tell ourselves; nor can they engage in conversation, hear announcements, use the telephone. The deaf person moves about, it seems to us, encapsulated; there's a barrier between us. Hence the deaf person is isolated. Ivan Turgenev's character Gerasim, for example, was "shut off by his affliction from the society of men," as was Carson McCullers's deaf protagonist in *The Heart Is a Lonely Hunter*.

In the parlance of hearing people, ordinary deaf people can't really communicate; for them to attempt it is to engage in a *dialogue des sourds*—a deaf dialogue, meaning mutual incomprehension. Hearing people are called deaf, by metaphorical extension, when they refuse to listen, especially to moral advice. If great flourishes in English are associated with a refined mind, simple, awkward speech and gesticulation are associated with a simple mind. Because language and intellect are so linked in our representations of people (we are surprised to hear a towering intellect expressed—unless by deliberate intent—in a Southern drawl or in ungrammatical sentences), deafness seems a defect of intellect. The "dumb" of "deaf and dumb" appears to refer not only to muteness but to weakness of mind. Joanne Greenberg's deaf couple in *In This Sign* are ignorant even about childbearing. Paradoxically, in a reaction formation, deafness may also seem ennobling: the very simplicity of mind, the child-likeness, bespeaks a pure soul, one free of the artifices of civilization. Dickens's Sophy seems to have descended from heaven; Maupassant's Gargan is speechless, an ignorant shepherd, but strong, upright, pure in his misery.

In fact, we imagine two kinds of deafness. The more usual kind is linked in our minds with blue-collar jobs or even poverty. Eudora Welty's deaf couple in "The Key" are poor, naïve, "afflicted," and childlike. A deaf person may sell cards inscribed with the finger alphabet; or work in the manual trades, say as a printer. But then there is the exceptional deaf person who can speak and lip-read— who is just like you and me, except for some slight difference. (What a relief!) This person does not sell cards or labor with his hands; he is not poor or even middle-class in our imagination, but distinguished, elegant. Henry Kisor, book editor at the Chicago *Sun-Times*, confirmed this comfortable image of the deaf person in his 1990 autobiography, *What's That Pig Outdoors*. (The title was chosen to illustrate the perils of lip-reading.)

Our society is sufficiently rich and enlightened that we are prepared to sympathize with marginal people who endorse our norms but, for reasons beyond their control, cannot live up to them. The deaf actress Marlee Matlin won the admiration of many hearing people when she chose to speak aloud on national television, rather than through an interpreter, on receiving the Oscar for her role as a culturally deaf person in the film *Children of a Lesser God*. By the same act she incurred criticism from some members of the American deaf community. For them, in those few halting words she negated the principles of the story she had so brilliantly enacted; she chose symbolically not to accept the award as a member of the deaf community; and she seemed to endorse the view that any amount of English is better for deaf people than the most eloquent American Sign Language.

Late-deafened people who make an effort to speak English and lip-read, to overcome the hurdles of their handicap, are much less discomfiting to hearing people than the members of the deaf community, with their distinctly different ways and language. What is unforgivable is that members of the deaf community insist they are fine— for example, two-thirds of deaf adults interviewed in a 1988 survey thought their social life was better than hearing people's—when in fact we can give them a thousand reasons why they can't be. Goffman points out that the stigmatized are expected to keep a bargain: "they should not test the limits of the acceptance shown them, nor make it the basis for still further demands." Thus, the person who is disabled (in our eyes) is expected to *be* disabled; to accept his role as such and to conform, *grosso modo*, to our representation of him. In return we will class him not among the bad (prostitutes, drug addicts, delinquents) but among the sick. The sick and the infirm have a claim on our tolerance and, even more, on our "reasonable accommodation," our compassion, our help.

But we've got it all wrong. Come with me to the annual convention of the Massachusetts State Association of the Deaf, for example. Friends, frequently former schoolmates, embrace at the joy of seeing each other after long separation. There's a lot of catching up to do, and throughout the hotel there are groups of deaf people conversing intently in ASL. At the same time, there are workshops in various meeting rooms to explore issues of common concern, such as the political, social, and athletic program for the year; the governance of the association; outreach to hearing parents; wise personal investing; new technology of interest to deaf people; and deaf awareness— including the roles of various deaf organizations in community service like teaching ASL or counseling unemployed deaf people. At dinner, there will be a banquet speaker—the last time I attended, it was the deaf president of Gallaudet University, the world's premier institution of higher learning in the liberal arts for deaf students. Speakers commonly urge on the audience some course of organized social action—protests at the statehouse in behalf of funding for interpreters; activism in the schools in favor of ASL; letters to the networks to promote captioning—action to enhance the lives of deaf children and adults.

The pageant to choose Miss Deaf Massachusetts has been part of the annual convention in some years. Young women sponsored by various Massachusetts high schools (or high school programs) for deaf students are judged by a committee of deaf community notables for their knowledge of state and national deaf history, for their presentation of their background and career goals, and for the sheer delight of looking at them. The winner becomes a contestant in the national competition held during the convention of the National Association of the Deaf. It has been my pleasure to come to know Miss Deaf New Jersey of some years ago, now a colleague at my university, and Miss Deaf America of 1989, both extraordinarily keen and beautiful young women. When I left the packed auditorium where the 1989 winner was being selected, a deaf student leader hailed me and asked what I thought of the pageant. I told her I liked parts of it but felt a little uneasy at seeing young women displayed like so many pounds of beef on the hoof. "You've a lot to learn about deaf culture," she replied. "I think it's just fine!"

In the course of the state convention there may be events that the deaf clubs in towns and cities across the nation also feature traditionally: a theatrical performance, a raffle, games, a dance, a sporting match. The state convention ends with numerous awards in recognition of service to the deaf community. The master of ceremonies (the last one I recall was B. J. Wood, who directs the state Commission for the Deaf and Hard of Hearing) recounts the many achievements of each recipient, who is given a plaque and asked to say a few words—they're usually about how he (or she) could not have done it (organized a successful tournament, put on a show, conducted a fund-raiser, run the summer camp for deaf children, published the community newspaper) without the help of A, B, and C. The recognition of service and the warm congratulations all around continue for hours, until friends bid each other a reluctant good night.

So the members of the American deaf community are not characteristically isolated, or uncommunicative, or unintelligent, or childlike, or needy, or any of these things we imagine them to be. Why, then, do we think they are? This mistake arises from an extrapolative leap, an egocentric error. To imagine what deafness is like, I imagine my world without sound—a terrifying prospect, and one that conforms quite well with the stereotype we project onto members of the deaf community. I would be isolated, disoriented, uncommunicative, and unreceptive to communication. My ties to other people would be ruptured. I remember my parents censuring me with silence; it was bearable for four hours, and then I implored their forgiveness. I recall the "silent treatment" of offenders in the Army. The Tunisian novelist Albert Memmi, author of several sociological studies of oppression, observes in his book on dependency: "The person who refuses to communicate severs the psychological ties that connect him to the other person. In so doing he isolates the other person and can drive him to despair." A world without sound would be a world without meaning. What could be more fundamental to my sense of myself than my sensory milieu—unless it be my spoken language.

What motivates the extrapolative error in disinterested laymen is existential dread. There but for the grace of God go I. "Contact with someone afflicted with a disease is regarded as a mysterious malevolency," writes critic and author Susan Sontag. Some of my hearing friends say they are uneasy around deaf people for a different reason, because they don't know how to communicate with them; but then I ask them if they give blind people a wide berth and look away from physically handicapped people, and they acknowledge that they do.* Each meeting with a person we perceive as handicapped is an invitation to make the extrapolation—and to experience dread. They are deserving of our sympathy because we are deserving of our sympathy. Nineteenth-century authors catered to such sentiments by idealizing their deaf characters. The American poet Lydia Sigourney sang of "the silent ecstasy refined" displayed by a pupil at the first school for deaf children in America, and Alfred de Musset's beautiful deaf Camille "had admirable purity and freshness."

Mothers in one central African nation report that on discovering that their child was deaf, their first thought was to verify that their ancestors had been properly buried. Mothers in many societies consider the cause of their child's deafness to be spirit aggression. We are fragile and dependent beings, they seem to imply, and deafness can be retribution for a moral failing. So, too, American mothers experience inexplicable guilt on discovering that they have a deaf child. There is a persistent belief, Sontag notes, that illness reveals, and is a punishment for, moral laxity. It is somehow reassuring when contracting a disease like AIDS is the result of doing something "wrong"; that hemophiliacs contract it through no act of their own arouses our rage at an immoral universe. It would be better if there were a reason for contracting deafness, something we could do, or refrain from doing, to avoid it. Such a reason might also justify our holding deaf people at arm's length, even justify our treating them badly. But there generally isn't one; so deafness or some other physical handicap may happen to us, as it were, whimsically, and that is dreadful.

The hearing person's extrapolation to what deafness must be like—a world without sound, without facile communication—is not entirely without a counterpart in the real world, for each year thousands of people lose substantial hearing because of illness, trauma, or old age. A few may take steps to enter the deaf community, to learn ASL, make friends in that community, join deaf organizations, attend a deaf club, and so on; most do not.

Growing up deaf, as have most users of ASL, is quite another matter. To evaluate that world of the deaf community, extrapolation from the hearing world is of no use at all. Is it better to be deaf or is it better to be hearing? Anthropologist Richard Shweder asks, "Is it better to have three gods and one wife or one god and three wives?" Of course, the question makes no sense except in relation to a cultural "frame." To know what it is to be a member of the deaf community is to imagine how you would think, feel, and react if you had grown up deaf, if manual language had been your main means of communication, if your eyes were the portals of your mind, if most of your friends were deaf, if you had learned that there were children who couldn't sign only after you had known dozens who could, if the people you admired were deaf, if you had struggled daily for as long as you can remember with the ignorance and uncommunicativeness of hearing people, if . . . if, in a word, you *were* deaf.

The extrapolative error is an error twice over: True representations of the members of another culture cannot be had without a change in frame of reference, which requires, at least, understanding and empathy. It is naïve to imagine otherwise, and it is self-defeating. There will be no successful relations between hearing and deaf people, no successful education of deaf children, until the extrapolative error is set aside.

The Infirmity and Cultural Models of Deaf People

The first time I saw ASL—really looked at it—was in 1973 at the Salk Institute for Biological Studies in La Jolla, California. On the sunlight-splashed terraces overlooking the Pacific, amid eucalyptus groves, a man and a woman were engaged in rapt silent conversation, their hands flying, their faces projecting fleetingly a hundred human emotions. Although I was in La Jolla as visiting professor of linguistics at the University of California, my first assumptions about this scene were quite wrong. I thought the couple must be deaf and their hand movements some sort of mime. Dr. Ursula Bellugi, who directs the Salk Institute's Laboratory for Cognitive Neuroscience, set me straight: The man was a hearing linguist who had learned ASL as an adult, the woman was deaf, and I was witnessing a natural language, one that was quite unlike English, although it had features that could be found in various spoken languages around the world. In one way it was different from all oral languages, for it was manual and visual; and in one way it was like all of them, for it had rules for combining elements into words and rules for combining words in sentences—a grammar.

It is hard to explain to a nonlinguist my emotion: I felt as Balboa must have felt on first seeing the Pacific! Language could be expressed, it appeared, by movements of the hands and face just as well as by the small, sound-generating movements of the throat and mouth. Then the first criterion for language that I had learned as a student—it is spoken and heard—was wrong; and, more important, language did not depend on our ability to speak and hear but must be a more abstract capacity of the brain. It was the brain that had language, and if that capacity was blocked in one channel, it would emerge through another.

Linguistic research on ASL, which began in the 1960s with the work of William Stokoe and colleagues at Gallaudet University, mushroomed in the following decades and soon led to research describing the sign languages of other deaf communities—in Britain, Sweden, France, China, and Thailand, to mention a few examples. As many speakers of oral languages are aware, spoken words are made up of a small inventory of vowels and consonants strung out in a row according to rules. Signs, it turns out, also consist of a small inventory of elements—handshapes, their locations on or near the body, their orientations, and their movements. These components of signs occur simultaneously. Using a fully spread hand, touch your thumb to the side of your forehead twice—that's the ASL sign for FATHER. Repeat the sign but with your thumb touching your breast and you get FINE in ASL. Repeat the sign for father but replace the two taps with an arcing movement away from your forehead; that's GRANDFATHER. Put the spread handshape on both hands facing out in front of your waist, cup your hands a little, and wiggle your wrists; that two-handed sign means TO-CHAT-IN-SIGN.

Just as there are rules in English that restrict the allowable sequences of vowels and consonants (e.g., if a word begins with three consonant sounds, the first must be *s*), so there are rules that restrict the simultaneous combinations of the four elements of signs—and apparently for the same reasons: simplicity of execution and of perception. One such rule in the structure of ASL requires that if both hands are moving in a sign, then the handshapes, locations, and movements of the two hands must be the same. To illustrate, sign BICYCLE; close both hands into fists and move them in alternating circular movements in front of your chest. If the two hands in a sign have *different* handshapes, then one must be stationary and, furthermore, only six of the score of allowable handshapes in ASL are permitted on that stationary hand. An example is DISCUSS, where an extended index finger strikes an open palm.

In a classic experiment, Dr. Bellugi and linguist Susan Fischer had hearing children of deaf parents, who were fluent in both English and ASL, tell the same story in each of the two languages. Since it requires much more time to move the large limbs of the body than the small articulators of the mouth, you might expect that signs will take longer to articulate than words, and that therefore a story will be longer in sign than a corresponding spoken one. You would be only half right; signs do take longer than words, but in Bellugi's and Fischer's experiment the two versions of the same story generally lasted about the same amount of time. The reasons for this bring us to the heart of the differences between signed languages and spoken ones, and between ASL and English in particular.

Signed languages exist in space and naturally take advantage of spatial reasoning to convey messages. In ASL, for example, I-SHOW-

YOU is one sign moving outward from the signer; YOU-SHOW-ME moves inward toward the signer. Where English would require three words in each case, there is only one sign with its incorporated movement. If I sign MY BROTHER and point to the left and MY SISTER and point to the right, "My brother met my sister" can be rendered by a single sign moving from left to right. I can then attribute qualities unambiguously to my brother or my sister by making the signed attributions either to the left or to the right. Many ASL verbs, such as GIVE, NAME, PREACH, SAY-NO, ASK, HATE, MOCK, are executed with movements that incorporate who is doing the action to whom. Since that information is in the modified sign itself, ASL, like many spoken languages, such as Russian, does not have to restrict word order, as English does. For example, the three signs HORSE, COW, and KICK (or the equivalent words in Russian) might be arranged in any order in ASL (or Russian), and there would still be no doubt about which animal was kicking which. Word order is available, therefore, to serve other purposes; thus, it is common for an ASL sentence to put the topic first and then the comment, as in the sentence with two signs: GIVE-HIM-THE-BOOK, I-DON'T-WANT-TO.

Changes in the movement of the sign also convey information about time that requires adding adverbs in English, such as "frequently," "repeatedly," "over a long time." Thus, SICK and SICK-FOR-A-LONG-TIME-OVER-AND-OVER-AGAIN (repeated lengthy bouts of illness) are each one sign. Movements meaning "to each of them," "to selected ones at different times," "to any and all at different times," are imposed on sets of verbs to give single complex signs, such as PREACH-TO-SELECTED-ONES-AT-DIFFERENT-TIMES. Changes in the shape of the sign can incorporate information; thus the sign DAY can be made into TODAY, the sign GIVE into GIVE-A-BOOK. Movement can also convey grammatical categories; where English would add a suffix to the word to indicate that it is a noun or verb, ASL uses tense or relaxed movement and repetition.

This brief description of a little of the grammar of ASL, based on the work of Dr. Bellugi and colleagues at the Salk Institute, may make it clear how stories told in ASL can reach the same rate of propositions as stories told in English—about a proposition every second and a half. English words are, on the average, twice as fast to articulate as signs in ASL, but it takes many more English words and word endings than it takes ASL signs to say the same thing. To convey the logical relationships in a sentence, as any language must do, ASL incorporates the information into its signs; they are layered and richly configured, as appropriate to the sense of vision. English, on the other hand, accomplishes the same ends by stringing many words and word endings out in a row. This is a strategy more suited to a spoken language than a visual one. Hence, the two languages clearly bear the impress of their different modalities, visual and auditory, and are very different languages indeed.

The literature of American deaf culture, told in ASL, consists of history, stories, tall tales, legends, fables, anecdotes, poetry, plays, jokes, naming rituals, sign play, and much more. Since the literature of the American deaf community recounts the deaf experience, much of it concerns, directly or indirectly, hearing oppression of deaf people. For example, in its performance of the play *My Third Eye*, the National Theater of the Deaf calls attention to some of the more laughable features of hearing people's behavior: our endless conversations on the telephone, our acute fear of being touched, our visual inattentiveness, our frigid faces, where only the jaw moves, faces that deny by their impassivity what our words declare.

Mastery of ASL and skillful storytelling are highly valued in deaf culture. There are success stories, in which the deaf person triumphs over adverse conditions—bluffing one's way into a job with the help of deaf accomplices, for example. There are also stories about starting a deaf club, buying a clubhouse, beating the other team. There are stories about the material culture of the deaf community—grandfather clocks rigged with weights that fall at the appointed hour and awaken the deaf owners with their vibrations—and tall tales (the weights waken all the deaf people in the town). Storytelling develops early in residential schools for deaf children, where youngsters recount in ASL the plots of cartoons, Westerns, and war movies, and the idiosyncratic mannerisms of hearing teachers. There is also formal storytelling, for example, bearing witness to the acts and character of great deaf figures. Clear communication is highly valued; stories should be rich in detail, start at the beginning and end at the end, and contain plain talk; hinting and vague talk in an effort to be polite are inappropriate and even offensive. As might be expected, members of this culture have quite distinct rules for attention-getting, turn-taking, polite discourse, name-giving, and other behaviors related to language.

Through ASL literature, one generation passes on to the next its wisdom, its values, and its pride, and thus reinforces the bonds that unite the younger generation. Since ASL is not a written language, publications in English—newspapers, magazines, and books written by and for deaf people—have played an important role historically in the bonding of American deaf culture. Another striking feature of this culture is its high rate of endogamous marriage: An estimated nine out of ten members of the American deaf community marry other members of their cultural group. Particularly important cultural institutions, the sites of much cultural transmission, have been the network of residential schools and the numerous deaf clubs throughout the nation. Deaf athletic, political, religious, and fraternal organizations also play an important role.

What are some of the salient values of this culture? Residential school ties are exceedingly important, and graduates are likely to return frequently for alumni events. When asked where they are from, deaf people will often reply with the name of the residential school they attended; it invariably comes up in introductions. Interviewed at a deaf club, an octogenarian eloquently testified to the importance of school ties: "You see those people sitting over there? Those are my classmates from the Berkeley School. When I was nine, my mother took me out of hearing boarding school and put me in the institution. They all befriended me, and we have been tight ever since. Of course, once we all started families, we didn't always see each other as regularly as we do now that everyone is retired. It's hard on my husband; he's from out of state and didn't grow up with us, so he feels kind of left out."

Deaf identity itself is highly valued; deaf people seem to agree that a hearing person can never fully acquire that identity and become a full-fledged member of the deaf community. Even with deaf parents and a native command of ASL, the hearing person will have missed the experience of growing up deaf, including attending a deaf school, and is likely to have divided allegiances. Speech and thinking like a hearing person are negatively valued in deaf culture. Deaf people who adopt hearing values and look down on other deaf people are regarded as traitors. "We are all in the same family," said one deaf leader, and, indeed, the metaphor of family is fundamental and recurrent. It is by hearing standards a heterogeneous family: the salience of deaf identity overshadows differences of age, class, sex, and ethnicity that would be more prominent in hearing society. Likewise, there is a penchant for group decision-making, and mutual aid and reciprocity figure importantly in deaf culture. Favors are more easily requested, my deaf friends tell me, more readily granted, and there is less individual accounting than in American hearing society. From a hearing person's perspective, this "family" engages in a great deal of hugging. Deaf people frequently hug on meeting and invariably hug on parting—real hugs! They mock the ritual hugs that hearing friends sometimes engage in. Partings can take a very long time and proceed in stages. Abrupt departures and even temporary unexplained departures are unacceptable.

There is fierce group loyalty, and this may extend to protectively withholding from hearing people information about the community's language and culture. Members of the deaf community believe, as do members of other cultural minorities, that one should marry within one's minority: marriage with a hearing person is definitely frowned upon. The deaf community collectively values deaf children highly; deaf adults in rural areas, for example, will drive great distances to see deaf children, especially if the children might otherwise lack such contact.

Clearly, we are concerned here with a language minority; a community that consequently has a rich culture and art forms of its own, a minority history and social structure. What is in dispute intellectually is the use of one type of description rather than another for this language minority, a cultural description rather than one based on infirmity. What is in dispute pragmatically is power and money.

To apply an infirmity model to members of a group is to regard them and interact with them particularly with respect to our cultural conception of bodily defect. This conceptual framework, which one normally acquires in the course of acculturation, is implicit; it entails issues, values, and reference to societal institutions. Some of the issues that naturally arise when a certain way of being or behaving is construed as an infirmity are: By what criteria and by whom is this construed as an infirmity; how did the infirmity arise; what are the risks and benefits of the available treatments, if any; what can be done to minimize the disabling effects of the infirmity? The values invoked are largely negative; we may admire someone's accommodation to his infirmity or his courage in struggling with it, but the infirmity itself is generally considered undesirable; at best we are ambivalent. The institutions that are part of this conceptual framework include notably the biological sciences and the health and social welfare professions.

To apply a cultural model to a group is to invoke quite a different conceptual framework. Implicit in this posture are issues such as: What are the interdependent values, mores, art forms, traditions, organizations, and language that characterize this culture? How is it influenced by the physical and social environment in which it is embedded? Such questions are, in principle, value neutral, although of course some people are ill-disposed to cultural diversity, while others prize it. The institutions invoked by a cultural model of a group include the social sciences; professions in a mediating role between cultures, such as simultaneous interpretation; and the schools, an important locus of cultural transmission.

I maintain that the vocabulary and conceptual framework our society has customarily used with regard to deaf people, based as it is on infirmity, serves us and the members of the deaf community less well than a vocabulary and framework of cultural relativity. I want to replace the normativeness of medicine with the curiosity of ethnography.

The contrast between deafness-as-disability and deafness-as-culture is sharpened when we consider the views of leaders of the disability rights movement in the United States and Great Britain. Those leaders and some scholars in the field of disability have presented a persuasive case that people with physical and mental disabilities are oppressed. They reject the "personal tragedy" view of disability and point to the ways in which society has discriminated against people with disabilities in education, in the employment market, and in physical access to public facilities. Indeed, they argue, society creates the conditions that lead to much of disability in the first place, such as war and poverty, and society determines to an important degree who shall be categorized as disabled and who not. For example, earlier in this century, educational psychologist Henry Goddard, using the new tests of IQ, "discovered" morons and announced that a new and dangerous form of disability, rampant among the poor and requiring custodial care, was in our midst. When it comes to mild mental retardation, the evidence is compelling that society has a large role in determining who is disabled and who is not.* In 1984, the U.S. Court of Appeals affirmed a finding that California's use of IQ tests to classify black children as mentally retarded discriminated against them intentionally on the basis of race.

According to disability theorist Paul Abberley, the view of disability as oppression rests on two fundamental assertions: first, that disability is in part a historical product of social forces, not merely a biological necessity; and second, that the disabled mode of living has value in its own right, even as we condemn the conditions that gave rise to the impairment. Consider people with physical handicaps, for example: They affirm that the design of the environment often disables them; in better-designed environments they are disabled less, or not at all. And they ask that their particular way of being and of living be respected and valued, even while we regret the lack of good medical care, or industrial safety, or the war that led to their disability. This model seems to apply to a wide range of disabilities, including hearing loss from aging, accident, or illness. It does not apply to members of deaf communities.

True, members of the American deaf community, like Americans with disabilities, African-Americans, and Hispanic-Americans, among others, are disadvantaged by the beliefs and practices of the majority in the United States. But the ambivalence called for in the case of disabilities—respecting that unique organization of life while regretting the conditions that create it—is not appropriate in the case of deaf culture. Deaf parents' joy at the birth of a son or a daughter is not commonly diminished by their finding that the child is deaf. The experience of the "Hanleys" is typical: Mrs. Hanley sat by the window on the Fourth of July, she recounts, watching children set off fireworks while her baby slept undisturbed. "I thought to myself, 'She must be deaf.' I wasn't disappointed; I thought, 'It will be all right. We are both deaf, so we will know what to do.'" Joan Philip Meehan comes from a large deaf family, all of whom had hoped that her baby would be born deaf. "I want my daughter to be like me, to be deaf," she affirmed in an interview with the Boston *Globe*. In the words of British deaf leader Paddy Ladd: "The deaf community regards the birth of each and every deaf child as a precious gift." American experts expressed the same view in a 1991 report to the National Institutes of Health; research in genetics to improve deaf people's quality of life is certainly important, they said, but must not become, in the hands of hearing people, research on ways of reducing the deaf minority.

What makes the American deaf community more like Hispanic-Americans than disabled Americans is, of course, its culture, including its language. Membership in the deaf community is not decided by diagnosis; in fact, it is not decided at all, any more than membership in the Hispanic community. Various culturally determined behaviors, and foremost among them language, reveal whether an individual belongs to a language minority or not. Each disadvantaged group has its unique characteristics, as well as features in common with other such groups. Women, gays, Americans with disabilities, and, arguably, African-Americans are not linguistic minorities, as are Hispanic-Americans, Native Americans, and members of the American deaf community. Gays and members of the American deaf community, on the other hand, have in common that most members of the minority do not share their minority identity with their parents and cannot develop it at home. The residential schools for deaf children provided a vital link in the transmission of deaf culture and language, which is why the deaf community finds abhorrent the dismantling of the residential schools, while the disability lobby finds abhorrent segregated schooling of disabled children in special residential schools. If a child's language and identity are bound up with mainstream American culture and that child can thrive in the local school, it is hard to see why he should not be enrolled there. This includes some partially hearing children. But nine out of ten deaf children are, or shortly will be, members of the American deaf community. They have a unique birthright and will require some measure of grouping in order to enjoy the benefits of that patrimony. That is why the grouping of deaf children and adults has always been voluntary, while the segregation of children and adults with disabilities was generally involuntary.

Anthropologist Roy D'Andrade observes that significant cultural concepts, like marriage, money, theft, are not givens but require the adherence of a group to a "constitutive rule." Different cultures have different constitutive rules. Debates about abortion (at what age is a fetus a person?), about what age defines a minor, and the like are debates about constitutive rules—they can be pursued only within a given cultural frame. "Smart" is such a concept; so are "on time," "successful," and "disability." Because there is a deaf community with its own language and culture, there is a cultural frame in which to be deaf is not to be disabled; quite the contrary, it is, as we have seen, an asset in deaf culture to be deaf in behavior, values, knowledge, and fluency in ASL. If we respect the right of people in other cultures, including those within our borders, to have their own constitutive rules, which may differ from ours (and we can refuse to do so only at the risk of being impossibly naïve), then we must recognize that the deafness of which I speak is not a disability but rather a different way of being.

Some deaf leaders will say that by insisting on the distinction between members of the deaf community and members of the hearing
community who have a hearing disability, I am serving the interests
of those who would "divide and conquer." It is true that by allying
with other groups, the deaf community can make gains difficult to
achieve on its own. But to embrace the representation of the members
of the deaf community as infirm is to endorse the very principle of
oppression the community has so long struggled to overthrow; it is
to undermine the community's efforts in behalf of some of its most
cherished goals, such as bilingual and bicultural education; it is to
render inexplicable the joy that deaf adults and their hearing friends
experience when they see a deaf child signing; and it is to go against
the common sense of most members of American deaf culture, who
are simply baffled when told they are disabled. The Massachusetts
Deaf Community News, for example, reporting on the 1991 Americans
with Disabilities Act, had to explain to its readers: "Deaf people are
defined as 'disabled for purposes of the ADA.'"*

We have come to look at deaf people in a certain way, to use a
certain vocabulary of infirmity, and this practice is so widespread
among hearing people, has gone on for so long, and is so legitimized
by the medical and paramedical professions that we imagine we are
accurately describing attributes of deaf people rather than choosing
to talk about them in a certain way. If we but consult history or deaf
people for five minutes, however, we will be reminded of the error
of this "common sense" position.* There was a time in American
history (as in European history) when hearing people viewed culturally deaf people predominantly in terms of a cultural model. It went
without saying at that time—the better part of the last century—that
you needed to know the language of the deaf community to teach
deaf children, that deaf adults and deaf culture must play a prominent role in the education of this minority. Deaf people published
newspapers and books and held meetings that were focally concerned
with the deaf community, and they discussed the pros and cons of
having their own land, where deaf people would live and govern
themselves, perhaps some land grant from the federal government
in the newly settled West. There were proportionately many more
late-deafened children then, and it seemed a pity not to maintain
their skill in speaking English, so those children who could profit
from it were given an hour or so of speech training after school a
few times a week. There were no special educators; the requisites of

a good teacher were a good education and fluency in ASL; nearly half of all teachers were deaf themselves. There were no audiologists, or rehabilitation counselors, or school psychologists, and for the most part, none apparently were needed. The deaf child was not "formulated, sprawling on a pin," by those professions: so many decibels of hearing loss at such and such frequencies; a profile on the Minnesota Multiphasic Personality Inventory; an IQ score. Instead, deaf children and adults were described in cultural terms: Where did they go to school; who were their deaf relatives, if any, and deaf friends; who was their deaf spouse; where did they work; what deaf sports teams and deaf organizations did they belong to; what service did they render to the deaf community?

We discover a similar conceptual framework if we consult the deaf community today. But, remarkably, those professing to serve deaf people do not consult the deaf community—remarkably because the values of our larger society demand that hearing and deaf people arrive freely at agreement on how to accomplish common purposes and, furthermore, that the overriding common purpose of all of us, hearing and deaf, should be, to use philosopher Richard Rorty's terms, "to let everybody have a chance at self-creating to the best of his or her abilities." Thus, deaf people themselves should be crucial participants in the discussion and agreement concerning the lives of deaf children and adults and the roles of the professions that serve them, but they have been excluded—socially, by law, and by oppressive education. They are excluded by statute or connivance from educating most deaf children. Their counsel, which the parent of a newborn deaf child needs more than any other, is excluded from the home and the clinic. Their services as a language model for the deaf child are eschewed and the responsibility unconscionably given to the child's hearing mother, who cannot fulfill it. Indeed, their very existence is all but denied. They are not participants in the programs of research on deaf people funded by our government annually at a cost of millions of dollars; they are merely the passive objects of that research. Their role in programs that provide services to deaf people is severely restricted.

How does the medicalization of deaf people take place? How is an infirmity model of deaf people promulgated when it is grossly inappropriate? Let us shift the focus from the person labeled infirm and his or her etiology to the social context in which the infirmity label was acquired.

If we ask culturally deaf adults how they first acquired the label "handicapped, disabled, impaired," we commonly learn that some circumstance of heredity, of birth, or of early childhood marked the child as different from its parents and created an initial breakdown in communication between parent and child. The parents then saw this as deviant relative to their norms and took the child to the experts—the pediatrician, the otologist, the audiologist. It was they who legitimated the infirmity model. Why do they do it? Because that is precisely a core function of their profession: to diagnose infirmity.

How do the experts medicalize the child's difference into deviance? First, they characterize the difference in great biological detail and often only in stigmatizing ways. Much will be said about impairment of spoken language, little may be said about acquisition of ASL. Much will be said about hearing loss, nothing about gains in visual perception and thought.* Second, while pursuing the infirmity model, the experts commonly remain silent about the cultural model; they may not even mention the community of adults who were once children much like their client. Otologists and audiologists are often poorly informed about the deaf community and its language; that knowledge is not a required part of their training. Moreover, the audiologist works for a clinic under the jurisdiction of an ear doctor. At the 1991 meeting convened in Boston by the Cochlear Corporation to promote childhood implants, a deaf leader asked an otologist at the rostrum whether his implant team informed parents, whose deaf children were candidates for surgery, about the deaf community and ASL as alternatives to implantation. The otologist replied with admirable candor: "We tend to present things from our point of view." The parents meanwhile are in crisis and unlikely to be critical of that view. If the professional person does describe the deaf community, it may well be in terms that are so concise that the parents do not really grasp an alternative conception of their child's status and destiny. The professional expert and the parents generally share the same hearing culture; they tend to evaluate and label the deaf child from that perspective.

The labeling is a prelude to profound, life-changing events, to special practices at home, to a "special" education, to training in some skills and not others, to studying some subjects and not others, to specific patterns of social relations, to the wearing of technological stigmata (electronic devices and wires), possibly to surgery, to the development of a certain self-image as a consequence of all these forces; naturally, the labeling has its own "ritual of power." The child is seated, wearing earphones, in a small steel room. The audiologist inspects and directs him through a large glass window. A test is about to begin. One wants to succeed on tests; but the child knows that this is a test not relating to what he is best at, or capable of, but precisely concerning what he is incapable of, an alien field. The audiologist gives instructions to the child in the soundproof room: Raise your hand when you hear a sound. The child tries to obey, all the while knowing that at any moment he may be in the process of failing; there may have been a sound—of course you don't know what you haven't heard. At the end, grave pronouncements are made: According to the child's response to certain pure tones at certain frequencies and intensities, he is declared "profoundly" hearing-impaired, or "severely" so; a small percent are assigned other labels, and there are numeric cutoffs for each category. What is important is the quantification, the process, the sentencing—it has little predictive or practical value; neither "totally" nor "profoundly" nor "severely" deaf children can understand normal speech, even with powerful hearing aids. Much as another ceremony of sentencing, that of the courtroom, it exists largely to perpetuate a certain social order.*

Having measured and labeled him, the audiologist passes the healthy deaf-child-become-patient to the special educator; the child is now tagged with an infirmity model and has acquired a second persona, the one described in the accompanying dossier. The job of the educator is not to educate; it is to find an educational treatment for what the otologist and audiologist could not treat, the child's failure to acquire English normally. A difference has been identified; now a massive campaign begins to eradicate it.

The medicalization of the deaf community is marked by a long history of struggle between deaf people and the hearing people who profess to serve them, for the right to define a problem and to locate it within one social domain rather than another—to construe it as a problem of medicine, education, rehabilitation, religion, politics—is won by struggle. Toward the end of the last century, hearing teachers seized control of schools for deaf children and banished ASL and deaf teachers. With the cultural frame changed, the deaf pupil was now an outsider. Spoken language in the classroom and speech therapy failed to make him an insider, while it drove out all education, confirming that the child was defective. Unsuccessful education of deaf children reinforced the need for special education, for experts in counseling of the deaf and in rehabilitation of the deaf. Finally and most devastatingly, deaf children in America, starting in the late 1970s, were increasingly placed in local hearing schools. Having cut off the deaf child from his deaf world, having blocked his communication with parents, peers, and teachers, the experts have disabled the deaf child as never before in American history. The typical deaf child, born deaf or deafened before learning English, is utterly at a loss as he sits on the deaf bench in the hearing classroom.* What is the teacher saying? How can I make my own thoughts clear to her? What can I do to be accepted by the other children? Is there someone here who could explain things to me after school? The infirmity model has become more plausible applied to the young deaf child; with academic integration, the medicalization of cultural deafness gained major ground while the technological "miracle" of childhood cochlear implants evolved. This latest development illustrates a principle of oppression articulated by Jean-Paul Sartre: "Oppressors produce and maintain by force the evils which, in their eyes, render the oppressed more and more like what he should be to deserve his fate."

Modernity seems frequently to be the enemy of deaf people and their community. The movement, late in the last century, to banish the traditional signed languages of deaf communities in favor of the national spoken languages was created by hearing teachers (who commonly knew no manual language) as a "modern" initiative. It was also consistent with efforts to forge linguistic and cultural unity, particularly in the new nation-states. The professionalization of teaching deaf children in this century was a "modern" development—but one that largely excluded deaf adults. Modern psychological measurement, called psychometrics, has been grievously misapplied to deaf children and adults, as I shall show. The modern invention of the telephone placed deaf people at a disadvantage; the hearing aid and the audiometer, while invaluable for hearing people with hearing losses, have arguably proved of little or no value for members of the deaf community. For deaf people, silent movies were better than the modern "talkies." Of course, with modernity imposed, some inventions mitigate the harm of others; teletypewriters used by deaf people and the captioning of television and movies are two examples. But the newest high technology concerning hearing also poses the greatest threat to the welfare of the deaf community; I mean that same technological "miracle": the microsurgical insertion of electrodes in the deaf child's inner ear.

"The best way to cause people long-lasting pain," Richard Rorty writes, "is to humiliate them by making the things that seemed most important to them look futile, obsolete, and powerless." What is most important to deaf people?

• *Their dignity* as deaf people, who, more fully than hearing people, operate in a visual-spatial world—their unique identity. Otologists and audiologists affirm that identity to be an illness and conduct heroic surgery on deaf children in a futile effort to change it.

• *Their language.* Hearing educators mangle it, attempting to make it express English on the hands, or they refuse to use it at all; they deny its standing as a natural language.

• *Their history*, which hearing people stole from them. Much as Abraham Lincoln was long presented as the leading figure in African-American history, such mention of history as occasionally occurred in textbooks for teachers of deaf students extolled hearing teachers of deaf children, such as Thomas Gallaudet. But deaf history is almost never taught to deaf children, for that would be a step toward legitimating a cultural model of the deaf way of being; deaf adults learn their cultural history today with surprise and delight.

• *Their social organization and mores*, which education and medicine declare inappropriate and obsolete.

• *Their political agenda.* But hearing experts continue to disempower deaf leaders in many of the areas most important to them.

A French deaf couple describe their disempowerment and humiliation:

> We were born deaf. We have been married ten years. We work like hearing people, live in a hearing neighborhood, drive our car like hearing people and take our vacations in the same places they do. The only difference in our lives is that we are deaf. Our two children, five and seven, were born hearing. Since their birth, their mother tongue is sign. Long before they could use words they spoke with us in our language. From their earliest childhood we made an effort to put them in touch with as many hearing people as possible, because we knew that the hearing world would be theirs one day. Now they are bilingual. Why don't hearing parents do the same thing when they have a deaf child? Why not teach them sign? Why not help them meet deaf people since it is the world they are destined to live in? When we were children, our parents prohibited our using sign. Because

the doctors, the professors, the deafness specialists, told them to do that. Throughout all our studies, we were taught speech and lip-reading and hearing culture. But when we started our jobs, we realized that it was all a failure: as far as hearing people were concerned, we had always been and were deaf. They said we were hard to understand and that we didn't understand them. It was hard, humiliating. . . . Other deaf children should never live through the mutilating experience we have been through.

Yes, we have humiliated, we continue to humiliate, deaf people. But deaf people are "us." We need to recognize our common susceptibility to humiliation. Each time the powers-that-be succeed in applying the infirmity model to any one cultural and language minority, all such minorities are in greater danger. If members of the deaf community can be declared defective and treated accordingly, it is that much easier to do the same to African-Americans, gays, Jews. Perhaps the reader himself or herself runs a risk. Unless, of course, you are Goffman's one complete unblushing male.

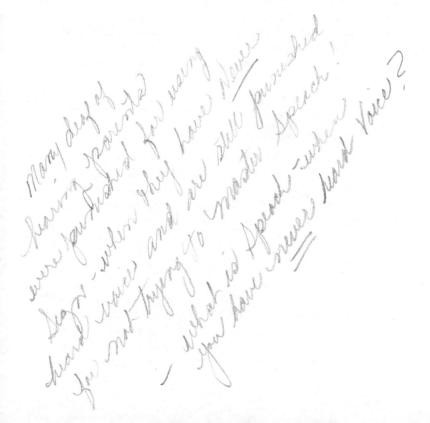

PART TWO

Representations of Deaf People: Colonialism, ''Audism,'' and the ''Psychology of the Deaf''

The Colonization of African and Deaf Communities

Colonialism is the standard, as it were, against which other forms of cultural oppression can be scaled, involving as it did the physical subjugation of a disempowered people, the imposition of alien language and mores, and the regulation of education in behalf of the colonizer's goals. My life has become intertwined with the lives of some deaf and hearing people in central Africa, in the Republic of Burundi, which long suffered under the yoke of colonialism and only gained its independence in 1962. I had traveled in western Africa in the late 1960s, examining the teaching of English in teacher-training colleges sponsored by UNESCO in several English- and French-speaking countries. That was before my fateful encounter with Ursula Bellugi, ASL, and deaf people. When I returned to Africa in 1976, I had come to know the struggle of deaf people, and I naturally saw in Africa's colonial history (and its aftermath) terms of comparison for the oppression of deaf communities.

I was invited to Burundi to examine a celebrated young boy who was believed to have lived with animals in the wild for some years. A year earlier, I had written a book, *The Wild Boy of Aveyron*, about the best-known and -documented wild child, long of interest to psychologists, who had been ensnared by civilization in France at the close of the eighteenth century. Thus, the eminent American psychologist B. F. Skinner suggested that I look into this latest case of a putative wild child in Burundi. The investigation that led me and a colleague to conclude that the boy was instead brain-damaged as a result of a childhood disease was described in our book on childhood autism, *The Wild Boy of Burundi*. Since there was no provision for the education of handicapped children in Burundi at that time, the boy, whom the priests named John after John the Baptist, was left in the care of an orphanage, where he died in 1985.

Although my central concern in Burundi was the boy John, his behavior, and his history, I could not fail to be struck by the legacy of colonialism and the sad plight of hearing and deaf people there.

Burundi has about five million people, occupying an area the size of Maryland; most subsist on small family farms scattered throughout the highlands. Exports consist almost entirely of coffee, and famine is a real threat if the weather is bad during the growing season. The only cities are Gitega and the capital Bujumbura, founded by the German and the successor Belgian colonizers, respectively. There are two major ethnic groups, the Hutus (85 percent) and the Tutsis (14 percent), with a common language, Kirundi, and a second official language, French. According to the World Bank, in 1981 a quarter of the adult population was literate, and about one child in three was enrolled in primary school. Apart from the efforts of a few missionaries, there was no education of deaf children; the Burundians viewed deaf people as mentally retarded, an opinion that echoed at least some former colonialists' views of Burundians in general. "The natives are incapable even of laying three bricks straight in a row," I was told authoritatively by one embassy official.

Not long after my visit to Burundi, the president of my university gave a reception for a group of African diplomats, and I met the counselor to the ambassador from Burundi. We spoke about my visit to his country, and, somewhat presumptuously, I lamented the lack of schools for deaf children there. As a student of deaf education and deaf history, I knew how the founding of schools for deaf children in Europe and America in the last century had allowed their manual languages to flourish and allowed deaf people to become fully contributing members of Western societies. I knew, too, that deaf education had drifted badly off course in this century, was now largely failing in its task, and urgently needed the inspiration and guidance of a successful program, a fresh start. If deaf and hearing people working together in Burundi could create a school where mutual respect and communication were paramount, as they once were in American schools for deaf children, this could be an important lesson not only for Burundians but also for Americans. So when the counselor said it was easier to criticize than to construct, I offered to assist the government of Burundi in establishing national education for deaf children, and he and I shook hands on it.

I thought that day I was merely undertaking a difficult managerial task, familiar terrain for a former academic administrator. In fact I was beginning a journey that would lead me to appreciate the profound commonalities between the cultural oppression suffered by the colonized peoples of Africa and that suffered by deaf communities. I was to learn that the answer to the question "What sort of person is a Burundian?" or "What sort of person is a deaf man?" is both a beginning and an ending. A beginning, because all our relations to the Africans and to the deaf community are predicated on our representation of their members, the way we perceive them to be. An ending, because the very act of posing the question, and the means employed to take the measure of the African or the deaf man, reflect an imbalance of power that in the end dictates the answer to the question.

Whenever a more powerful group undertakes to assist a less powerful one, whenever benefactors create institutions to aid beneficiaries, the relationship is frought with peril. After the League of Nations placed Burundi under the protective mandate of Belgium, early colonizers found in place a unique and elaborate system of government that had evolved over many centuries. They chose to imagine, however, that Burundi society was a feudal society such as their own had been at an earlier stage of development. This was foolish: they were not in Europe in the Middle Ages; they were in equatorial Africa in the twentieth century. Burundi society did not have a strict hierarchy that extended from the king, through the nobles, down to the peasants, as in feudal Europe. Instead, the monarch shared authority with the chiefs, with dignitaries in the royal entourage, with local elders who rendered justice, with religious authorities, and with a network of loyalists throughout the land.*

The Belgian colonizers' perception of Burundian society was defective not only because it imposed the familiar on the unfamiliar but also because it was self-serving. They hoped to find a tightly hierarchical, aristocratic society such as theirs had been because they intended to make the king their puppet and rule through him. Likewise, it suited them to see the "natives" as children, for this confirmed the Africans' need of Belgian guidance and control. As the Belgian colonists saw it, the Burundians were evidently uncivilized, their customs clearly immoral, but European intervention could raise the natives to the status of civilized men and women. And if colonial rule did not bring about a better way of life, it was the primitive nature of the society, which needed ten more centuries to mature, that was responsible for the failure.

The Belgian colonizers have written of Burundians: "The natives are children . . . superficial, frivolous, fickle. The chiefs are suspicious, cunning and lazy." As long as white men had charge of the affairs of the Africans, this was the condescending and demeaning conception of them that reigned in government.

I kept a list, as I read about Burundi and other countries in Africa, of the characteristics of Africans, good and bad, according to the Europeans who were in charge of them before their independence. Here is that list, without terms that repeat others, and arranged for convenience into four groups.

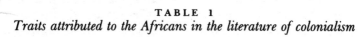

TABLE 1
Traits attributed to the Africans in the literature of colonialism

SOCIAL	COGNITIVE	BEHAVIORAL	EMOTIONAL
Barbaric	Arts: none	Alcoholic	Carefree
Bloodthirsty	Business: none	Animalistic	Emotional
Cannibalistic	Cunning	Childlike	Excitable
Coarse	Fast learners	Diligent	Fatalistic
Conscienceless	Frivolous	Dirty	Fickle
Cruel	Ignorant	Feeble	Fierce
Depraved	Improvident	Ill-fed	Hilarious
Discouraged	Intelligent	Impulsive	Proud
Economy: none	Irrational	Lazy	Servile
Gregarious	Mentally lazy	Orgiastic	Unrepentant
Insolent	Superficial	Passive	Unstable
Secretive	Suspicious	Restrained	Vengeful
Submissive	Unimaginative	Shy	
Treacherous	Unintelligent	Stunted	

For the most part, it is an ugly list. It is, it seems to me, a reflection of the Europeans' desperate need to impose their will on the Africans and to justify that imposition as civilizing an uncivilized people.

I found the list deeply disquieting for a further reason: It was all too reminiscent of what hearing experts have so often claimed about deaf people. Faced with the unique languages, cultures, and histories of deaf communities, hearing professionals frequently see only stopped-up ears and a desperate need for their services. In an American psychiatric publication from 1985, I read: "Profound deafness that occurs prior to the acquisition of verbal language is socially and psychiatrically devastating." Because nearly all deaf children today became deaf before they could learn English, and most are labeled profoundly deaf, that would make most deaf children "psychiatrically devastated."

And indeed, a reputed authority on deafness writes in an American psychiatry journal: "Suspiciousness, paranoid symptomatology, impulsiveness, aggressiveness have been reported as typical of deaf adults. . . . More recent reports tend to confirm these judgments." Here is another expert's published perception of deaf people: "The deaf are more impulsive and aggressive than the hearing, they have deficiencies in language skills, their intellectual development is delayed. . . ." Likewise, a summary of published research on the "psychology of the deaf" that is frequently cited in the United States finds "rigidity, emotional immaturity, social ineptness."

I decided to prepare a list of the characteristics of deaf people according to the hearing experts in charge of their affairs, who give these descriptions in their professional journals and in their textbooks. The list is a distillation of twenty years of psychometric research on the so-called psychology of the deaf.* Each time I came upon a characteristic of deaf people according to the experts, whether favorable or unfavorable, I wrote it down. In the end I had a very long list, one based on some three hundred fifty articles and books concerned with the traits of deaf children and adults as revealed by psychological evaluations. I eliminated terms that meant the same thing, arranged the rest into four groups, and alphabetized them. The list appears in Table 2; it, too, is a disturbing list—all the more so as these descriptions come from studies published in professional journals, studies that say they used impartial scientific testing.

This is how we portray deaf people to the young men and women who are in training to become their teachers, their doctors, their social workers, and so on. The list describes the deaf client that the experienced practitioner imagines is seated across the table: socially isolated, intellectually weak, behaviorally impulsive, emotionally immature.

Many of the traits that hearing authorities attribute to deaf people

TABLE 2
Some traits attributed to deaf people in the professional literature

SOCIAL	COGNITIVE	BEHAVIORAL	EMOTIONAL
Admiration, depends on	Conceptual thinking poor	Aggressive	Anxiety, lack of
Asocial	Concrete	Androgynous	Depressive
Childlike	Doubting	Conscientious	Emotionally disturbed
Clannish	Egocentric	Hedonistic	Emotionally immature
Competitive	Failure externalized	Immature	Empathy, lack of
Conscience weak	Failure internalized	Impulsive	Explosive
Credulous	Insight poor	Initiative lacking	Frustrated easily
Dependent	Introspection: none	Interests few	Irritable
Disobedient	Language: none	Motor development slow	Moody
Irresponsible	Language poor	Personality undeveloped	Neurotic
Isolated	Mechanically inept	Possessive	Paranoid
Morally undeveloped	Naïve	Rigid	Passionate
Role-rigid	Reasoning restricted	Shuffling gait	Psychotic reactions
Shy	Self-awareness poor	Stubborn	Serious
Submissive	Shrewd	Suspicious	Temperamental
Suggestible	Thinking unclear	Unconfident	Unfeeling
Unsocialized	Unaware		
	Unintelligent		

reflect the struggle of those authorities to impose their will on deaf children or adults. They say: "The deaf have poor social awareness"; they mean: "I wish my deaf pupils or clients would do what hearing people do in this situation." They say: "The deaf are isolated"; they mean: "They can't understand me or other hearing people, and they can't communicate with us." They say: "These deaf children are disobedient, immature, impulsive"; they mean: "I wish they would do what I tell them to do; it's hard enough teaching them anything without their disobeying."

The list of traits attributed to deaf people is often inconsistent: they are both "aggressive" *and* "submissive"; they are likewise naïve *and* shrewd, detached *and* passionate, explosive *and* shy, stubborn *and* submissive, suspicious *and* trusting. The list is, however, consistent in one key respect: it is entirely negative—virtually all the traits ascribed, even in pairs of opposites, are unfavorable. Africans and deaf people appear to have one more thing in common: they are incompetent socially, cognitively, behaviorally, and emotionally.

The inconsistencies of the trait attributions and their negativity must lead us to suspect that we are dealing, in both cases—the "psychology of the native" and the "psychology of the deaf"—not with objective descriptions but with stereotypes. Thus, the trait attributions may reveal little about Africans or deaf people but much about the colonial authorities or hearing authorities and the social contexts in which they operated. In both cases we are dealing with "a system under which an authority undertakes to supply the needs and regulate the conduct of those under its control"—the definition of paternalism.

Like the paternalism of the colonizers, hearing paternalism begins with defective perception, because it superimposes its image of the familiar world of hearing people on the unfamiliar world of deaf people. Hearing paternalism likewise sees its task as "civilizing" its charges: restoring deaf people to society. And hearing paternalism fails to understand the structure and values of deaf society. The hearing people who control the affairs of deaf children and adults commonly do not know deaf people and do not want to. Since they cannot see deaf people as they really are, they make up imaginary deaf people of their own, in accord with their own experiences and needs. Paternalism deals in such stereotypes.

Stereotypes are not only a result of paternalism, they are also a cause, and they have effects of their own. The British acting on these

stereotypes in East Africa caused the bloody Mau Mau rebellion—
and then failed to see the bloodshed coming. "I say without hesita-
tion," the senior British officer there wrote, "that the native is, on
the whole, fully satisfied with our native policy." Acting on these
stereotypes, hearing administrators of schools for deaf children have
needlessly turned away countless normal deaf children; psychiatrists
acting on these stereotypes have needlessly institutionalized countless
deaf adults in American mental hospitals; teachers acting on these
stereotypes daily set absurdly low goals for deaf children and approach those goals with inept means.

Paternalism's ignorance, I have explained, is self-serving. It is designed to reassure benefactors of the rightness of what they are doing,
to protect them from the need for change, and to protect their economic interests. If the profession of deaf education acknowledged
that deaf children have a language and that manual language is the
best way to educate these children, then deaf adults would once again
enter the profession (as they did in the last century), and hearing
people would lose their monopoly. Paternalism and money are insep-
arable—this is another of its universal traits. When King Leopold
assembled a few hundred officers from up and down Europe and
sent them to central Africa, his goal was to ensure quick profits in
rubber, ivory, and palm oil, collected as tribute or by forced labor.
He created a downtrodden working class, extracted unimaginable
wealth, and triggered a European race for spoils that ended with the
lives and fortunes of a quarter of the world's population under the
control of Belgium, France, Great Britain, and Italy.

True, the Belgian colonizers established some schools in Burundi,
but this was also self-serving; they wanted Africans trained as tax
collectors and administrators, who were, moreover, fluent in French
so that the Belgians could deal with them. Likewise, the colonial
authorities opened an agricultural college so that Burundians could
work the coffee plantations effectively. Although the colonizers saw
the colonies at first as a source of labor and of raw materials that
could be turned into manufactured goods and sold on European
markets, later many colonies became markets themselves—for European military goods, clothing, and even food—and they remain European markets today.

Paternalism, whether that of the colonizers in Africa or that of
hearing professions concerned with deaf communities, is benighted,
unsuccessful, and selfish, but the catalog of its evils does not end

there. Paternalism places its beneficiaries in a dependent relation and keeps them dependent for its own psychological and economic interest. Paternalism deprives its beneficiaries of their history and therefore of the possible lives they can envision. Paternalism corrupts some members of the oppressed minority, forming a class who conspire with the authority to maintain the status quo. Paternalism evades responsibility for its failure by affirming the biological inferiority of the beneficiary. Allowed to endure, paternalism instills the benefactor's values in the beneficiary—the oppression is internalized. And in the end, the beneficiaries despise the benefactors who have so long despised them, and the benefactors decry the thanklessness of their jobs.

How can I protest the harm that paternalism does and in the same breath prescribe a course of action for Burundi? I cannot. I can only point out the limitations of our own system, as I perceive them, and the lessons of our own history. Even in this I am caught inescapably in the fabric of relations between deaf and hearing people in America. I am a product of its history, a participant in a debate that never ends because it concerns the enduring desire of deaf people for self-determination and self-actualization.

The Paternalism Indictment

I have suggested that the traits attributed to deaf people by the "psychology of the deaf" reflect not the characteristics of deaf people but the paternalistic posture of the hearing experts making these attributions. Thus, the education, counseling, and institutionalization of deaf children and adults may rest on no more solid foundation than a set of paternalistic stereotypes. The contrary position is that these attributions are by and large true of deaf people; they are the reliable and valid results of giving scientific tests to deaf children and adults; they capture ways in which deaf people as a group differ from hearing people more than the individuals in either group differ among themselves. Only in this case may we claim that there is indeed a "psychology of the deaf."

Four kinds of evidence seem to support my indictment of the "psychology of the deaf" as an expression of paternalism. In the first place, the traits attributed by diverse benefactors to their beneficiaries are likely to overlap because of the overlapping social context of paternalism, and this provides one test of my claim. True, there are differences between Africans under European domination earlier in this century and deaf people under hearing domination in the present day, and the two lists of traits reflect those differences. Africans were not precisely called "psychotic" or "paranoid" by the colonizers; contemporary paternalists prefer those epithets to "barbaric" and "cannibalistic." Historical specificity shapes the form that oppression takes; it took different forms under different colonial powers in different parts of the world. I call deaf communities colonized, using the term in an extended sense—as when French philosopher Michel Foucault speaks of the "colonization of the body" by the state— because deaf communities have suffered oppression, in all its forms and consequences, in common with other cultures that were literally subjugated by imperial powers. The universal properties of paternalism do show up in the stereotypes the colonial authorities and hearing authorities create for themselves to rationalize and justify their predicament. Consider some adjectives common to the lists in Tables 1 and 2—characteristics attributed to Africans that are also attributed to deaf people. For Africans and deaf people to be characterized in common as *childlike, shy, submissive,* and *unintelligent* suggests that their benefactors are indeed concerned with justifying their role; if Africans (or deaf people) were seen as mature, self-assured, assertive, and smart, their "benefactors" would be seen in another light.

It also appears that paternalists find their charges difficult to manage—*aggressive, treacherous, disobedient, impulsive, suspicious.* This may be because the benefactor's goals differ from the beneficiary's. For example, a spokesman for the French colonization of North Africa maintained that "the conversion of Algeria to speaking French is in accord with the true needs of its peoples, and if not always with their sentiments, certainly with their aspirations for a better life in the modern world." Likewise, hearing benefactors want deaf pupils to sign in English word order; in 1987, eighty-five students of the Tennessee School for the Deaf were suspended for resisting this decree. The benefactor finds his charges difficult to manage not only because of a divergence in goals but also because he does not know their language, culture, and values—he has only self-serving stereotypes to misguide him.

A second test of whether a representation of a certain group of people is paternalistic arises from the fact that a paternalistic authority is likely to give a very different description of its charges than the one they would give of themselves—provided they have not internalized the stereotype promulgated by the authority. Applying this "parallax test," we find, indeed, that Africans and deaf people present quite a different characterization of their groups than those recorded in Tables 1 and 2, respectively.

Deaf people have long been giving an account of their language and culture, an account of themselves radically at variance with the representations put forth by hearing people. The deaf account has traditionally been found in the "silent press," newspapers and magazines, such as *The Deaf American,* printed for and by deaf people. It continues to be found in plays and poems by members of the deaf community that are performed in American Sign Language or, sometimes, written in English. And it appears in stories, biographies, and autobiographies of deaf leaders, such as *Notable Deaf Persons* and *A Deaf Adult Speaks Out.* I will venture a generalization about the deaf person portrayed in this literature, sizable since the Enlightenment: he is proud of who he is, proud of his language and culture, and angry at the injustices heaped on him by a hearing world.

Of late, there has been such an outpouring of accounts of the lives, language, arts, and community of deaf people that it constitutes a veritable renaissance of deaf culture—and not in the United States alone. In July of 1989, five thousand spokesmen from deaf communities around the world—scholars, artists, and political leaders—gathered in Washington, D.C., at a congress called The Deaf Way, to celebrate deaf culture with lectures, exhibits, media events, and performances. We have been witnessing the flourishing of deaf arts; there was a spectacular display of those arts—mime, dance, storytelling and poetry in manual languages, crafts, sculpture, video and fine arts—at the Deaf Way congress. There are plays by deaf playwrights and many deaf performers and performing groups,* including the National Theater of the Deaf in the United States. Perhaps the best-known example of a contemporary work of art concerning deaf people is hearing playwright Mark Medoff's play, later a movie, *Children of a Lesser God*; award-winning performances by deaf actresses Phyllis Frelich, in the play, and Marlee Matlin, in the movie, apprised Americans (and Europeans) of the struggle between deaf people and hearing professionals. Deaf actress and producer Juliana Fjeld won American television's highest award for *Love Is Never Silent*, a poignant story of a deaf couple raising their hearing children. Beginning in 1991, Matlin appeared in a nationally televised serial, "Reasonable Doubts," in which she played an attorney. Although the role was not focused on deafness—a breakthrough for a deaf performer— Matlin's use of sign language and interpreters, her artistic gifts, and the status of the character she played all contributed to making a large public more aware of deaf people, their abilities, and their language.

We are witnessing the burgeoning study of manual languages, particularly in Sweden, Great Britain, France, and the United States. American Sign Language is taught in nearly a thousand colleges and universities in the U.S. Recent laws affirm that ASL meets high school requirements for study of a foreign language in numerous states across the nation. Journals, articles, books, and conferences teach us about ASL structure, use, history, dialects, registers, poetry.* New and better materials are available for studying the language; books and videotapes abound.* Much the same is true for British Sign Language.

Deaf people are increasingly taking the helm of programs that provide educational and social services to deaf children and adults. There has been a surge in activism of organizations of deaf people. Many states in the U.S. have established commissions on deafness to act with and for deaf people. The appointment in 1988 of I. King Jordan as the first deaf president of Gallaudet University, in Washington, D.C., following the revolt of the deaf community known as the Gallaudet Revolution (of which more below; see pages 186–91), and the selection of Robert Davila as assistant secretary of the United States Department of Education are further signs of deaf leadership in America, as is a threefold increase—from four to twelve—in the number of deaf superintendents of schools for deaf children in the period 1987 to 1991. (Ninety-six schools for the deaf, however, and hundreds of day programs were, as of this writing, still supervised by hearing people.)

The shroud of silence that hearing educators placed over deaf history for nearly a century has been cast off, and this branch of minority history is thriving. Jack Gannon's *Deaf Heritage* is required reading in college classes across the nation, and his *The Week the World Heard Gallaudet* narrates the major events of the Gallaudet Revolution. I have traced the history of deaf communities in the Western world since the Enlightenment in *When the Mind Hears: A*

History of the Deaf. The Gallaudet Encyclopedia of Deaf People and Deafness is a major new resource for students of deaf culture. Important historical studies of deaf communities around the world have been appearing, and in June of 1991 the First International Congress on Deaf History convened at Gallaudet.

There is a growing awareness of deaf community and culture among scholars and laymen: there are courses in many colleges and a shelf of scholarly books, such as *Deaf in America: Voices from a Culture; Seeing Voices; American Deaf Culture; At Home Among Strangers: Exploring the Deaf Community in the United States*; and *The Sociolinguistics of the Deaf Community*.

But very little of this renaissance in deaf culture, not even the shadow of this representation of deaf people, is allowed in the corridors and classrooms where the hearing establishment serving deaf people is perpetuated—in the schools of education, of human services, of medicine. There paternalism reigns.

It will be convenient to have a name for the paternalistic, hearing-centered endeavor that professes to serve deaf people; borrowing a term from American deaf educator and author Tom Humphries, I will call it "audism." Audism is the corporate institution for dealing with deaf people, dealing with them by making statements about them, authorizing views of them, describing them, teaching about them, governing where they go to school and, in some cases, where they live; in short, audism is the hearing way of dominating, restructuring, and exercising authority over the deaf community. It includes such professional people as administrators of schools for deaf children and of training programs for deaf adults, experts in counseling the deaf and in deafness rehabilitation, teachers of deaf children and adults, interpreters, and some audiologists, speech therapists, otologists, psychologists, psychiatrists, librarians, researchers, social workers, and hearing aid specialists.

The audist narrative of what it is like to be deaf, captured in the literature of the "psychology of the deaf" and in other hearing fiction, is the acceptable one. The deaf narrative, rarely committed to paper, is not acceptable; it can be published, but its rebuttal of the hearing narrative carries no weight. What literary critic Edward Said has observed about anthropology applies with equal force to the family of disciplines constituting audism. The native point of view is not only an ethnographic fact, he wrote, "it is a continuing, sustained adversarial resistance to the discipline and the praxis of anthropology (as representative of 'outside' power) itself, anthropology not as textuality but as an often direct agent of political dominance." Similarly, deaf leaders here and abroad have been resisting the alinguistic, acultural model of their minority culture and the undeaf methods of studying deaf people that give rise to it, not merely as ignorant ravings of dangerously powerful people but as the intellectual underpinning of hearing intervention, in forcibly imposed educational isolation, in institutionalization, in ear surgery, and in all the forms that audist imposition takes.

Like the colonizers and the colonized, the hearing establishment serving deaf people and deaf people themselves have two different points of view, two different conceptions of deaf people, and two radically different agendas in America.

The hearing leadership of special education has maintained that the local school offers the least restrictive environment for deaf education; deaf people themselves think it is the most restrictive environment.* Hearing authorities commonly view American Sign Language as a crutch, refuse to learn it, and discourage its use; the half million or more deaf Americans for whom this is a primary language believe it is the equal of English as a natural language and clearly superior for instructing and communicating with deaf people. The hearing experts are frequently opposed to deaf teachers and conspire to block their entry into the profession by denying them access to training programs and selection for job vacancies.* Organizations of deaf people think they would be as good as or better than hearing teachers and seek their admission into the profession.

This is but a partial list; the startling and disturbing truth is that there is deep conflict between deaf people and those who profess to serve them in America and in many other nations. The fundamental divergence is this: hearing experts generally do not concede to deaf people a major say in the conduct of deaf affairs, especially as their ideas are so contrary; deaf people do not see why hearing people should have the determining say in matters that concern deaf people. So it is ever with the colonizers and the colonized.

The trait lists do seem, then, to incorporate paternalistic universals and paternalistic parallax; I come to a "White Man's Burden test" for ethnocentrism. In a paternalistic relation, the benefactors have, among other roles, that of educators, and they prove to be educators who subscribe to the *tabula rasa* view: Their beneficiaries have no language, culture, institutions—or none worth considering—and the benefactors have the burden of supplying them with their own. Ethnocentrism is one way, an intellectually unreflective way, of coming to grips with the diversity of humankind and human culture. It takes its own, generally unexamined, values as a universal norm; when these are patently not subscribed to by a culture that it is obliged to consider, the ethnocentric view frequently embraces evolutionism: The subject culture is at an earlier stage of development, it is more barbaric and animalistic (Table 1). The benefactor may see this as an immutable fact of intrinsic nature. But when there are economic and social rewards for beneficence, he is more likely to see the primitivism as remediable by his intervention.

· Thus it was that the civilizing task of the colonizers in Africa required them to supplant the natives' languages, religions, institutions, with those of the European mother country. A British leader in the colonization of West Africa described a native uprising in Sierra Leone as showing "the nature of the Negro in all his primitive savagery and barbarism which generations of missionaries failed to eradicate." A president of the American Historical Association wrote at the end of the last century: "Without disparagement it may be said there is a cruel streak in the Mexican nature. . . . It may, and doubtless should, be attributed partly to the Indian blood." Scholarly writing of this sort served to justify the Texas Rangers' violence toward Mexican-Americans: "vigorous methods" were necessary in dealing with such "savage adversaries."

The test for ethnocentrism is also positive when we examine the relations between the hearing establishment and deaf people. Deaf people are seen as occupying a lower rank of development: concrete in thought, impoverished in language, unsocialized, immature, morally undeveloped (Table 2).

Consider audist policies concerning the language of the American deaf community. This is a telling point, for language is not only a means of communication; it is also a repository of cultural knowledge and a symbol of social identity. In hearing people's milieu, languages are spoken; since deaf people rarely speak, hearing professionals have long contended that deaf people command little or no language. The classic American book on the psychology of the deaf, a primer for generations of experts on deafness, states: "Sign language cannot be considered comparable to a verbal symbol system." A 1978 French textbook for training teachers of deaf children asserts: "Mimic grammar is characterized above all by simplifications. There are no articles.

The adverbs and adjectives are indistinguishable. There are only three tenses and no passive." This lack of differentiation, the author explains, leads to thinking ambiguities. "Chair" and "to-sit-down" are expressed by the same gesture, he claims, as are "knife" and "to-cut"; in the end, the deaf child can't distinguish between them and countless other similar pairs. Likewise, a 1976 British textbook contends: "The argument against the traditional sign language, that it is nongrammatical and impedes the development of correct language forms, is valid." A Dutch book on signed languages and psycholinguistics, published in 1986, ignores an extensive scientific literature concerning those languages and claims: "The informative power of the natural sign language of the deaf is extremely weak." A major survey of research on cognition and deaf children holds that "[t]he deaf child grows up essentially without any language. . . . Lacking language, they have been exposed to few sophisticated ideas." Indeed, teachers of deaf children commonly say they are teaching their charges "language" when in fact they are trying, and failing, to teach them English: most of the children are already as fluent in their primary, manual language as the teacher is in his or her oral one.

Just as there are no skilled users of ASL who denigrate deaf language and culture, so it is difficult for someone who has not learned the language to compass the richness of American Sign Language, the shared body of knowledge of America's deaf people across the generations. Beginning in the 1960s and developing in the decades that followed, linguists and psychologists provided an avalanche of evidence that the world's manual languages were natural languages with autonomous vocabularies, grammars, and art forms all their own. American Sign Language has received particular study, and much is known now about its grammar, its literature and poetry, its evolution, its cognitive processing and how the brain works to accomplish it, its acquisition as a first language by children with deaf parents, its registers and dialects, and so on.* In 1985, a UNESCO report on deaf education stated as a principle that "We must recognize the legitimacy of the sign language as a linguistic system and it should be accorded the same status as other languages." Nevertheless, most educators and administrators in programs for deaf children and adults are proceeding as if ASL simply did not exist and as if the deaf community were not a language minority.

Educators of deaf pupils believe the most negative claims about manual language, even in the face of linguistic evidence to the contrary, because their concept of deaf people, like the colonizers' concept of Africans, requires deaf people's linguistic and intellectual inferiority. Most educators of deaf children worldwide speak to their profoundly deaf pupils. Yes, speak. Sometimes they write, as well, or accompany their speech with signs, but all these forms of communication presuppose a knowledge of the national oral language, which these children do not have. As if it needed scientific proof, many studies have shown that deaf children cannot understand their teachers' language on their lips or speak it intelligibly.* Nevertheless, it is the teachers' language that is used in class, and so education fails miserably.

Hearing educators place the source of the problem elsewhere—they blame the deaf students themselves. Their pupils are intellectually deficient, the educators claim, because they lack true language. These highly insulting assertions about deaf people and their language are quite false, as it was false, and dangerous, for the European colonizers to dismiss the African village debates, which they could not comprehend, as native palaver.

This ethnocentric misunderstanding about the nature and status of manual language has led some hearing educators to try to "fix up" the children's "arbitrary gestures" to make them more like English. Thus, they invent new signs for English function words and suffixes, which have no place, of course, in American Sign Language, and the grammatical order of the signs is scrambled in an attempt to duplicate English word order. No deaf child has ever learned such a system as a native language, nor indeed could he, for it violates the principles of the manual-visual channel of communication. No deaf adult uses such ways of communicating. No one has ever tried to teach French by using Franglais. But Signed English is widely used in classrooms for deaf children, on the pretext that it assists the deaf child in learning English. Deaf children characteristically do not succeed in learning English, however, so that cannot be the real reason for imposing a manual form of English on them; the ethnocentrism of paternalism is a more likely explanation.*

Finally, there is the issue of money: many political theorists maintain that the driving force in paternalistic relations is self-interest—economic self-interest, in particular. The issue is structural and not primarily a matter of the motives of individuals. The question is, are the relations between the audist establishment and deaf people constituted in such a way that they operate to the economic advantage of audists? The answer is, yes indeed. Audist education of deaf children has for a century equipped them primarily to enter the manual trades and not the professions serving deaf children and adults, to which many are naturally inclined. Deaf people are also consumers: they buy many of the things hearing people buy, but, in addition, they buy hearing aids, captioning devices, teletypewriters, speech therapy, audiology, rehabilitation and interpreter services, special education, and more. Some of these services and products for deaf people are bought by government. I estimate that the market of products and services aimed specifically at hard-of-hearing and deaf children and adults in the United States is about two billion dollars annually.

Consider the hearing aid share of the deafness market, for example. The Hearing Aid Industry Association estimates that all eighty thousand deaf children in school in America own one or more hearing aids—after all, their teachers can require the purchase. This "educational" policy, promoted by audiologists as well as educators and the hearing aid industry, has a slogan: "Every deaf child has a right to a hearing aid." Yet virtually all these children became deaf before they could learn English, and nearly half of them cannot hear and understand any speech at all,* so it is doubtful whether most deaf children derive any educational value from their aids, which may be why they are continually taking them off. Given such facts, it is natural to suspect that social and economic issues have played some role in determining this educational policy. Deaf parent and teacher Guy Vollmar recounts that the school for deaf children where he was employed and where his son Justin was enrolled required the boy to wear hearing aids, although both father and son protested they were costly and of no value at all. Informed of the dispute, the principal insisted the boy must wear the aids, but the school would lend him a pair. When the aids broke on account of Justin's negligence, his father was forced to buy them. Justin continued to resist and was held after school. Guy Vollmar appealed the school policy unsuccessfully, and at the end of the year he was dismissed.

Over one million hearing aids are sold annually in the United States, I am told, but perhaps only half of them to persons who purchase other products or services in the deafness market. The average cost of an aid is five hundred dollars. This comes to an annual market of a quarter of a billion dollars. Before being fitted for a hearing aid, the client sees an otologist and an audiologist. Add, conservatively, another half billion dollars. Then there are the educators, administrators, psychologists, counselors, interpreters, and more.

This market is controlled by hearing people. It is said to be conducted in the interest of deaf people, but the profits go almost exclusively to hearing people. A hearing person entering one of the professions that serve deaf people is expected to take on a way of perceiving and relating to deaf people that operates to the social, psychological, and monetary advantage of hearing people. Moreover, the future of this very large audist establishment depends on the continuing desire of the hearing community to view culturally deaf people as hearing-impaired and to aim to mitigate this impairment as far as possible. Audists have the strongest inducement to believe that deaf children and adults are indeed in need of hearing aids, speech therapy, rehabilitation, and the like, and in need of hearing administrators to manage their affairs and to educate deaf children.

What would become of the audist establishment if deaf people were allowed to educate deaf children using their most fluent language, the language of their nation's deaf community? What would become of the audist establishment if deaf children who chose not to wear hearing aids were no longer required to do so; if deaf people were so well educated that they required rehabilitation services as infrequently as hearing people? The answer is that if cultural deafness were accepted by hearing professionals, the practices of some would be only slightly affected; many otologists, audiologists, and hearing aid specialists, for example, treat primarily hearing people who have become deaf, frequently late in life. Other audists, however, would be more crucially affected: This group includes teachers of deaf children, school psychologists and administrators, and rehabilitation specialists.

Four different kinds of evidence thus support the claim that the traits attributed to deaf children and adults by the psychological literature are an expression of paternalistic stereotypes. As I have shown, there are paternalistic universals and parallax in the attributions, and a claim to a civilizing burden that fails to mask the benefactor's economic interest.

Audist "Psychology of the Deaf"

It seems, then, that there are fundamental commonalities between the relations of colonizers and colonized on the one hand and those of audists and deaf people on the other. The struggles of two different kinds of communities, separated in space and time, and with quite different historical specificities, seem to be embraced, nevertheless, by one set of principles. Yet if the experience of colonization is to be more than an analogy and actually a template for the experience of audism, we must reconcile the conclusion that the "psychology of the deaf" consists of paternalistic stereotypes with the fact that it is the distillation of an imposing body of scientific literature, the results of innumerable programs of research, whose findings were published after peer review in professional journals. Recall that the traits attributed to Africans in Table 1 were merely racist venom, whereas those attributed to deaf people that I listed in Table 2 I took without sifting from scientific publications. Is there, as the audist establishment maintains, a body of scientific knowledge concerning the psychology of deaf children and adults? Are the trait attributions trustworthy? Can we screen students, develop curricula, prepare teaching materials, train teachers, design environments, treat and institutionalize patients, and so on based on this information?

Let us start at the beginning. The deaf schoolchild takes his seat, and the psychologist or teacher distributes a test booklet and an IBM answer sheet. The child must read the first item on the test form, select an answer from among several plausible possibilities, most of them false, encode his choice as the corresponding letter or number, mark the corresponding place on the answer sheet, and promptly move on to the second item. Some deaf clients have been tested a lot, others not at all, but however sophisticated they may be in test-taking generally, they cannot know what is required by the particular test confronting them; they are commonly baffled, and the examiner is forced somehow to convey what needs to be done without dropping any hints on how to do it.* Some specialists believe that group testing of deaf clients is ruled out by the dual problems of their unfamiliarity with tests and the examiner's inability to communicate the instructions for taking the test. The beleaguered examiner, who rarely knows ASL, commonly resorts to ad hoc pantomime to convey what the deaf child or adult should do with the test in front of him. But the pantomime of such examiners is undependable, often unclear, and incomplete. Hearing people lose about five IQ points when given pantomime instructions for taking an IQ test, so some investigators have suggested that five points be added to all deaf IQ scores. The hearing psychologist with a deaf client is damned either way: If he (or she) uses pantomime, the score will be misleadingly low; if he uses English, he probably will not be understood at all, and the score will be even less valid. The manner of administering intelligence tests to deaf children can affect the child's "measured" IQ by fully thirty points.

Consistent and clear administration of personality tests is even more of a problem. For example, when one personality test was given to deaf people using elementary English and again using ASL, the results were so different that the investigators concluded it was like giving two different tests. Several studies of deaf people's personalities and mental health have used tests such as the Rorschach and the Thematic Apperception Test, called projective tests because the subject "projects" the unconscious forces at play in his personality onto the ambiguous figures presented. The Rorschach consists of ten ink blots on cards that are presented one at a time to the client, who is to tell what each form brings to mind, what parts of the blot are involved, and what makes him see it that way. The TAT consists of nineteen black-and-white pictures, and the client must make up a story for each one. With deaf subjects, it is difficult to know whether they understand the instructions or not.

One psychologist responsible for widely cited early results on the mental health of deaf adults frankly expresses his wonder that his patients were never irritable with his primitive signing as he struggled to convey to them what they were supposed to do on the Rorschach test and the TAT. Many deaf clients, not understanding the instructions and limited in their command of English, simply describe what is in the TAT picture instead of making up a story based on the picture, as they are supposed to. Others say or write rather little when confronted with either test. Knowledgeable people agree that meaningful scoring of the Rorschach and the TAT requires an examiner fluent in manual language and informed about the communicative, cultural, and social aspects of the deaf community, a condition that is rarely fulfilled.* According to a 1987 survey, only 15 percent of professional people who serve deaf clients focused on deafness in their education. I presume that an even smaller percent of service providers are knowledgeable about deaf language and culture.

Psychologists who want to give their deaf clients tests designed for hearing people have a problem: If they change the procedures and language so the deaf person understands the test, then they cannot compare the results to the norms obtained with hearing people and thereby evaluate their client. But if they do not adapt the test for their deaf clients, the deaf persons' scores do not present a true picture of their knowledge or state of mind.

Since deaf test-takers in America frequently are not fluent in English, they not only fail to understand test instructions thoroughly, invalidating the results, but also fail to understand the test content itself, as most tests are presented in written English, and in rather high-level English at that. Nevertheless, psychologists continue to administer such tests to deaf subjects, to report the peculiar results in scientific journals, and to misclassify deaf children as, for example, learning disabled.*

One authority estimates that a tenth-grade knowledge of English is needed to take most personality tests meaningfully. Yet only one deaf student in ten reads at eighth-grade level or better, and the average deaf student on leaving school has only a third-grade command of English. Even if merely a third-grade reading level is necessary for some tests, half of the test respondents must then frequently answer on whim, since roughly half of test scores fall below the average. Hence, we must reject the results of most personality testing done with deaf people, and with them most of the unfavorable attributions I reported earlier.

A British study illustrates the problem of test comprehension with the responses of a profoundly deaf thirteen-year-old with average intelligence and a fondness for playing soccer, who took the Maudsley Medical Questionnaire on two occasions twelve months apart.

1. Do you find it difficult to get into conversation with strangers? *First administration: Yes / Second: No*
2. Have you ever been troubled by a stammer or stutter? *N / Y*
3. Do you have nightmares? *Y / N*
4. Are you an irritable person? *Y / Y*

5. Do you ever get short of breath without doing heavy work?
   Y / Y
6. What are you going to be when you leave school? *16 years / Builders or joiners*

Even more dependent on interpreting language nuances are clinical interviews and the diagnostic decisions and data that arise from them. Several studies have shown that psychotherapists prefer clients who are middle-class, articulate, and well educated, and assign such clients more hopeful diagnoses than those who are not. Many deaf clients would not be accepted into therapy and would receive adverse diagnoses based on these criteria. Centers for psychiatric treatment of deaf adults in Illinois and in New York reported that only one deaf patient in four could make himself understood through speaking. How, then, is the diagnostician to distinguish among the bizarre delusional language of schizophrenia, the retardation of thought of psychotic depression, and the pressure of talk in mania? Generally, hearing specialists cannot, and this has led them to misdiagnose deaf people and to label deaf children and adults as emotionally disturbed or mentally ill without good evidence.*

In 1987, a superior court judge in Washington, D.C., ordered Matti Hoge, a seventy-five-year-old deaf woman, to be released from the institution for retarded persons where she had been placed by foster parents in 1930. Institution officials claimed that she had an IQ of 34 when tested on admission, but recent testing showed her IQ to be near normal. For the last fifteen years of her incarceration, Ms. Hoge was in the cottage with the most retarded patients; she knew ASL but was unable to communicate with other residents or staff. In California, the family of Alberto Valdez, a thirty-three-year-old deaf man, filed suit against Orange County officials for mistakenly placing him in a mental institution, where he has spent most of his life. Mr. Valdez, one of six children in a Spanish-speaking family, became deaf following an illness when he was a little over a year old. At school age, he was refused admission to school because officials believed him mentally retarded. Subsequently, he was placed in the Metropolitan State Hospital.

In a study of one mental institution with four thousand patients, only one of the two hundred patients listed as deaf was in fact deaf, while there were five patients on a single ward in that hospital who were deaf and not on the list. Had no one ever tried to talk to the deaf patients in all their years in that hospital? Or had doctors tried and failed and put the problem out of their minds? In another hospital, some five hundred children with behavioral problems were given diagnoses, first by one clinician, then by another working independently. The first examiner found twelve deaf children in the hospital, the second, thirteen. But these two groups did not overlap; not one child was diagnosed as deaf by both specialists, who were hearing.

Misguided arrangements for testing deaf children and adults do not prevent the audist psychologist or psychiatrist from publishing, for publish one must, but they do make him anxious. Preposterously, the deaf person's mental health is judged by his ability to alleviate the psychiatrist's anxiety. According to an authoritative work on deaf people and mental illness, if the client can "gauge his communication to the manual language abilities of the interviewer, this shows the deaf person's social empathy and insight." Clearly, the first priority of benefactors is the management of their beneficiaries. If the psychiatrist finds he can communicate with his deaf client because the patient comes to his rescue with written English or pantomime, then the deaf person must be mentally healthy. If, on the other hand, the psychiatrist cannot communicate fluently with the deaf person, then the deaf person is no doubt ill. His lack of language (that is, English) has distorted his personality. "As hearing children grow up," a 1978 textbook on the "psychology of the deaf" explains, "they replace physical violence with verbal aggression. But the deaf cannot do this as they have no language." And in the *British Medical Journal*, I read that "It is not difficult to understand how deafness might facilitate [a persecution complex because] where there is a failure of reality testing, an edifice of paranoid disorder may be erected upon this foundation of misunderstanding." It is, of course, the hearing stereotype of deaf people and not real deaf people who have no language, who cannot test reality, and who are, as a consequence, isolated, aggressive, impulsive, and so on. Unfortunately, however, psychiatrists, psychologists, rehabilitation counselors, social workers, and other professional hearing people have power over real deaf children and adults.

The Illinois center for psychiatric treatment of deaf adults found depressive illness common among its patients, but the New York center found it rare. The former group interpreted all the depressive signs as evidence that deaf people generally internalize thoughts of failure; the New York group interpreted the lack of depressive findings as evidence that deaf people generally externalize failure, attributing it to anything but themselves. Other studies of the incidence of mental illness among deaf people find schizophrenia a common diagnosis in the United States but rare in Denmark, where deaf adults are more likely to be found suffering from paranoia, a rare diagnosis for deaf Americans. Such diagnostic mayhem not only leads to irresponsible characterizations of deaf people; it prevents effective planning of the services deaf people need, and it deprives deaf children and adults of proper care. Heaven help the deaf man or woman who really is mentally ill; earthly help is not likely to be forthcoming.

Do deaf adults differ from hearing people in the types and frequencies of their mental disorders? No one knows. On the one hand, deaf children are commonly portrayed in the psychological literature as emotionally disturbed, and some psychiatrists believe that this must lead to increased mental illness in adulthood. On the other hand, most investigators maintain that deaf adults are no different from hearing adults when it comes to mental illness—somehow, all those severely disturbed deaf children become healthy adults.*

Researchers who believe that deaf people cannot be normal in cognition and behavior, that "common sense [suggests] the deaf would have an increased risk of developing schizophrenia," are clearly biased, and most experiments with deaf children and adults are wide open to the charge of conscious or unconscious bias against deaf people. To aggravate the problem, a child or an adult who is acting up and who also does not respond to English commands represents a double threat to the examiner, parent, or teacher. When the assessment of the deaf person is subjective, as it is with projective tests, rating scales, checklists, and interviews, a biased examiner can unwittingly influence the scores and therefore invalidate the results. One study duped examiners by presenting them with personal histories that identified some subjects as lower-class and others as middle-class along with their (fabricated and matched) Rorschach responses. In nearly every scoring, biases were apparent in favor of the "middle-class" patients.

In short, the Rorschach is a projective test for the examiner as well as the patient. Nevertheless, just such subjective scoring methods are used by many personality tests whose findings make up the literature on the "psychology of the deaf." Most studies not only use these kinds of measures but also fail to concern themselves with the problem of bias, and fail to take the elementary precaution where possible of withholding from the scorer the hearing status of the child or adult whose test results he (or she) is evaluating. The results collected and biased by audist psychologists are then used by other audists to make educational decisions. To illustrate: Two psychologists present a case against residential schools for deaf children based in part on Rorschach scores of doubtful validity obtained from children in those schools. The children's responses to the inkblots, the authors claim, give evidence of "immaturity, egocentricity, distorted perception, lacking empathy, more dependency on others, and deficiency in intellectual functioning" and thus show that "one's personality may be negatively affected [by the residential school]."

One type of study of deaf children that is particularly subject to the examiner's biases, and whose results are therefore particularly untrustworthy, uses ratings of behavior or checklists. (Example: Does Johnny come when called? Check one—Always, Sometimes, Never.) Yet the results of such studies carry great weight with the audist establishment. For example, an expert on psychiatry and deaf people, Hilde Schlesinger, writes: "It has been found that deaf school age children, when compared with their hearing peers, have five times as much emotional disturbance." This is a significant claim from an authoritative source who, like many other authors, cites her study with psychologist Kathryn Meadow, conducted fifteen years earlier. In that study, eighty-five teachers and counselors at the state school for deaf children in Berkeley, California, were asked to rate all of their students as: "severely emotionally disturbed and have been or should be referred for psychiatric help"; or "not severely disturbed but whose behavior necessitates a disproportionate share of the teacher's time, or requires other special attention"; or neither. The staff considered that 12 percent of their pupils (figures rounded) were severely disturbed and another 20 percent demanded too much attention. Teachers in the Los Angeles County schools, however, found only 2.5 and 7 percent of their pupils disturbed and disturbing, respectively. Comparing the 12 percent of deaf pupils to the 2.5 percent of hearing pupils rated "severely disturbed," Schlesinger concluded that deaf children "have five times as much emotional disturbance" as hearing children.

Such teacher ratings are widely used in the "psychology of the deaf" despite the research of, for example, Robert Rosenthal and colleagues, which has long led psychologists to expect bias in teacher ratings. In the famous experiment called "Pygmalion in the Classroom," teachers who were told untruthfully that a certain 20 percent of their students were ready to bloom intellectually later rated those children superior to their classmates in personal qualities such as cooperativeness and adjustment, although the children singled out had been chosen at random.

Like the teachers at the Berkeley school, teachers of deaf children nationwide frequently label their pupils as having an "emotional/behavioral problem," a "specific learning disability," and "mental retardation"; they report nearly a third of their students have a handicapping condition beyond deafness. A British study of all deaf high school leavers, however, found that only one deaf child in ten had an "additional" handicapping condition. And when a British psychiatrist examined a group of deaf children transferred to a special school for mentally ill youngsters, he found that one third were improperly referred and were simply a little difficult to manage in their regular schoolroom. American special educators, who are mostly female, labeled twice as many male deaf students "emotionally disturbed" as female students. African-American deaf children and those with the least English skills are also promiscuously labeled emotionally disturbed.

Reviewing records at the California School for the Deaf, Riverside, a leading American authority on the "psychology of the deaf," McCay Vernon, concluded that 23 percent of the children had "severe psychiatric problems," while another 21 percent were "poorly adjusted"—44 percent in all—nearly half again as many as Schlesinger and Meadow found at Riverside's sister school in Berkeley. The highest incidence of emotional disturbance among deaf schoolchildren was reported by one (anonymous) teacher who sent her entire class to the Berkeley school project for therapy. We are tempted to conclude, in the words of two researchers who studied teacher ratings of deaf children, " 'Disturbed' to the teacher means 'disturbing to the classroom situation.' "

The incidence of emotional disturbance reported for deaf children fluctuates wildly across the fifty states—from 2 to 28 percent in schools of comparable size. In some school districts, a report of higher rates of emotional disturbance translates into a larger budget; in others, it means smaller classes as children are transferred to specialized facilities. In the words of two demographers who have studied the question: "Both the fiscal climate and the organization of human services [in each state] affect the process of identification and labeling."

If the deviance of deaf children is exaggerated, so, too, it appears, is the normalcy of the hearing children to whom they have been compared. Schlesinger and Meadow claimed that only 2.5 percent of hearing schoolchildren were emotionally disturbed (in contrast with 12 percent of the deaf children at the Berkeley school), but this is a gross underestimate of the incidence of emotional disturbance among hearing children, according to two authorities: "Estimates from knowledgeable sources in education and mental health fields range from 10 to 20 percent or more." I find it reasonable to suspect that some estimates of emotional disturbance among hearing children are also inflated, so let us retain the lower end of the range—that proves to be about the same incidence as Schlesinger and Meadow attributed to deaf children. How, then, can we explain the peculiarly low rates of emotional disturbance that they reported for the Los Angeles County schools? I was curious, so I obtained the reports from the county that Schlesinger and Meadow used as a benchmark. A closer look at the percentages of hearing pupils in the Los Angeles County schools who were rated emotionally disturbed offers some surprises. Data were not included for any pupil with an IQ less than 75, nor for some four thousand disturbed hearing children whose grade level was not reported, nor for hearing pupils in more than ninety county schools for "exceptional children." Moreover, in some fortunate schools there were, according to teachers, virtually no disturbed children, while in others the rate of emotional disturbance was far above the average. Seven percent of the hearing children in the inner-city schools were considered so seriously disturbed by their teachers that they were not merely labeled disturbed; they were sent to professional staff for mental health testing.

The higher concentration of ethnic minorities in the inner-city schools has probably contributed to the reports of emotional disturbance by biased teachers. Another study of California schoolchildren showed that Mexican-Americans and African-Americans were much more likely to be labeled "retarded" and sent to special programs than Anglos with the same (low) IQ scores.

That the weight of the evidence impugns the accuracy and impartiality of teacher ratings should not surprise us. As Dr. Meadow-Orlans has noted, teachers of deaf children carry a "tremendous emotional load [and the teacher's] frustration, impatience, and anger can create additional classroom problems." Likewise, parents of deaf children "feel powerless and become increasingly angry and shrill," according to Dr. Schlesinger. Only one parent in ten could communicate with his or her deaf child in the Berkeley school study, but there is good evidence that the more parents can communicate with their deaf child, the better their opinion of the child. The capacity of the teachers to communicate fluently with their pupils was unreported but doubtlessly low.

Ratings are not only of doubtful validity but unreliable—raters often disagree. Much of the time parents do not agree with teachers or among themselves on their deaf children's emotional disturbance. Psychologists consider two judges reliable in evaluating whether a child has or has not a set of traits if most of the time they make independent judgments that agree. A rule of thumb is that they must agree 95 percent of the time. One study found that mother and father disagree about 15 percent of the time whether their deaf child is emotionally disturbed; mother and teacher disagree 25 percent of the time, and father and teacher disagree 40 percent of the time. For most deaf children, neither their mother's nor their father's opinion of their emotional disturbance agrees with the psychologist's test results. And teachers generally do not agree with each other about the emotional or behavioral problems of their deaf pupils; they so rarely agreed in one study that "these ratings had to be discarded." When Meadow and Dyssegaard found that deaf students in Denmark were rated better adjusted than their peers in America, they acknowledged that "Possibly the Danish teachers are less willing than American teachers to make negative statements about their students"; but they go on to conclude that the American children's high ratings for "impulsivity" are supported by psychiatrist Kenneth Altshuler's theories, "Schlesinger's clinical practice ... Levine's projective testing, Vernon's clinical evaluations [and the experiment on impulsivity] of Yugoslav and American deaf and hearing adolescents by Altshuler."

Impulsivity is the type of psychological disturbance most often ascribed to deaf children in the psychological literature. The reasons for this ascription need scrutiny. As early as 1964, Altshuler hypothesized that without auditory experience, the deaf child develops an inadequate conscience, has difficulty internalizing rage, and handles tension by a kind of primitive riddance, reflected in impulsivity. The Schlesinger and Meadow study at the Berkeley school seemed to add credence to this ascription. Altshuler later claimed to have confirmed his theory of deaf impulsivity in the only study comparing hearing and deaf children on this measure that did not use ratings; he administered tests to hearing and deaf adolescents here and in Yugoslavia.

One of the tests was the Rorschach, which was scored for impulsivity in numerous ways—for example, by counting the number of inkblots that the deaf child said resembled animals. In a second test, the deaf student had to trace his way out of a series of paper-and-pencil mazes—the more errors, the more impulsive. In a third, he was asked simply to draw a line as slowly as possible—the shorter the time, the more impulsive. A fourth test used pictures of emotionally charged situations, and the deaf child was to choose one of three pictorial resolutions or to give titles to the situations. There were still other tests.

It is unclear, however, how much the deaf students understood of the instructions for performing these tests and of the content of the pictured situations; how the experimenter and subject communicated for the projective tests; how much bias was introduced by the experimenters, who knew the hearing status of each subject. To further confound any interpretation of the results, no information is provided on the validity of the tests as a measure of impulsivity in deaf students. Suppose the average deaf child did draw lines more quickly than the average hearing one. Does that mean that deaf children are more impulsive than their hearing counterparts or that they are more adept at visual tasks? Many of the tests used in this experiment must be invalid, because the scores of none of the tests agreed (correlated) with those of any other. If the children's scores on line drawing and on animal responses to the inkblots are unrelated, for example, so that some fast drawers gave few animal responses and slow drawers many, then both tests cannot be valid measures of impulsivity; for if one affirms that the results on the draw-a-line test are valid measures of impulsivity, the unrelated results on the inkblots cannot be, and vice versa.

Finally, the investigators failed to provide evidence that the differences in test scores between hearing and deaf groups were reliable and could not have arisen by chance. After all, testing either group twice would yield different average results. This proof of reliability is usually accomplished with statistical tests showing that the difference between two groups is large in comparison with average differences among people within the groups. Probably, some of the differences between the groups did not meet accepted standards of reliability; the article indeed implies that several of the differences between the hearing and the deaf subjects were not much larger than differences frequently to be found among the hearing and among the deaf subjects.

Estimates of learning disability among deaf children are as unreliable as those of emotional disturbance. In the first place, there are no reliable and valid criteria for making these ascriptions to deaf children; and in the second place, the teachers who commonly make them are untrained for the purpose and possess a scanty knowledge at best of the language and mores of the children they are judging. The answers to questions such as "Is Johnny an emotionally disturbed child?" or "Is Susan a learning disabled child?" depend more on the values of the person making the judgment than they do on the child. Sally Tomlinson, a British sociologist studying special education, has pointed out that children from all social classes appear in the categories of handicap for which there are clear criteria, such as physical disability, but the lower classes and ethnic minorities dominate in categories for which the criteria are unclear, like emotionally disturbed and learning disabled. One American survey found 7 percent of deaf children in a large sample had been labeled "learning-disabled" and, therefore, "multiply-handicapped." Vernon reported that 25 percent of the deaf children in a large sample were learning disabled; he actually called them "aphasic"—that is, impaired in language processing due to brain damage. He was apparently unaware that many of the children were fluent in ASL. Vernon, too, merely took ratings by teachers at face value. A Canadian study, however, found only 2.5 percent of deaf children learning disabled. A 1989 review of the published research on this topic, such as it is, concludes, reasonably enough, that the incidence of learning disability among deaf children is uncertain. The review goes on to argue, however, that where there's smoke, there's fire: These surveys provide evidence that educators believe such a problem exists and therefore evidence that "a significant proportion of the hearing-impaired population falls within the learning-disabled hearing-impaired group."

It may come as a shock to the many educators who think that "a significant proportion" of deaf children are learning disabled to hear that deaf children have outperformed matched hearing children on several cognitive tests: Some six independent studies have found that deaf children of deaf parents score reliably above the mean on nonverbal IQ tests; the means are based on a large sample of hearing children of hearing parents.* Likewise, Bellugi and colleagues at the Salk Institute gave deaf children of varying ages tasks involving face and pattern recognition and found they outperformed hearing children matched in age. Other studies have shown that deaf children recall spatial arrays better than matched hearing children and that adults born deaf are faster and more accurate in detecting movement out of the corners of their eyes than are hearing adults.

All things considered, is it reasonable to trust teacher and parent ratings of the deaf child's emotional disturbance and intellectual capacity and to publish their judgments as facts about deaf children? Shouldn't we demand some separate proof, besides the hearing person's subjective opinion?

Scores are assigned to deaf children by teachers, examiners, or parents using a rating scale; or the children themselves, unclear as to the procedures and the meanings of the questions, docilely answer test items as best they can. Now their answers must be compared to the "right" answers to obtain a score, and the score must be compared to those of a large group of children or adults. But the "right" answers are right for hearing people and not necessarily for deaf people, and very few tests have ever been used with large numbers of deaf people, so there is no way to compare one person's score with an average. Personality tests, for example, contain questions that were designed to spot hearing people with personality problems. When the scoring system designed for hearing people is applied to deaf people, the results often have little validity. Consider the widely used test that bears the imposing name Minnesota Multiphasic Personality Inventory: the MMPI, in the trade. It consists of more than five hundred statements, which the subject must answer with "true" or "false." Each answer potentially gains him a point for hysteria, paranoia, depression, schizophrenia, or five other disorders. Here is one of the statements: "At times I hear so well it bothers me." Psychiatric outpatients at the University of Minnesota Hospital who were diagnosed paranoid answered "true" to that question more often than the presumably normal friends who accompanied them to the clinic and were willing to do some of the test while waiting. What is a deaf person supposed to make of that question, however, or of "I would like to be a singer"? Some questions are more subtly biased: "I enjoy reading love stories"; "In a group of people I would not be embarrassed to be called upon to start a discussion or give an opinion about something I know well." I read all the questions on this test designed for and by hearing people and concluded that about a fourth are inappropriate for deaf people. Should it count as paranoid if a deaf person confirms that "People often stare at me in restaurants," when indeed they do generally gape at his signing?

Although it is a major source of the literature on the "psychology of the deaf," the MMPI suffers from all the invalidating weaknesses I have described; difficult to administer, to read, to interpret, with content and norms inappropriate to deaf people, it should never have been used with this population, and certainly the results should not have been published. Nearly all of the other tests whose results constitute the literature of the "psychology of the deaf" have likewise not been revised for and standardized on deaf populations.

Finally, I will note that the research on the "psychology of the deaf" commonly fails to describe the group of deaf people who are evaluated. This, too, is a paternalistic error—regarding all members of a minority as fundamentally alike. Average results are reported for groups made up of very different kinds of deaf people. Deaf people differ in sex, age, and social class; in the age at which they became deaf; in whether their parents and relatives are hearing or deaf; in the ways they communicate at school, at home, and with peers; in the type of schooling they receive; in their command of oral and written English and of ASL; in their membership in minority groups, including the American deaf community; in whether they had physical or mental handicaps prior to and following deafness. All of these factors (and others) can be important in determining how a deaf person performs on a test.

The common failure to select subjects on these characteristics ruins experiments in two ways. If a sample of deaf people contains all these different kinds of deaf people, it becomes unlikely that differences between deaf and hearing subjects can be discovered that are large compared to the average differences among individuals within the two groups; thus, there can be no confidence in the apparent difference between hearing and deaf subjects if one is uncovered.

Second, if the investigator does not know what kinds of deaf people responded to his tests, he does not know to which kinds of deaf people his results apply. He cannot generalize his findings. Clearly, research that fails to distinguish the characteristics of its test population is uninterpretable and without value for educational policy, even if the tests themselves were appropriate for deaf clients. For example, when Schlesinger concluded from the Berkeley school ratings that "deaf school age children" are five times more emotionally disturbed than their hearing peers, she was assuming that a group of deaf children from a residential school was representative of the national population of deaf children, which is decidedly not the case.

Some deaf people to whom I have shown the list in Table 2 have told me that it seems natural for deaf children to be disturbed when you consider how long most were frustrated in their efforts to communicate with parents and teachers. Parents who refuse to adapt to their deaf children, and teachers who refuse to learn and use manual language, are responsible, they say, for the abnormal thinking and behavior of deaf children. McCay Vernon, on the other hand, suspects that the cause of behavioral and emotional disturbance in deaf children, as well as their difficulty in learning "language" (he means English), may be undetectable lesions of the central nervous system that accompanied the child's loss of hearing.

Before we debate explanations, however, we should be sure we have something to explain. We have seen that the studies that gave rise to the trait attributions in Table 2 are invalid: Tests were administered to deaf children and adults in ways that were certain to be unclear and to yield unreliable results; the language of the tests must surely have been incomprehensible to many of the deaf persons tested in the research; the scoring of results proved to be undependable, subjective, and easily influenced by the prejudices of the examiner; there was poor agreement among hearing evaluators judging the same deaf children or adults; rarely was there any evidence that the tests employed actually measured what they claimed to measure; the content of the tests, designed originally by and for hearing people, was often unrelated to deaf experience and schooling; the interpretation of results obtained from deaf people was usually based on hearing people's scores; and most research reports gave very sketchy descriptions of the kinds of deaf people tested. With the benefit of hindsight and the knowledge of deaf people's culture and language acquired since the 1970s, I found in this literature, which continues to grow, an object lesson in how not to conduct psychological measurement and a mockery of science that dangerously lays claim to be science.

We must have tests that are designed for deaf people from top to bottom, from administration to content; we must have tests that provide reliable and valid measures of the thinking and behavior of deaf children and adults; we must have evidence of the performance of large groups of deaf people of all kinds so that any individual's score can be evaluated with respect to the larger population. This is just what we do not have. What we have, instead, are stereotypes recast as science, stereotypes that blame the victims in order to obscure the failings and self-interest of the audist establishment.*

There is no psychology of the deaf. It is, in fact, not clear that there *can* be one. The term may inevitably represent the pathologizing of cultural differences, the interpretation of difference as deviance. Of course, there are interesting things to be learned and reported about deaf culture, deaf language, and deaf people; the same can be said about many minorities. This knowledge may be found in the literature of that minority, or in works of anthropology, sociology, and sociolinguistics focused on that group. These descriptions are not, however, a "psychology" of the minority and are not offered as such. There is no text or body of scientific studies on the psychology of African-Americans or Hispanic-Americans, and if there were one, we would suspect the author in advance of racism. True, there are books and courses called "the psychology of women"; perhaps that misnomer came about because women do not constitute as distinct a cultural subgroup as, say, Hispanic-Americans.

Attempts to articulate the psychology of a minority group play into the hands of those who manipulate the members of the group for their own ends. Neither the blatant shortcomings of the research on the "psychology of the deaf," nor the incongruity of its findings with the achievements of countless deaf people, nor cries of alarm from a few renegades in the audist establishment, have inhibited the proliferation of slapdash studies purporting to show the character flaws of deaf children and adults. Indeed, the perceived incompetence of deaf people may be not the result of research on the "psychology of the deaf" but rather its cause; it is an interpretation that has a disturbing resemblance to stages in the crystallization of the colonizer's racist stereotypes, as Albert Memmi described them: (1) Discover differences; (2) assign them values to the advantage of the colonizer and the disadvantage of the colonized; (3) make the differences inherent: affirm that they are definitive, and act to make them so.

How did such a tragedy occur in the professions serving deaf people, at great cost in human suffering, scholarly effort, and federal funds? Why doesn't much of the research in this field meet elementary standards of scientific rigor? I believe it is because social science research is a social institution itself. As a hearing activity devoted to characterizing the deaf minority, it came under the sway of the basic tenet of hearing-deaf relations in our society, paternalism. Experts who are hearing and are commonly ignorant of the language, institutions, culture, history, mores, and experiences of deaf people could only be guided in the first instance by the stereotypes to which we have all been acculturated and by their training within the audist establishment. I submit that when their investigations tended to confirm these seemingly logical a priori beliefs, they pursued them and published them without niggling, as it seemed, about procedural details. And as I will show, there are close links—political, social, and economic in nature—between the measurement of deaf children and adults, their education or rehabilitation, and the control of their bodies by the audist establishment.

How can we protect research on deaf children and adults from the structural paternalism that dictates the training of professional people, the funding of their research, their access to subjects, publication, and so on? The single most effective remedy would be to involve deaf people themselves at all levels of the undertaking. Federal agencies such as the Department of Education and the National Institutes of Health, which support most research on deaf people in the United States, should formulate a strategy to recruit and qualify many more deaf principal investigators. Those agencies should require the projects they sponsor to turn preferentially to the deaf community for advisers and collaborators in research design and implementation, for assistance in data collection and analysis, for guidance in interpretation of results. Federal agencies should refuse to fund, and universities to conduct, research on deaf people that does not involve deaf people, as these institutions would refuse, I trust, at least in these enlightened times, to sponsor research of vital concern to African-Americans without their involvement. Likewise, Africans contribute to social science research on Africa with cogency, originality, and insight, and they hold their non-African colleagues to account. The old paternalism of the European Africanists is no longer tenable. Shouldn't it be the same way with studies of deaf people?

PART THREE

Representations of Deaf People: Power, Politics, and the Dependency Duet

Representation and Power

To portray a group is to engage in a political activity. If the native is a child, he needs the European's guidance. If his actions are immoral and heathen, he needs the missionary. If he is uncivilized, only European intervention can raise him up to the status of civilized man. Deaf children and adults, in becoming the technical objects of psychometric investigation, make the audist establishment possible and seemingly legitimate its control over them. The ways in which audists characterize deaf people are intimately bound up with the conduct of deaf education and training and the program of implanting deaf children with cochlear prostheses. The portrayal of deaf people as socially isolated, intellectually weak, behaviorally impulsive, and emotionally immature makes school psychology and counseling, special education and rehabilitation, appear necessary; the failure of deaf education makes desperate and ill-founded medical intervention more appealing. If there is to be a treatment, and a treatment establishment, there must be a "syndrome" to treat.

The audist establishment produces information, largely in schools of education that train teachers of the deaf, audiologists, speech and language pathologists, and educational psychologists, among others. Students are required to conduct research for master's and doctoral degrees; faculty are required to publish research in order to receive promotion, increases in pay, and "tenure," a guaranteed job until retirement. Researchers in schools of education tend to conduct studies that are consistent with prevailing educational policy and may even have as their purpose to legitimate that policy. The audist establishment is so constituted that a great many hearing people write a great many articles about deaf people. It would be unthinkable today for black studies programs to be composed entirely of white people who published articles about black people in professional journals; nor could there be an all-male women's studies program that published antifeminist literature. Our universities have yet to apply the same ethical (and practical) principles when it comes to the deaf community.

Thanks to the misbegotten educational programs operated by the audist establishment, deaf people are mostly illiterate—but they are the subject of a huge body of literature as the establishment disseminates the information it produces through the professional journals that it publishes, such as *The American Annals of the Deaf*, published by the Convention of American Instructors of the Deaf and the Conference of Educational Administrators Serving the Deaf. Papers submitted for publication in the journals or for presentation at the professional meetings must be approved by members of the profession in a process called "peer review," and generally the journal editor or the chairman of the meeting has some discretionary power as well. In this way the profession decides what information is legitimate and shall be disseminated and what is not and shall not be. It is in a position to influence professional, governmental, and public perceptions of deaf people and to shape the appropriate responses. Textbooks based on the published literature are selected by the establishment to train future audists, who will generate more literature. Courses are prepared and required of students that teach some things—for example, "the psychology of the deaf"—and not others—for example, ASL. The education of professional people to conduct research and provide services to deaf people is value laden, but the values are rarely discussed. So the profession controls what it disseminates to itself and its students and to practitioners as well. This has driven the substantive debate outside the profession and into other intellectual forums, such as *The New York Review of Books*, professional journals in linguistics, and autobiographies by deaf authors.

Hearing people require large amounts of money to conduct much of the research that they perform on deaf people. Money is needed to pay part of the professional person's salary; money is needed to pay for assistants and for travel to professional meetings to disseminate findings; money is needed for publication charges, for equipment and supplies, for telephone calls and postage and the like. And the university will tack on a large increment to the basic budget—it can run as high as 80 percent or more—for "overhead." So researchers frequently submit proposals for contracts or outright grants to government agencies such as the National Institutes of Health and the Department of Education, which have been given large amounts of money by the Congress for this purpose. When these agencies receive a proposal for research, they send it to the investigator's peers for review. My point is twofold: The money our government spends on enhancing the education and welfare of deaf children and adults goes almost exclusively to hearing people; and the members of the audist establishment review one another's proposals, with all the dangers of inbreeding that this arrangement entails.

Understandably, the establishment tends to support research and disseminate information that is consistent with its views and favorable to its own welfare and aggrandizement. There is exceedingly little of the deaf point of view to be found in the *Annals* or any other audist journal or in conference proceedings. This is not, generally, the result of conscious malevolent attempts to suppress information. Rather, views that have a deaf "center" seem to audists wildly at odds with prevailing views, unworthy of dissemination, and the credentials of the people who present these views or the methods they employ may seem unconventional: For example, the rejected study may have surveyed deaf people themselves rather than professionals who work with deaf people, or ethnographic methods may have been used rather than those arising from educational psychology. All in all, the system works to filter out what it most needs to incorporate, a perspective from outside the system—above all, one provided by the deaf community.

Preposterously invidious descriptions of deaf people issued with authority by hearing people in the audist establishment have thus enjoyed a long and protected history. The practice continues. The award for zaniest defamation may well have been earned by the educator of deaf college students who reported in 1988 a "failure of hearing-impaired [college] students to conceptualize changes over time and space," as if such students didn't keep appointments, couldn't find classrooms, hadn't used for most of their lives a language that requires subtle temporal and spatial discriminations, and had not relied on temporal and spatial understanding in much of their precollege education. Such invidious descriptions are designed to confirm the audist belief in the deaf child's "special needs"—above all, his special need for the audist establishment. The notion of need, as the need for food and the need for love, has been extended metaphorically here.

"The needs of the blind," writes sociologist Robert Scott in his classic *The Making of Blind Men*, "[are those] blind people must have if they are to fit into and be served by programs that have arisen for other reasons." We have seen that there are no trustworthy measures of deaf children which can establish that a particular deaf child has certain extended needs. Instead, the construct, with its biological overtones, serves to deflect attention from educators' abuse of power—for example, in the choice of instructional language, in the exclusion of deaf teachers, in the denial of deaf culture. Conceptualizing minority education as a matter of the deaf child's "special needs" aims to make individual and medical what is communal and cultural, so it is an act of mystification designed to obscure the true power relations that are involved. When an educator affirms the pupils' special needs, he may also be gaining funds for the school (state allocations are often based on the number of "special needs students"), justifying a child's poor academic progress, or legitimating the exclusion of a child from a regular classroom and his or her incarceration in a "special" facility. As special education is a safety valve for the regular classroom, the designation "multiply handicapped" is the safety valve for special education. Writes one distinguished sociologist of special education: "Special needs is a euphemism for failure."

The failings of deaf people exist always in relation to the strengths of hearing people; moreover, deaf people are fantastically flawed in nearly all respects (Table 2); so it is clear that the purpose of the devaluation of the deaf person is to enhance the apparent value of the audist professional. The definitive text on deaf education in the last century was written by Baron de Gérando, Napoleon's vice-minister of the interior, and administrative director of the Paris National Institute for Deaf-Mutes, the first school ever founded for this class of citizens. He described deaf children as "isolated, detached, fickle, capricious, superficial, unimaginative, complacent, irritable, ungrateful," and so on and so forth. Comparison with Table 2 reveals that hearing authorities have not fundamentally changed their view of deaf people in a century and a half. The parallel with colonialism continues. Albert Memmi has put it this way: "The oppressor is on a balance scale with the oppressed; if his level is high economically, socially, in power, it is only because the other's is low." In an auto-defense doomed to fail, "He may insist on the extreme deficiencies of the oppressed, or on his own distinguished abilities, or both." Hearing people reason abstractly, morally; they are social and even-handed, whereas deaf people are concrete, amoral, isolated, and impulsive. Well then, if hearing society is so splendid, why not work exclusively among hearing people? "But the colonist is a god in the colony and a nobody in the metropole."

Deaf intellectuals of the last century, such as the French educator Ferdinand Berthier, wrote books rebutting hearing calumnies against deaf people, citing behavioral evidence of the moral sensibilities of deaf children, recording the intellectual feats of deaf adults (the books themselves gave the lie to the hearing claims), affirming the limitless possibilities of French Sign Language—but all this was utterly ignored in the corridors of power, as today deaf outrage is still ignored by the audist establishment.

The autodefense of the balance scale doesn't help. In the end, the colonizer knows he is guilty, has little confidence in his personal case, and espouses instead the case of his class, which he grandly calls "society"—restoring the deaf to society is what the audist also claims to be about.

Thus, in 1800, shortly after the dawn of deaf education in the French Enlightenment, Abbé Sicard, head teacher at the Paris school and author of the first textbook for systematically educating children born deaf, wrote there: "Such a child is a complete nonentity in society, a living machine, a statue. . . . He does not even possess animal instincts. . . . His mind is empty. . . . The moral world does not exist for him. Virtue and vice are unreal." Life begins for the deaf child when the audist establishment takes charge: Only with hearing tutelage do "the world, people, duration, life, time . . . begin." When the deaf child's education is complete, he is restored to society: "He was a wild and evil animal; now he is a reasonable being." The founder of otology, author of the first book on diseases of the ear and hearing, Jean-Marc Itard, described congenital and early deafness in these terms: "It condemns the victim to moral isolation, impaired speech, and incomplete intellectual development. The deaf-mute appears like a civilized man, but inwardly there is the barbarity and ignorance of a savage. Indeed, a savage is superior to him if he has a language, however limited it may be." Itard's medical experiments on the deaf children of the Paris school were aimed at providing them some hearing and thus the opportunity to acquire speech and "language" and become fully civilized.

The metaphor of the deaf person as a savage has had particular staying power. What the savage and the deaf person have in common most of all in this fantasy is a lack of development, a certain childishness. Abbé Sicard wrote: "If we call the deaf-mute a savage, we understate his sad condition, for he is below the level of the savage as regards morality, which they possess up to a point, and far below them when it comes to communication." De Gérando wrote: "The deaf-mute is also a savage," and thought the similarity so great that he urged the newly founded Society of Observers of Man, the first anthropological society, to master manual language as a means of entering into communication with the savages they would encounter on their voyages. And when a true wild child was discovered and captured, it was evident to all concerned that the place to educate the Wild Boy of Aveyron was the National Institute for Deaf-Mutes.

The colonizers frequently described Africans as childlike (Table 1). For example, a leading British general wrote: "The natives are like children of nature and in many points resemble the wild animals of the forests." David Livingstone went to Africa in 1841 and spent more than thirty years there, some of them in Burundi. "The Africans are mere children," he wrote, "as easily pleased as babies." The fantasy of the African as an uncorrupted child—spontaneous, impulsive, morally undeveloped—is, as Pascal Bruckner points out in *The Tears of the White Man*, a form of contempt. More than that, the benefactor's ignorance of the African, on the one hand, or the deaf person, on the other, makes of each an excellent screen onto which to project his own fantasies. When we are told that the natives are orgiastic or that deaf people are innocent and impulsive, just whose world are we invited to glimpse? When a psychologist or an educator tells us that deaf people are aggressive, is it because he himself feels threatened— perhaps by an inability to communicate with the deaf person? Ethnographer Octave Mannoni sees the white man as divided between a desire to "correct" the errors of the savage—that is, to project his conscience onto him—and his desire to identify himself with those uncivilized ways—that is, to project his id onto them.

Recall how much ambiguity there is for the colonizer who confronts the colonized or the audist who confronts the deaf person. Both regard a mask that has been put on for this encounter. Both are unfamiliar with the customs that lie behind the mask (the inscrutable Arab; the mysterious Chinese). Both colonizer and audist are frequently unsure how to communicate, and not clear on the meanings (even less the nuances) of their partner's communications. The colonizer is an expatriate. The audist, too, has in some sense ventured out of familiar territory. There are gestures half understood, the presence of urgent needs communicated but their nature unclear, behavior evident enough but motivations and contextual meaning difficult to discern; this is naturally anxiety-arousing for the psychologist or teacher who cannot do his job under the circumstances and who in any case is aware of vague stirrings in his feelings, aroused above all by the grimaces of the living mask. Is it any wonder that in this ambiguous situation, all kinds of traits are read into the deaf person's appearance and actions? The teacher recognizes at some level that he has to contend, not with the guileless, docile child whom he hoped to fill up as a vessel with his superior knowledge, but with a definite human being marching to another drummer; this may be experienced as an aggression, or as a sign of emotional disturbance. The teacher is in the predicament of Abbé Sicard, who was shocked to find that the Wild Boy of Aveyron did not conform to his image of a docile child of nature at all—and he chooses the same way out. There must be something wrong with the boy; turn him over to a doctor.

If hearing professionals see deaf children and adults as needy, we must remember that beyond projecting their own needs onto their deaf clients, they live by their clients' needs—that is, they need neediness. A retired professional has written: "It was not until I relinquished the power that I had as an educational psychologist that I realized how much power I had, and how much I missed it." The audist and the deaf person dance what Memmi calls a "dependency duet." In some cases, hearing professionals and deaf people enter a dependency relationship mandated by law, as when a deaf child is sent to school or a deaf adult to an institution. In other cases, the dependency duet is mandated by circumstances: for example, a deaf college student engages an interpreter. But whenever either of the parties enters the relation by choice, it is because the one seeks to be a provider and the other seeks to be provided for.

Why do the audist and the deaf person enter into this elective mutual dependence? Memmi says it is human nature to seek the dependency duet. But why has one person chosen one role and one the other? Octave Mannoni claims that the provider is responding to a complex of inferiority, he is compensating; while the dependent is guided at bottom by a fear of abandonment. This dependence is encouraged by the system. In fact, the more the provider plays the parental role, the more the recipient is encouraged to play the dependent role. There are, of course, also economic and social forces at play. The deaf person is unlikely to be a health care provider, because dependency relations are at work throughout deaf education and he will find it difficult to rise to such professional heights—the more so as there are frequently barriers erected specifically to keep him out. Many deaf people understand all this, especially as the germs of each partner's behavior are in each of us; and the deaf person who is in a dependent role vis-à-vis his rehabilitation counselor, say, may be in a provider role vis-à-vis his children.

What kind of person elects the provider's role in the dependency duet? Mannoni reasons as follows: In childhood fantasy, there are grotesque and wild beings on the one hand and gracious beings bereft of will and purpose on the other. Colonial societies were the closest thing to the desert island with its innocent natives; the colonials who were drawn there were drawn to an infantile world without men— that is, they were misanthropes. It is true that often the colonizers were people who had been rejected by the mother country, people who evinced a certain lack of adaptation to life in the metropole. It is true that the residential schools for deaf children, which until the 1980s sheltered most such children and a large part of the audist establishment, were like little desert islands, communities apart, with their own rules and regimens, spacious grounds, and surrounding walls. In any case, working among deaf people exclusively is meta-phorically working in a place apart, the so-called world of the deaf.

Are many people in the professions serving deaf children and adults drawn there by this dreamlike vision of innocence, are they people fundamentally out of tune with their own society? Certainly Jean-Marc Itard was a misfit, even a misanthrope. Irascible and soli-tary all his adult life, he wrote in the final sentence of his will: "Man cannot escape the sad circumstances of his existence, which are to suffer and to die." Abbé Sicard, too, had much greater difficulty in the world outside the enclave of the National Institute for Deaf-Mutes than within it; he was in and out of prison because of his political naïveté; in and out of carelessly contracted debt; in and out of safe places, hiding from the law.

Flight from the hearing world is not the only reason, of course, that hearing people choose to work in the deaf world. Baron de Gérando, for example, suffered from a veritable mania for benefi-cence to achieve the well-ordering of society; deviation in any form was undesirable. He opened a home for fallen women, founded a savings bank for the poor, a society for industrial training, and one for elementary instruction; he adopted the seven orphaned children of his wife's sister, and his five nephews when his brother died. He wrote twenty-five volumes on doing good. In the last days of his life, he wrote in his diary, speaking of the deaf people who had come to detest him for his opposition to their language and community, "Let it be said they loved me as a father."

Nine out of ten teachers of deaf children in America today are women. It seems likely that women choose to be the provider in this dependency duet so much more often than men in part because of their conventional role as the nurturers of children in our society. But whatever the reasons or deeper motivations, whoever enters the field of deaf education, or any other branch of the audist establishment, generally enters on the understanding that there will not be mutuality between the benefactor and the beneficiary. An imbalance is inherent whenever an adult teaches a child, because of the difference in age and power, but that difference is multiplied many times over in deaf education, counseling, and rehabilitation, for the client is generally not perceived as even potentially a provider one day. There is no equality in any dependency duet, but there is not even potential equality in the audist duet. And this the professional has chosen.

The politics and economics of the audist's paternalism (or maternalism) are masked by the audist's language; he is in the human-services professions, he is there to serve deaf people's "special needs." The valuable good that services deliver is care, and even if that care is remunerated and self-interested, even indeed if it is harmful, we cannot fully discharge its surplus meaning of loving care, the care tendered in the first place by our parents and our loved ones. As love is not a political issue, so care and service wear a mask that screens them from scrutiny. Behind the mask of benevolence is the professional engaged in the human-services market, staking out his particular claim in the fastest-growing sector of our economy. The more these professionals can identify unmet needs, the more they can prosper in servicing those needs. They need an increased supply of human deficiencies. They need a broad "client base," so that the defection of any one group does not threaten their viability. They need to supplant individual and group solutions to human problems in favor of recourse to human-services experts. Ultimately, they need the client to identify his needs with theirs, to see the dependency duet as self-contained and successful by its very existence, without reference to any external criteria.

It is the manifest destiny of hearing people, the audist would have us believe, to come to the rescue of deaf people; it is our "errand in the wilderness." "What more noble activity than to go among them, living proof of our happiness, our wealth, our superiority. . . . Perhaps they will call us to their midst to show them the road that can lead them to our condition. What joy! What conquest!" So de Gérando wrote, speaking of the "savages," but the same philosophy guided his relations to deaf people and continues to guide audists today.

According to the audist, the deaf child or adult is in the dependency duet not because of audist practices or legislation but because of the deaf person's intrinsic nature. Not only is the deaf person different from us, and different in starkly negative ways, according to psychometric science, but also those differences are absolutized, they are inherent—further mystification to obscure the distribution of power. The Mexican was aggressive not because his lands were taken from him but because of his Indian blood. Similarly, the purposes of imperialism and evangelism were served by portraying the African as less than fully human. An East African medical journal reported in 1943: "A highly technical skilled examination of a series of one hundred brains of normal natives has found naked eye and microscopic facts indicative of inherent new brain inferiority . . . quantitatively, the inferiority amounts to 14.8 percent." A belief in the intrinsic nature of African-American inferiority, fueled by eugenicist interpretations of Darwinian evolutionism, also seemed to justify the treatment of African-Americans as slaves. Contemporary claims of the native inferiority of African-Americans arise in the context of the manifest educational and social inequalities between the majority and African-American populations in our nation. Political scientist James Q. Wilson and psychologist Richard Herrnstein, in their 1985 book *Crime and Human Nature*, contend that men of a certain body type—square-shaped, barrel-chested, muscular—are predisposed to crime, and that more young black males fit this type, called mesomorphy, than do young white males. They cite the pioneering work of physician William Sheldon, who claimed a relation exists between three body types and patterns of criminal behavior. In 1949, Sheldon and colleagues pored over the bodies, photographed nude, of two hundred Boston delinquents and assigned each several ratings, including one for "thoroughbredness (t)." Here, illustratively, is Sheldon's description of case 113:

Somatotype 3.5 − 6.5 − 1; Primary t 3; Secondary t 1. A sixteen-year-old extremely mesomorphic Negro . . . Coarse, primitive features . . . "a throwback to aboriginal ancestors" . . . Teachers were afraid of the boy. . . . Infantile mentality . . . Now very sex conscious . . . His recently stated ambition is to "lead his race out of the wilderness." . . . He presents a difficult problem from the standpoint of crime control. There is no ground on which he could be regarded as a criminal or detained as a psychotic, yet he is dangerous as dynamite.

In the same vein, psychologist Arthur Jensen has contended that African-Americans systematically score lower than Caucasians on IQ tests for reasons related to the biology of their race. Extend this line of thinking and you get physicist William Shockley's proposal on how to remedy the problem, which he articulated on the television program "Firing Line": "I have this voluntary sterilization bonus plan . . . depending upon genetically carried disabilities . . . $1000 for every point you score below 100 on an IQ test."

"The native is natively incapable," observes Memmi. And so it is with the audist's characterization of deaf people. Either their sorry state is the result of the practices of the audist establishment, which is unthinkable, or it is the result of the deaf person's innate inability to profit from those practices. The tenet of the native inferiority of deaf people shores up the entire audist establishment. Thus psychologist McCay Vernon writes: "It is now apparent that behavior noted as characteristic of deaf children [is] often an interactional effect of both the loss of hearing and of other central nervous system lesions associated with the condition causing the deafness." No wonder deaf personality, socialization, and cognition are in such poor repair! No wonder the professionals of the audist establishment are so urgently needed! No wonder deaf education is largely failing at its task! These children have brain lesions! Not demonstrable brain lesions, mind you: a tiny percent have those (2.1 percent in one survey); but inferred brain lesions, the same as may be inferred from the allegedly poor performance of African-Americans on IQ tests. With the same line of reasoning, a British psychologist reviewing *The Deaf Experience*, a compilation of classics in deaf education translated from the French, which I edited, rejected my claim that deaf children were better educated in the nineteenth century, when a cultural model of the deaf community guided educational practice: "It is not the lack of [sign language] in the schools," he wrote, "which is responsible for the deaf experience of social isolation and impoverished opportunity: it is deafness itself."

Audism has a supplementary reason for believing in the constitutional inferiority of culturally deaf people, beyond self-legitimation and mystification. For the audist establishment, unlike the colonialists and white supremacists, has a sector devoted to treating this constitutional flaw, to measuring it, modifying it, surgically correcting it; this is the medicalization of cultural deafness, and it requires a biological theory of deaf inferiority. Audist claims that deaf people are constitutionally flawed not only are aimed at validating the impairment model of all deafness, and hence the large role of hearing people in shaping the lives of culturally deaf people, in the face of grave doubts and poor results; they also serve to undermine the deaf community's claim to the status of a legitimate linguistic and cultural minority with a right to shape its own present and future. Research on minority influence has shown that the image of the minority is fundamental in its ability to effect change. Those in power can resist change by presenting the minority in a negative light and, in particular, by showing that minority members have some idiosyncrasy that naturally leads them to their peculiar, nonconformist position. When I suggested to the chairman of a projected conference on childhood cochlear implants that some deaf leaders should be invited among the speakers since implanted children are deaf and are likely to rely on ASL and the deaf community, the otologist replied that it was impossible to have a reasonable conversation on this topic with deaf adults—they were irrational.

Psychologizing is one strategy for undermining the influence of a minority; individuating is another. Hearing people are the majority group. "It's a hearing world," they say, meaning, deaf people should conform to our ways. Deaf people, on the other hand, are an aggregate of individuals, according to this view. Each is different. It is very important to know the degree of "hearing impairment"—important for the child to know it, the teacher to know it, the parent to know it. It can be total, profound, severe, moderate, or mild. These are approximate terms, and the audiogram will chart the unique pattern of just perceptible loudnesses for the deaf individual, depending on the pitch of the sound. Deaf individuals differ in their etiology: maternal rubella; heredity; trauma at birth; prematurity. They differ in the presence of handicapping conditions. They differ multidimensionally on the psychometric battery, the MMPI, the TAT, the SAT, etc. Here is the list of tests administered in the dossier of Claudine Umuvyeyi, a deaf Burundian girl now enrolled at Gallaudet University's Model Secondary School for the Deaf: the Stanford Achievement Test; Wechsler Intelligence Scale; Hiskey Nebraska Test of Learning Aptitude; Detroit Test of Learning Aptitude; Test of Nonverbal Intelligence; Raven's Progressive Matrices; Bender Visual-Motor Gestalt Test; Woodcock Reading Inventory; Boehm Test of Basic Concepts. Claudine, like deaf children throughout our land, has become a "case." Michel Foucault observes that once it was a prerogative of power to have one's life documented. But "the turning of real lives into writing is no longer a procedure of heroization; it functions as a procedure of objectification and subjection."

Countless hours and a great deal of money are spent specifying these audiologic and psychometric differences, though frequently they make little difference in what we do to or for the deaf person. Because, as we have seen, the practitioner knows the data are not a valid basis for action. Because frequently there are no educational strategies that link up to various test outcomes. Because of limited resources. Then why all this individuation? It masks and denies the communal reality of this linguistic and cultural minority. It affirms that they are not legitimately different but pathologically deviant.

When asked why there are all these distinctions among deaf people, a French deaf leader replied: "Because our numbers frighten hearing people, and they prefer to divide and conquer, rather than respect our rights. It's the same with apartheid: from black to white with numerous gradations. Biological and racist arguments are used for social ends; with them, it's the degree of their skin color; with us, it's the degree of our deafness."

Foucault points out that the psychological examination not only imposes its mark on its subjects, "holds them in a mechanism of objectification," but also is itself the ceremony of this objectification. I am reminded of the photograph, sent me by the Kenya Society for Deaf Children, of an eight-year-old deaf boy whose schooling I had agreed to sponsor. Although he goes to a little country school for deaf children, with no electronic equipment—indeed, with no windows—Gideon appears in the snapshot wearing enormous headphones; the two phones combined occupy a larger surface than his face. The psychological test, the headphone, and the other paraphernalia of audism—especially the hearing aid—are symbolic objects. That is why French deaf leader Jean-François Mercurio opened the International Conference on Sign Language held in Poitiers in July 1990 by smashing a hearing aid with a sledgehammer.

Cultural history is the enemy of psychologizing and individuation. In a typical Burundi home, the family would gather around the fire after sunset and listen in Kirundi to the wisdom of the father and the accumulated wisdom, called history, of his fathers before him. Similarly, deaf children growing up in the deaf community learn in manual language from older deaf children and adults what it means to be a deaf person, the lives that deaf people have lived before them and therefore the possible lives for them to lead, the wisdom of this minority, peculiar to its situation and accumulated across the centuries. In African historiography, however, "Quotes [by the natives] were diminished to summaries. . . . In the end it was the foreign observers themselves who were quoted, as if they were the authors and witnesses of an entire culture." Likewise, the hearing authors of books on deaf education or psychology cite only other hearing authors. Written English replaced the spoken narrative of the Africans as it has the signed narrative of the deaf. In the end, Africa's own sense of historical dimension was negated, as has been the deaf community's. Africa has no history or only that of the Europeans. Political scientist Ali Mazrui argues that white Americans totally destroyed the capacity for cultural nostalgia of most African-Americans until late in this century.

The audist establishment is concerned with neither the deaf child's cultural heritage nor his language, which is an embodiment of that heritage. They are denied. What is important instead, required by law, is a plan, an Individualized Educational Plan, called an IEP for short. All the test results go in the IEP folder; these are supposed to predict what the deaf child can become. But the decision to construe and shape his fate in psychometric terms rather than historic ones is the most powerful determinant of that future it claims to predict. Thus, as Foucault has argued, power not only excludes and oppresses; it produces reality. Identification, testing, classification, institutionalization, and surgical intervention are successive steps in increasing expropriation of the deaf child's body, the "colonization of the body." The sequel to certain test results is that the deaf child is institutionalized with emotionally disturbed or mentally retarded children, and deaf adults are improperly sequestered in mental institutions. High test scores can be equally devastating. Many local schools, for example, refuse parents' wishes to have their deaf child attend a school expressly for deaf children; the test results show, they insist, that their child can make it in the local public school.

They refuse to put a special placement in the IEP. The most general deleterious result of audist power, however, is that it fails to educate deaf children.

There are striking parallels between the operation of regulatory authority in the case of the prisoner, as Foucault describes it, and in the case of the deaf pupil. The prison receives a convicted person; it is not really concerned with his offense, nor even exactly with him as an offender; rather, he is a different object, one defined by variables not taken into account at sentencing, for they are relevant only for corrective technology. Likewise, the parent delivers a deaf child to the school. The school is really concerned not with the child as such but rather with the object of a different set of variables that we may call the pupil. The school is concerned with classifying, training, and disciplining the pupil; to accomplish this, and to legitimate the actions taken, the school determines the "dimensionality" of the pupil on some constructed scales. We might say the school seeks total knowledge of the pupil but not the child. The pupil is an isolated "case," whereas the child is characterized by his social relations in his family, in his community, and in his school. From Claudine Umuvyeyi's point of view, some of the most salient issues are her growing mastery of ASL, which links her to her peers and the American deaf community; the incessant novelty of her environment; her romantic attachment to some of her schoolmates; the friendships she has formed with classmates and some deaf adults; her homesickness for her parents and friends in Burundi; her distaste for the food; her dislike of the regimentation. . . . None of this is measured and entered in her dossier. Of course, she is also concerned with herself as pupil, and there her concerns overlap with those of the school. She enjoys learning some things. She wants to be "a success."

The knowledge that the child Claudine possesses includes considerable knowledge of "the way things are" in her country: the roles of women and the rituals attached; the preparation of food; agriculture; the role of fathers, tribal leaders, ritual leaders; the attitudes of hearing people toward deaf people; and much more. But this is not the pupil. The child and the pupil are twins, as it were, the one existing in subjectivity and in nexus to the family and community; the other a technological creation existing in relation to the school.

"Discourses . . . systematically form the objects of which they speak." Foucault's observation has truly terrifying relevance for members of the deaf community who accept the rewards offered by the audist establishment in return for wearing the emblem of disability. If the deaf community denies its cultural, linguistic, social, and historic reality and embraces instead an infirmity model, if it acts in systematic ways that validate and reinforce current practices of measurement, which decree its psychological and sensorial impairment, current practices of sham education, which aims to teach the impaired child his role in unimpaired society, and current practices of heroic medicine, which works its ferocious technological prowess on that child—if the deaf community chooses to add its powerful legitimacy to the disability discourse about deaf people, then that community will indeed become disabled. Negative stereotyping in the guise of psychometric science *is* disabling. Education conducted in a way that negates the child's identity, fails to use his language, and isolates him from peers *is* disabling. Surgery and technology that reinforce these behavioral practices of individuation and medicalization *are* disabling.

Naturally, the deaf community resists the antihistorical, individuating denial of its existence. That is why the National Association of the Deaf, early in the era of silent films, recorded the nation's greatest deaf orators as they recounted their struggle and their times in eloquent ASL. That is why it sponsored the preparation and publication of the influential *Deaf Heritage: A Narrative History of Deaf America* in 1981. That is why deaf organizations never tire of decrying the infamous Congress of Milan where, in 1880, hearing educators of deaf children resolved to banish manual language from their schools worldwide. That is why the NAD proposed to the centenary of that congress that it renounce the Milan resolution (contemporary leaders of deaf education, true to *their* heritage, refused to allow a vote on the proposal, or to reprint it among other resolutions in the congress *Proceedings*). That is why the NAD has assailed the unrestricted marketing of surgical implants for young deaf children.

Michel Foucault has analyzed the historical evolution in which the control of people's bodies came to be seen as a legitimate concern of government. What he calls "bio-power" extends its reach into our civilization in such diverse fields as criminality, psychiatry, education, and family planning. In bio-power, knowledge and power form a regulatory technology whose purpose "is to forge a docile body that may be subjected, used, transformed, and improved." Foucault affirms the connection in bio-power between the attribution of traits and the regulation of bodies: "A power whose task is to take charge of life needs continuous regulatory and corrective mechanisms. . . .

Such a power has to qualify, measure, appraise, and hierarchize, rather than display itself in its murderous splendor ... it effects distributions around the norm." Those who participate in the exercise of this power contend, first, that technology can isolate deviance and, second, that other, related technology can correct that deviance. Henry Goddard's IQ testing, with its alarming results, helped to lay the foundations for special education; it computed a distribution around a norm and assigned those children who fell a specified number of units below the norm to specialized institutions, on the grounds that technology had revealed their inner deficit, though that deficit lacked any outer sign. That the norm was more than a little arbitrary can be seen from the fact that, to judge by his test, the average mental age of recruits for World War I was thirteen, and more than half of the children he labeled as morons requiring institutional care would have been classed as normal by other IQ tests. The aggrandizement of the new "special education" proceeded apace in the following decades, encouraged by regular classroom teachers who were delighted with the homogenization of their classrooms.

The French psychologists Alfred Binet and Theodore Simon, whose test Goddard had modified, noted at the outset the connection between the new technology of measurement and the expansion of special education: "Ever since public interest has been aroused in the question of schools for defective children, selfish ambition has seen its opportunity. The most frankly selfish interests conceal themselves behind the mask of philanthropy, and whoever dreams of finding a fine situation for himself in the new schools never speaks of children without tears in his eyes. This is the everlasting human comedy." The proportion of children enrolled in special education has grown a hundredfold in Finland over the last five decades; in some states in Australia, it has grown fifteenfold; in Great Britain, the Warnock report, a comprehensive survey of special-education "needs" in 1978, concluded that as many as one in five children would need those services and called for a major expansion of the special-education establishment.

Thus is the majority protected from social deviation. But are we not all impoverished and hindered by this kind of "defense" from the diversity of humankind? "We need to liberate ourselves both from the state and from the type of individualization which is linked to the state," Foucault writes. The political task is to criticize these institutions—audism in the present case—so as to strip away the veil of neutrality, revealing their political violence for what it is, so it may be countered. Edward Said has observed that Orientalism (Middle Eastern Studies) hid the imperial contest for territory and wealth "beneath its scholarly and aesthetic idioms." I have similarly argued that the disciplines constituting the audist establishment have hidden a contest for power beneath the idiom of psychometrics and the claim of disinterested humanitarianism. What audists seek, contrary to the will of deaf people, is the perpetuation of the audist establishment "serving the deaf," with its guiding antideaf philosophy and with the exclusion of deaf people from its ranks. That is the contest that the "psychology of the deaf" seeks to hide.

As the denial of the colonized is injurious to the colonizer, so the denial of the deaf community and their world has grave consequences for the audist. Since he does not recognize deaf history, deaf culture, deaf language, he cannot partake of them. In any case, his allegiances are to hearing culture, spoken language, and hearing values. So he cannot truly communicate with the people among whom he has chosen to spend his professional life. Naturally, he senses a certain lack of gratitude for his efforts. Has he not always respected deaf people's dignity and rights, even worked to ensure that others did so? He would like a little more reward. But a right is inherently due respect; there is no reason to show gratitude if it is accorded, there is only reason for indignation if it is not. If the audist becomes aware that he is usurping the role of a deaf person, if he sees that his structural relationship to deaf people is that of oppressor to oppressed, he may come to resent the people whose very existence places him in that situation. "Overall, teachers of the hearing-impaired are not happy with teaching," finds one study that assessed the attitudes of some two hundred teachers of deaf children. Those teachers, compared with colleagues in general education, express greatest dissatisfaction about their workload and the pressures created by community expectations. Audists frequently complain of "burnout," and Kathryn Meadow finds it a serious problem among educators of deaf children, according to a survey she conducted. Interestingly, the major "key" to prevention and cure she recommends is that hearing professionals develop their own support networks. I am reminded of enclaves of old colonialists I have visited, huddled together in alcoholic bonhomie in Dakar or Ouagadougou.

To show that the relations institutionalized between two groups are oppressive is to reveal ways in which social structures operate to the detriment of both parties. There are many victims but few victimizers. When we analyze the matrix of force relations in such institutions, Foucault has written, "the logic is perfectly clear, the aims decipherable, and yet it is often the case that no one is there to have invented them, and few can be said to have formulated them." The participants cannot control those relations and are often unaware of them. "People know what they do; they frequently know why they do what they do; but what they don't know is what what they do does." There are, of course, individuals who try by their actions and statements not to behave paternalistically or otherwise oppressively, but it is in the nature of things that they can be only partially successful. Within one frame of reference, on the micro level, we can distinguish between intentional and unintentional paternalism, and between degrees of paternalism—not all individuals and groups are intentionally paternalistic, nor are they paternalists to the same degree. At a greater distance, however, at the macro level, we can see that there are no villains and no heroes. The oppressive structural relations are the result of historical forces such as the appropriation of the body by the state; the increasing empowerment of medicine; social Darwinism, eugenics, and the rise of psychometrics; ethnocentrism and the formation of new states; the unequal distribution of wealth and power. As Memmi points out, a person may choose not to be involved with the oppressed, but once he accepts that involvement he cannot refuse its conditions, which predate his birth and will probably outlast his life. Thus, there are no good and bad members of the oppressing class—only those who accept their reality as oppressors and a few who do not. One of these few, a renegade, may struggle for a more equal distribution of power, "but the privileges he denounces are those he enjoys." I apply this to myself: where would I be without deaf people? If deaf people were not oppressed by hearing people, this book would be pointless. Moreover, there would have been many valid histories of deaf people, most of them written by deaf people, and it would have been superfluous for me to write *When the Mind Hears*. The oppressors are furious with the renegade. His actions question the validity of theirs. He can take further steps to enter the class of the oppressed, but he is not one of them and does not really want to be; they are different people. What, then, can a hearing person of goodwill do? Karl Marx said that the role of the bourgeois intelligentsia was to hasten the revolution.

The Role of the Oppressed

I have focused on the audist, the provider in the dependency duet. However burned out he may be, however frustrated, he would never change places with his dependent; it is clear who has the better part of this bargain. The behavior of the oppressed person responds to the context of oppression. Hostility finds safe channels and is redirected. Deaf humor frequently includes the theme of the deaf person using his deafness to outwit hearing people. A deaf couple receives a surly reception from a motel owner when they check in late. They retire to their room, whereupon the wife discovers she has left her cigarettes in the car. The husband goes to fetch them and then can't recall which of the nearly identical rooms, all dark, he had left minutes before. He leans on the car horn; lights go on throughout the motel—except in one room, where he enters and goes to bed.

Another "safe" rechanneling of the hostility born of repression is to victimize other oppressed people. As I write, two factions of black South Africans are killing each other rather than attacking the whites who manage apartheid. In a sequel to the slave trade and the colonization of Texas, African-Americans blamed the Mexicans rather than the landowners for their poverty and raided the Mexicans' quarters, for example in Beeville in 1894. With the colonization of Burundi, intertribal warfare was inflamed, and carnage on an unprecedented and genocidal scale resulted. When deaf frustration is directed horizontally, explains British deaf leader Jeff McWhinney, "it often takes the form of gossip-mongering, back-stabbing and derision of Deaf leaders." Here are some of the terms deaf people use, when they have internalized audist values, to "put down" other deaf people, according to deaf author Ben Bahan: LOW-LEVEL, PEA-BRAIN, ENGLISH NG (weak in English), STRONG ASL, DEAF CLUB PEOPLE, NOT SMART BUT GOOD WORK, LOW VERBAL, M-L-S (minimal language skills, an audist designation).

The colonized seek to fit the colonizer's categories—black, colored, white, quadroon, octoroon; Mexican, Spanish-American, Hispanic, Latino, Spanish surname; Indian, half-breed, quarter-breed; underdeveloped, less developed, developing—so deaf people frequently and tragically seek to fit the audist categories. HIGH-SIGN, for example, refers to a way of signing that is least like ASL and most like English; LOW-SIGN, the core of deaf culture, the central heritage of deaf history, is ASL. If a deaf person calls himself HEARING-IM-PAIRED, he speaks volumes. The classification was coined and promoted beginning in the late 1960s by the audist establishment, with the claim that deaf children would be treated better if they were called hearing-impaired. The label has embedded within it the infirmity model that legitimates that establishment; and it exists only in opposition to hearing; in this it is like "non-men" as a label for women, "non-white" as a label for people of color, or "sexually impaired" as a label for gays. When a member of the deaf community accepts such a label, he surrenders his own identity and accepts definition by the dominant social group. From time to time, the dominant group will change the labels; what is important is that it has the power to do so.

Had the perpetrators consulted the deaf community, they would have learned that "deaf" is not negatively valued—"hearing-impaired" is. "Deaf" refers to shared culture, language, and experience; "hearing-impaired" seems to refer to a physical defect that someone outside deaf culture possesses. By what right, in any case, can outsiders tell members of the deaf minority their communal name? Is not the giving of names a precious right and ritual of a culture? May we replace the label "German," say, with another because at some moment in our history German people find disfavor with many Americans? This is not to deny that there are hearing children and adults with hearing losses. But most of the children that the audist establishment succeeded in relabeling were culturally deaf before the relabeling and culturally deaf after. They had become deaf before learning English, and ASL was their primary language; they had joined or would join the deaf community. So the linguistic shell game, the inverse of identity-affirming labels like "black" or "Chicano," could not have created new possibilities for the deaf child but rather fewer ones.

The more the deaf person internalizes the identity of "hearing-impaired" proffered by the audist establishment, the more he lends himself to its designs. "The classifications are taken up by the deaf community itself," says a French deaf leader. "Remarks like: 'He's late-deafened and hangs out with hearing people.' 'He wears a hearing aid, so he's hard of hearing.' 'He prefers lip-reading and speech to sign, so he's not part of our world.' " The system as a whole is structured to establish and perpetuate the dependency of deaf people on the audist establishment. If the deaf student internalizes a self-image as infirm, if he is indeed incapacitated by oppressive education and thus limited vocationally and economically, if his emotional growth is stunted through isolation in the local school for hearing children, then he is more likely to be seen as needing—and to receive—audist services such as rehabilitation counseling, psychology and psychiatry, outreach programs for deaf adults, and the like.

Because audists seek to sustain the dependency duet, they frequently treat deaf children and adults in ways that preempt their opportunities to learn self-reliance. In addition, they will deprive deaf people of needed information by conducting discussions in English and by presenting lectures without interpreters or with poorly prepared interpreters. Thus, they endeavor, unwittingly, to shape deaf people to be the way audists believe deaf people are. The deaf child or the adult deaf client learns what the school or other audist agency expects of him; in order to please those in power, and frequently as a condition of receiving benefits, the deaf person is compliant and may even make a positive and sincere effort to be who he is expected to be (but knows he is not). Among his own kind, his behavior is likely to be quite different. He is one man in the vocational rehabilitation agency and another man in the deaf club, as the deaf child of deaf parents is dependent in school and self-reliant at home.

As a consequence, a "complementarity principle," in which inspection of an event changes the event itself, applies to cross-cultural testing: when the oppressor evaluates the oppressed, the oppressed changes his behavior. A student of Spanish imperialism has written: "The Conquistador was thus caught up in two paradoxes: one ignored the continuity of an indigenous discourse outside the representation of the Conquistador. The other disregarded the transformation of the object in the process of gaining knowledge." In the 1960s, as director of a center for research on language at the University of Michigan, I sent a research assistant, a tall Jewish New Yorker, as it happened, to Tuskegee, Alabama, to make tape recordings of white and black students' speech at local colleges. The two sets of recordings he brought back proved nearly identical—not a trace of black dialect. I soon realized my error and sent a black assistant to interview black students. This time, they spoke quite differently.

"A dependent," writes Memmi, "is anyone who believes in the efficacy of his provider." "The men in my village," a Burundian friend once told me ruefully, "will sooner take the advice of a Belgian they have never seen before than of one of their own tribal leaders." The relation between deaf people and audists is created from early childhood to tap symbolically the power of the healer and the power of the scientist combined. Paramedical is, after all, practically medical: audiology and speech therapy are frequently conducted in clinics or hospitals; audists frequently wear white lab coats. The schools are most insistent that the deaf child wear scientific devices at all times, and urge the parents to maintain the school's surveillance out of class. The deaf child, aware of his weakness and of his stigma, may rely absolutely on a hearing teacher. When the child becomes an adult, he may rely absolutely on a rehabilitation counselor or a hearing neighbor, for example. Any sign of the hearing person's inadequacy is disconcerting and reminds us that the reliance is not on a real person but on an idealized one, born of the deaf person's needs and expectations, which are in turn a result of the imbalance in power. Those needs and expectations, Memmi observes, are always greater than the provider is prepared to provide; in the gap between the two grow the dependent's resentment and the provider's guilt. The provider tries to set limits; this hurts, and the deaf person is reminded that he is only one of many "clients"; so he is interchangeable but also necessary to the audist; without deaf people, there would be no audists. He was looking for someone he could count on, and he finds instead someone who is using him.

In my observation, deaf people are angry with audists and not with hearing people, just as the colonized drew a clear distinction between Belgian colonizers and Belgians back in the mother country. Deaf people are inclined to believe that hearing parents of deaf children are well-intentioned but ill-informed by hearing professionals. It is self-selection and ethnocentric training that make the innocent hearing layman into an audist.

The dependent's idealized focusing on one person diminishes his awareness of others and other solutions. Thus a rich interdependence with speech therapists rarely coexists with a rich interdependence with the deaf community. We cannot simultaneously entrust our hopes to several different people; all the less if they have divergent views. The deaf community is an abstraction; but at precisely that level it has language, mores, and history; its institutions—the deaf club, for example—may be a better provider than any one individual, deaf or hearing; they have symbolic content.

The deaf child or adult is not an ordinary dependent, as any hearing person might be who goes to a doctor, an audiologist, a psychologist. He is a stigmatized dependent. When isolated from others of his kind, the deaf child with hearing parents and a hearing school is bound to feel deviant. Why can't he be like other people and conform to the demands made on him—most of all, the demand of facile communication in English? Clearly, because he is handicapped. So the deaf person commonly believes he must adapt to hearing demands; he should yield, even when he thinks it wrong; in principle he has no standing with which to shape the majority. This arrangement suits the teacher; socially competent students are threatening, for they may challenge the teacher and even institutional practices. That is why the youngest children, who are the least socially competent, are often given the most latitude in the classroom. Children are at the bottom of any power hierarchy, observes Sally Tomlinson, but children in special education are the lowest of the low: their complaints are seen as less legitimate, and more physical control is exercised over them. Only such children can be placed in a school against their parents' wishes, without court intervention.* These children are thus the most vulnerable to administration of drugs and surgery.

The pliant and powerless deaf child receives messages, sometimes conflicting, about the nature of his self. Consider first the deaf child of deaf parents; his self is bound up with his likeness to his parents in activities, in language, in the treatment received from other people, notably deaf friends or relatives. Hearing children are weird to this child; they apparently have a different self. A deaf friend from a distinguished deaf family recounts how, as a child, he made friends with a little girl next door. He discovered, however, that he could not communicate with her as he could with his family; even the simplest gestures baffled her. So he was reduced to pointing and to bringing her to things, or things to her. He did not know what was wrong with her, but then something happened to confirm his conviction that she was strange indeed. Her mother walked up to them one day while they were playing and started moving her mouth furiously. Suddenly his playmate picked up her toys and left. My friend went to his mother and asked what this child's affliction was. His mother explained that she was HEARING; she didn't know how to SIGN, so she and her mother communicate with TALK.

The late president of Kenya, Jomo Kenyatta, has recounted that when white skin was first seen, it was assumed to be the result of some pitiful disease. Only in that moment did the black man conceive his blackness, as the deaf man becomes deaf only in hearing society. Psychiatrist Frantz Fanon tells about his boyhood: "I am a Negro but of course I do not know it simply because I am one. When I am at home my mother sings me French love songs in which there is never a word about Negroes. When I disobey, when I make too much noise, I am told 'Stop behaving like a nigger!' " One French deaf friend told me he realized he was deaf when, at age eight, he was placed in a home for hearing physically handicapped children. The deaf child's deafness is salient only among hearing people. Among deaf people, the trait loses its salience and other traits can come into focus. Thus, ironically, the child learns to be a true deaf person among other deaf people, just where the criterion trait of deafness is not salient.

How does the deaf child's sense of self develop in a hearing family? He observes that commonly one adult will approach another and move his mouth rapidly for a long time, and the other responds likewise, or perhaps engages abruptly and inexplicably in some activity. If there are hearing children in the home, they will behave in the same ways among themselves, and they will perform this seeming dumb show with adults. "I noticed people watching each other's faces," a deaf educator has written, recalling her childhood, "but I saw only a blur of lipshapes, mouths opening and closing, stretching and puckering into lines and circles. Why were mouths so interesting? Mouths bored me." "Lipshapes" are rarely directed at the deaf child, and when they are, they are indecipherable; his own mouthings go unnoticed. Sometimes the family seems able to presage events: They open the front door just when people are waiting there; they arrive from another part of the house just when the child has hurt himself and cried. These may be some of the first inklings that *something is wrong*. If the child is the object of extensive oral drills, which are painful and frustrating, the concept emerges: *Something is wrong with me.* When he goes off to a school or program for deaf children, where the urgency of understanding lip movements is greater than ever, what is wrong becomes localized. The behavior of the teacher and others, the conduct of school itself, project to the deaf child of hearing parents a certain image of his selfhood—the very representation that is guiding the audist establishment and is distilled in Table 2. If the child can be brought to internalize that image, he will fit better into a system that is guided by it. Less brute force will be needed; the child will be more manageable. If, for example, a deaf child who derives no benefit from his hearing aids comes to see them as an integral part of his persona, it will no longer be necessary for the teacher to implore, reprimand, and physically insist on the child's wearing them. And his wearing them is an ever-present reminder for the child and a reassuring symbol for the teacher of the fit between the system and the child.

Ben Bahan has pointed out that the hidden curriculum in the deaf school is oppressive as much by what is not there as by what is. There are often no deaf adults. Indeed, some deaf adults have reported that as children they thought they would die before reaching adulthood, since they had never seen any deaf adults. There are no deaf heroes. There is no ASL. The manual behaviors the pupils know are prohibited or useless, while those that seem alien—grasp chin, pull (in articulation lessons)—are endlessly demonstrated.

To the deaf child of deaf parents, the new focus of most interactions addressed to him in school must be surprising. It is as if everyone were interested in his thigh. He has never thought much about it. But many people insist on measuring it. X-rays are taken. He must always keep it exposed and wear an uncomfortably tight garter around it. His thigh becomes an important part of his selfhood—a negative part.

While the deaf child of deaf parents discovers the unnerving preoccupations of the hearing world upon entering a deaf school, the deaf child of hearing parents discovers with joy the solidarity of the deaf world, which replaces the incomprehension and alienation of his hearing home and, frequently, hearing school. The discovery of a deaf community is fraught with emotional and symbolic significance; it is a rite of passage that is told over and over in deaf autobiography: The most common metaphor is a coming home, a new family. For example, Edmund Booth, a nineteenth-century deaf journalist and one of the founders of the National Association of the Deaf, described his arrival at the American Asylum for the Deaf and Dumb in Hartford in 1827: "[My hearing brother] Charles and I went into the boys' and next the girls' sitting rooms. It was all new to me and to Charles it was amusing, the innumerable motions of arms and hands. After dinner he left, and I was among strangers, but knew I was at home."

Interviews (translated from ASL) with students at the National Technical Institute for the Deaf bear witness to this passage. One student explains that when he attended a residential high school for the deaf, "I didn't see my family much, but I felt that I belonged to the family at the institution. And still in my heart, I belong to the family at home too." Another tells what the local hearing high school was like: "Bad experience. I'm the only one deaf there and it's hard for me to get along with the people. Sometimes they would leave me alone, sometimes they would bother me, sometimes they'd pick on me, sometimes they'd laugh at me because I can't hear, my mumble-jumble and they didn't understand what I was saying." But a class-mate was more fortunate, having attended a high school that served several districts, "so most of my friends would be hearing-impaired friends. We would have our own home room. . . . So this is where most of my friends are, and I didn't have many hearing friends—I had a lot of deaf friends." One student joined a deaf teenagers' club: "I would go there and rap with them, so I was never excluded from the deaf. I was always involved with the deaf community in many different ways." Another recounts: "It was very lonesome for me through the [high] school years." Then he went to NTID. "I found happiness is to be with deaf people, rather than my lonely life. . . . I became so popular, I couldn't understand it. It was amazing. It was just from darkness to light." "When I went to [college for the deaf] I felt part of a family," another student recounts. "I was part of something and even though I have had friends and I have my ene-mies . . . we always still acted as a community. . . . One of the things that impressed me with the deaf people was that they cared for each other."

In youth, solidarity with the deaf community is confirmed by the child's rejection of incomprehension at home and at school, and his positive attraction to facile communication and friendships among deaf people. In adulthood, the repelling force is frequently incom-prehension and rejection in the workplace, and an important inte-grating force is marriage to another deaf person. "I hate to go back to work. I don't like to be the only deaf person. It's lonely," complained a working mother near the end of her maternity leave. And a deaf man explains his decision to marry a deaf woman: "If I married a hearing wife, what would happen to her? . . . Would she visit the deaf club? Hearing people go to the hearing club—they go to the clubs and dance. Am I going to be able to interact with the hearing? No way. They don't know me. . . . So, I'd be just sitting back doing nothing; I'd say, 'I don't want to go to a hearing club,' and my wife would say, 'I don't want to go to the deaf club.' We'd become opposites. Opposite cultures and opposite lives."

After years of acculturation in the deaf community, after countless shared social experiences, after exposure to cultural artifacts and art forms and history, the deaf adult may gain a mature sense of his or her own community and culture. In the following interview with a hearing educator (translated from ASL), a deaf adult tries to make explicit her feelings of belonging to a cultural minority:

Many people think that deaf and hearing are the same. It's true, yes, but it's different. Deaf culture is more deaf. [If] you're deaf, [and] I'm deaf—we're family. . . . How often do you see some of your old high school classmates? You don't see them for a long, long time, right? How often do I see my old classmates? Often! Deaf culture is always more involved with family, we're *deaf* family. . . . When you see hearing and deaf, they're the same, but in the way of family ties, they're two types of families and they're not the same. It's the same thing with Italians . . . Russians . . . different ethnic groups. Some of those people don't understand English, so they stick together. I can't have a good time with my [hearing] cousins. The brothers and sisters say, "Hey, come on, let's have a good time," and I say, "Uh. . . ." But with the deaf, there's always good things to do and [so] we go with the deaf.

This positive sense of deaf identity and community is not easily or widely acquired, however. For, as the deaf child grows up, two things become clear to him: that the hearing values purveyed by the audist establishment are different from his own; and that hearing people are generally successful. "The oppressed accepts the judgment of the other," Sartre writes, "incorporating into himself the very standard which decrees him a pariah. He actively consents to oppression. In response to the look of the other, he looks down." African-Americans long subscribed to the notion of African inferiority. For a long time, deaf people in countries like Britain, Germany, and France, all with very powerful audist establishments, have taken it as quite natural that deaf children will not receive a normal high school education, let alone have a chance to attend university. Many deaf adults in those countries also will deny that they have a language; or, rather, the only language they will lay claim to is the national oral language, which they cannot speak and do not read. When I insist with them that I am interested in learning about their manual language, they frequently dismiss it: "Oh, you're interested in my idioms?" they ask, surprised. By this they mean that their sign language has a word order that does not correspond to the national oral language and is therefore "idiomatic."

Deaf people must overcome this acceptance of the judgment of the other, Jeff McWhinney has argued, and must acquire a deaf consciousness "before we can achieve political equality. In other words, to destroy the dangerous relationship between hearing people's control and deaf people's learned inadequacy, we have to overcome our own fear of helplessness in the face of the apparent power of hearing people."

Some of the colonized so thoroughly accept those values which decree that they are inferior that they break away—from the deaf community, from the Algerian community, from the African-American community. They seek to emulate the colonizer. "There is a pyramid of tyranny," Albert Memmi has written. The turncoats will disdain the oppressed; their disdain is born of the disdain for them. Belonging to neither group, they will frequently fail, but they are too valuable to the colonizer to be allowed to fail, so they are shored up. From Saboureux-de-Fontenay in the eighteenth century, famous pupil of the "great demutizer," Jacob Pereire, to Mabel Bell in the nineteenth century, Alexander Graham Bell's pupil and later wife, right down to clients of the audist establishment today, there have always been deaf people who have been socialized to be hearing-impaired and who serve the audist agencies that socialize them by confirming that deaf people have the needs the agencies claim they have. A few years ago, the BBC televised a debate on the relative merits of British Sign Language and English as means of instruction for British deaf children. The opposing sides were seated in opposing bleachers on a stage; interpreters and the host stood in the middle. On the left were a group of deaf people from various walks of life—and I. On the right were hearing educators of deaf children—and one deaf young woman with rather intelligible speech. She was clearly ill at ease in her position, the more so as she could not understand directly either what was said or what was signed; she had her own oral interpreter, who sat facing her and articulated clearly the gist of what had just been said.

The colonized are given the model twice over: There is the colonizer, and then there is the assimilated, much like themselves. If the stigma is not too obvious, the assimilated may even try to pass as one of the powerful. Even if passing is not possible, techniques of covering help to remove the stigma from attention. Dark glasses for the blind man; Western dress and hypercorrect French for the African; turning away for the deaf speaker.

Passing can be exhausting; each situation requires its own brand of cunning and contains its own threats of disclosure. Some people must be avoided—especially similarly stigmatized people—while accomplices must be recruited. "I shrink from any reference to my disability," Mabel Bell wrote near the end of her life, "and won't be seen in public with another deaf person." "I have striven in every way to have [my deafness] forgotten and to be so completely normal that I would pass as one. To have anything to do with other deaf people instantly brought this hard-concealed fact into evidence. So I have helped other things and people . . . anything, everything but the deaf. I would have no friends among them."

Now members of the minority will tell the person who is trying to pass or cover that he is kidding himself. His real solidarity is with other deaf people. Instead of trying to be like the oppressor, he should take a militant stand. Flaunt his manual language (his black dialect, his gay behavior) instead of hiding it. Embrace the unique characteristics of his minority. But pass and cover, or fight back—either way his behavior is determined by the oppression he is subject to.

When the audist is unmasked for the deaf person, dependence is no longer tolerable. The dependent's inferior standing seems a gross injustice. There is a clear standard of justice: The treatment providers afford each other. The former dependent now insists on that treatment—equality. "The slave returns the look of the master. In this moment a man is born." The audist is faced with a terrible predicament: If he makes concessions, he risks his superior standing. Suppose, for example, deaf people were hired in substantial numbers at a school for deaf children. They might displace some hearing people. Their greater ability to communicate with the deaf children, and frequently to empathize with them and govern them, could embarrass the hearing faculty. And, as Mannoni points out, "every increase in equality makes the remaining differences seem the more intolerable." Reasonably enough: if the standard of just treatment is the way the providers behave toward each other, then the more you accord me equal standing, the more the rules you live by seem to apply to me and the more I demand that they be extended to me. So small concessions lead to larger ones and, in the end, the undoing of the oppressive relationship. That is why there are few moderates in such struggles. Then the former dependents conclude that they must resort to force to obtain their just demands, as the deaf students did in the Gallaudet Revolution of 1988, as many minorities and colonized peoples have done.

The Gallaudet Revolution came as a shock to America and Western Europe. We knew there were oppressed language minorities; we did not know the deaf community was one. We thought we were doing all that an enlightened society would do for deaf people. We find it unacceptable that deaf children are deprived of an effective education, that deaf adults are refused a role in that education and in other professions serving deaf people; that deaf people's counsel is neither heeded nor even sought in matters that vitally concern them; and that this all takes place before our very eyes and largely with our tax dollars. We are ill at ease because, without our collective indifference, the audist establishment could not carry out the deeds that damn deaf people and themselves, and shame the rest of our society. Jean-Paul Sartre's words seem to accuse us when he writes: "Your passivity only serves to place you in the ranks of the oppressors."

PART FOUR

Language Bigotry and Deaf Communities

The Oppression of American Sign Language

Most countries are multilingual. In the world's roughly two hundred countries, some six thousand languages are spoken. There are more multilingual people than monolingual people around the globe. Power, however, lies principally in the hands of the monolinguals. Multilingual people become so largely because they live in a country where their primary language is not the language of official discourse, and so they are obliged to learn a second language.

The members of these language minorities are usually realistic about language and power; they recognize that their children need to know the majority language to get ahead. They generally favor an education for their children in their most fluent language, the language of their minority, but an education that will make the children bilingual.

Majorities, on the other hand, generally regard monolingualism in the majority language as the normal and desirable state. They frequently protest that a society that speaks in too many voices is a society divided. Our daily newspapers record the power struggle between the world's various language minorities and the language majorities that engulf each of them. French speakers protest their oppression in Canada, Breton speakers in France, Tamil speakers in India, Georgian speakers in the Soviet Union, Kurdish speakers in Iraq, Armenian speakers in Turkey, Turkish speakers in Denmark, Basque speakers in Spain, Spanish speakers in the United States— the list goes on and on. Each entry on the list stands for lives taken and for countless more lives enfeebled by needless suffering and ineffectual education.

Listen to the Hispanic-American leader Cesar Chavez describe the common experience of Spanish-speaking children in the United States before the modern era of bilingual education:

In class, one of my biggest problems was the language. Of course, we bitterly resented not being able to speak Spanish, but they insisted that we had to learn English. They said that if we were American, then we should speak the language, and if we wanted to speak Spanish, then we should go back to Mexico. When we spoke Spanish, the teacher swooped down on us. I remember the ruler whistling through the air as its edge came down sharply across my knuckles. It really hurt. Even out in the playground, speaking Spanish brought punishment. The principal had a special paddle that looked like a two-by-four with a handle on it. The wood was smooth from a lot of use. He would grab us, even the girls, put our head between his legs, and give it to us.

Modern studies in multilingual countries such as Canada show that excluding minority teachers and their language from the schools and attempting to force the assimilation of minority children carry heavy penalties. Educators do indeed become disciplinarians as they pursue the aggressive steps required to stop the child from using his or her primary language—grades are lowered, physical punishment is inflicted, friends are separated—and the school becomes a place of incarceration. An Alsatian student: "When I was in primary school it was forbidden to speak Alsatian both in and out of class. Children were punished if they were caught." An Arab student: "In my boarding school the nuns forced us to speak French to one another, even when we were playing. We had a special [dog] collar that every violator of the rule had to wear." A Gaelic-speaking student: "Well you were made to feel small and embarrassed, y'see. I mean, if you were asked anything [in school] . . . it was always in English, and as often as not you would run home rather than stand it out." A student speaking French Sign Language (*Langue des Signes Française*, LSF): "Sometimes the old man made us speak with our mouths open, sometimes he made us pronounce the expressions written on the board. Then, having uttered that spoken language which we were a thousand leagues from understanding, we asked each other in sign language the meaning of what he made us say." In his 1982 book on bilingualism, *Life with Two Languages*, François Grosjean calls this "sink-or-swim" approach characteristic of many educational systems around the world and protests that, if some children learn to swim, frequently at the cost of losing their native language and culture, many other children sink: "they fail to master the majority language well, feel insecure, and often have negative attitudes toward both the majority group that rejects them and the minority group they have been taught to look down upon."

Language oppression is not a recent development. Language has long been an instrument of empire, used to create homogeneity and fealty to a central power, to minimize or eradicate diversity. Queen Isabella of Spain, for example, ordered that the people of her American colonies were to abandon their "crude barbaric tongues" in favor of Castilian Spanish, so they would become subject to God—and the crown. Two centuries later, the goal of linguistic domination had still not been achieved, and Charles II decreed that the Indians were to learn Spanish "and other good habits of reasonable men." They were to be schooled only in Castilian, which was to become the one and universal idiom, since "it belongs to the monarchs and conquerors." "This universal knowledge of Castilian," the decree continues, "is necessary in order to facilitate the governing and spiritual guidance of the Indians, in order that they may be understood by their superiors, conceive a love for the conquering nation, banish idolatry, and be civilized for purposes of business and commerce.... The natives' inclination to retain their own language impedes their will to learn another and foreign language, an inclination accentuated by the somewhat malicious desire to hide their actions from the Spaniards and not answer them directly when they believe they can be evasive."

Likewise, at the end of the Enlightenment, when the first French republic supplanted the monarchy, its legislators were told: "Governments do not realize, or do not feel keenly enough, how much the annihilation of regional speech is necessary for education, the true knowledge of religion, the ready implementation of the law, national happiness and political tranquillity.... Federalism and superstition speak Breton; emigration and hate of the Republic speak German; the counterrevolution speaks Italian, and fanaticism speaks Basque." The renowned *Encyclopedia* defined a patois as "a degenerate tongue such as is spoken in all the provinces.... The language of France is spoken only in the capital." The history of Scotland is in large part the history of English displacing Gaelic. Early in the seventeenth century, Gaelic chiefs of the Western Isles were forced to accept a set of statutes that required every gentleman to educate his sons in Lowland schools, so that they would be able to speak, read, and write English. John, thirteenth earl of Sutherland, was advised by his tutor: "Apply yourself to removing the Gaelic barbarity that still remains in your country.... To extinguish the Gaelic language, plant schools in every corner of the country to instruct the youth to speak English."

Education is the battleground where linguistic minorities win or lose their rights. Starting with an impressionable six-year-old child and continuing for a decade or more, the school shapes values, beliefs, and knowledge. Thus, those who govern look characteristically to the schools as a highly effective instrument of government. As majorities are more often disturbed than delighted by minorities in their midst, the schools are often the main means for minimizing or obliterating cultural differences and for fostering assimilation in the name of better governance. In Great Britain, for example, a six-year study of the education of children from minority groups, the Swann Report, published in 1985, came out strongly in favor of assimilation and opposed to incorporating linguistic diversity in the educational process. Bilingual education also has its vociferous opponents in the United States. There are groups lobbying for an amendment to the Constitution that would make it illegal to require the use of any language other than English (except for teaching English); bills have been introduced in Congress to this effect nearly every year, and seventeen states have passed this type of legislation. Thus, consciously or unconsciously, majorities seek to ensure continuing domination over minorities in their nation.

Where a minority has a strong say in the conduct of the education of minority children, where its adults are role models, where their language is used and hence children are educated in their primary, most fluent language, education is more successful, career aspirations are higher, the profession of teaching is opened to the minority, minority language and culture tend to be legitimized, children grow up adapted to—and proud of—their minority identity.* That is why the linguistic minority leaders interviewed for the Swann Report urged, in opposition to the main recommendation of the report, that the education of minority children include the maintenance of their mother tongue.

But if the minority language is not allowed in the schools, this reduces the self-image and the potential achievement of those who use it. It discourages minority members from entering the teaching profession, where they would serve as role models to the children and tend to perpetuate minority language, culture, and identity.

This outcome is often acceptable, and even appealing, to majorities in power. If education is ineffective, because it is conducted in a language foreign to the students and because no role models are available, the minority stays in the laboring classes. Hence, much of the minority is poor, illiterate, and unlikely to exert political influence in behalf of goals distinct from those of the majority. The Swann

Report states: "The role of education cannot be . . . to reinforce the values, beliefs, and cultural identity which each child brings to school." This is why education is a vital battleground for minority rights.

Many deaf Americans recount bitterly the oppressive language policies of their schools in terms much like those of Cesar Chavez. Witness the deaf painter and actor Albert Ballin: "I resented having my lessons hurled at me," he wrote in his autobiography. "It seemed as if all the [English] words, for which I never cared a tinker's dam, were invented for the sole purpose of harassing and tormenting me. . . . How I hated my teacher, my school, the whole creation!"

Deaf communities in the Western world have long been aware that education is the foremost concern of their minority. The first book by a deaf author, Pierre Desloges, published in 1779, is largely devoted to education of deaf children and the role of sign language. A torrent of information, protest, and proposals concerning education pours from the pages of the first newspapers by and for deaf people, as from the proceedings of the earliest congresses of deaf people in the last century. Indeed, my history of deaf communities in the Western world, *When the Mind Hears*, proved to be concerned most of all with education. Although education is a key issue for all minorities, it has even greater significance for deaf people. No doubt the reason is this: Throughout deaf history, the language and culture of this minority could not be transmitted primarily through the home. Since most deaf children have hearing parents, it has traditionally been in the residential schools instead that they found their "roots"— especially, of course, their minority language.

Few communities have as long and as tragic a history of language oppression as sign language communities. Many centuries went by before the world even recognized manual languages. At the dawn of deaf education in the seventeenth century, its founder in German-speaking lands, Jan Conrad Amman, could write: "The breath of life resides in the voice. The voice is the interpreter of our hearts and expresses its affections and desires. . . . The voice is a living emanation of that spirit that God breathed into man when he created him a living soul." And because signers did not use the voice, "What stupidity we find in most of these unfortunate deaf," Amman wrote. "How little they differ from animals."

How do we explain such linguistic bigotry? One might as well ask how to explain the resistance to French among English-speaking

Canadians, to Basque among Spanish speakers, to Tamil among Hindi speakers, and so on. The natural state of man is linguistic bigotry: my language is the only true language; all others are impoverished and cumbersome—in fact, not true languages at all.

Education alone is not a sure cure for linguistic bigotry. So distinguished a scholar as Denis Diderot argued that the study of French grammar could reveal principles of thought, because the order of words in French corresponds to the order in which they arise in the mind. Similarly, an instructor of deaf children at the New York School for the deaf wrote: "[We must] change signs into the English order. . . . I believe the adjective should come before the noun, that the substantive should come before the verb—just the same in sign language as the written language. . . . Let the signs be used as nearly as possible in the order in which we think." Napoleon exclaimed to Abbé Sicard that sign language had only nouns and adjectives; and Sicard's colleague Jean-Marc Itard vilified French Sign Language as "that barbaric language without pronouns, without conjunctions, without any of the words that permit us to express abstract ideas."

Linguistic bigotry will not explain, however, why signed languages are singled out for particular repression among minority languages. At least three other considerations come into play. First, if the language bigot is abetted by the mismatch between the structure of the foreign language and his own, how much greater is that mismatch, and how much more grievously will he be misled, therefore, when the foreign language is in another mode—manual-visual rather than oral-auditory? The organization of ASL is appropriate to its singular mode: Itard and dozens of other audists since him who have assailed manual languages as impoverished would have found their precious pronouns, conjunctions, and abstract words if they had only known the language well. Then, too, the delayed development of sign language interpreting as a profession allowed the illusion that there was nothing to translate in this strange pantomime, or, worse, that a series of English glosses for the signs was indeed a translation.

If the language itself was too alien to be accorded equal status with our own, its speakers, on the other hand, were too like us to be accorded their own language. Only two kinds of people, after all, fail to use your language properly: foreigners and the mentally retarded. The deaf clearly were not the former: They did not come from some other land or visibly constitute a distinct community in our own, like, for example, the Navajo Indians. Therefore, they could not have their own language, and their failure to use ours properly, like that of a person with mental retardation, could only be the result of faulty intellect. The errors that the deaf student makes in writing English were viewed not as a product of second-language learning—that is, a result of interference from his first language and overextension of the rules of the language he is acquiring—but rather as a sign of stupidity.

In order to trace the history of oppression of manual languages, we need to distinguish the two fundamental ways in which speakers of a dominant language can undertake to annihilate a nondominant language: replacing it outright or dialectizing it. In the latter case, the users of the nondominant language are led to believe that theirs is a substandard dialect of the dominant language, a "vernacular," which should not be employed for serious purposes such as education or government. It has generally been thought that the nondominant language could be dialectized only if it was related to the dominant language. The linguist Heinz Kloss contrasts the cases of Basque and Catalan:

> So the Spanish government, in trying to establish and maintain the monopoly of Castilian Spanish must (and does) try to blot out the Basque language completely, for there is no possibility that the Basques will ever lose consciousness of the fact that their language is unrelated to Spanish. The position of Catalan is quite different, because both Catalan and Spanish are Romance Languages. There is a chance that speakers of Catalan can be induced to consider their mother tongue as a patois, with Castilian as its natural standard language. As a matter of fact this attitude to Catalan is already to be found [in] the province of Valencia and in the Balearic islands. In a similar manner, nearly all speakers of Low Saxon (Low German) and the overwhelming majority of Occitan (Provençal) speakers have lost consciousness of their linguistic identity and consider their folk speech as naturally subordinated to German and French respectively, though linguists continue to group these folk languages with other Gothic and Romance Languages. The spiritual subjugation of speakers of Sardinian, and of Haitian Creole, is no less complete.

At first, it might seem improbable that people whose native language is American Sign Language could be induced to consider their mother tongue a patois, with English as their natural standard language; the two are as unrelated as any two languages could be. From time to time, the oral majority has, however, waged such a campaign, using schools for deaf children as the vehicle for indoctrination. The fact that such efforts have never had long-lasting effects has not prevented renewed attempts: what we learn from history, as George Bernard Shaw pointed out, is that we do not learn from history. Unhappily, we are currently witnessing such a program of dialectization, in which one or another version of Manual English is taught and used for instruction in many classes for deaf children. All versions have in common that they take some signs from American Sign Language as base forms and add invented sign suffixes for -*ing*, -*ly*, -*ment*, -*tion*, -*ed*, -*s*, and the like. Only the rare deaf student would dare object that this cumbersome invention is unnecessary, that he understands time, number, and so on perfectly well in the unaltered language, in ASL.

Manual English goes on to invent signs for pronouns, prepositions, conjunctions—all the appurtenances of the well-equipped language; never mind that the time to sign a message has been doubled; that there was no need for all this apparatus, ASL having its own genius to conduct its grammatical housekeeping: utilizing space, direction of movement, handshapes, and facial expression, among other means. Manual English requires that the order of the signs shall be in the order of English and that signs shall also adopt the semantics of English; no matter that often one word in English subserves several concepts, for which there are several signs, so that whichever single sign is adopted is generally incongruous. Can speakers of a visual language ever be induced to believe that such a contortion of their native tongue, annihilating its basic principles, is in fact a language of which they speak a substandard dialect when using ASL? Yes indeed. Some deaf people refer to their language (ASL) as "low verbal," "broken language," or "slang." A deaf friend of ours referred to her signing in ASL as "low sign"; for her, "high sign" was Manual English. Other informants have referred to ASL as "broken English" or "bad English."

The first attempt by the oral majority to dialectize sign language occurred with the founding of the first school for deaf children, in mid-eighteenth-century France, by Charles Michel, Abbé de l'Epée. On the one hand, Epée was impressed by the medium of communication that he had observed two deaf sisters use. When he was asked to instruct them, he undertook to learn from them. He offered them bread and obtained the sign for EAT; water, and obtained that for DRINK; pointing to objects nearby, he learned the names they applied to each. Soon he could hold a conversation with them. As the class of his pupils grew, the signs used by the two deaf sisters, probably French Sign Language in the form in use in Paris at that time, came to be used by all of Epée's pupils. On the other hand, Epée did not understand that his pupils used a true language which could have served for their instruction. He believed he had to endow their signs with grammar—he called the new system "methodical signing"—and what better grammar to use than that of French? "We choose first," he explains, "the signs of the three persons singular and plural because that is easiest. Then we go on to the tenses and moods and assign to each of them signs which connoisseurs find simple and natural, hence easy to remember." The connoisseurs, significantly, are his deaf pupils, as his description of how he chose signs to indicate tense makes clear:

> The pupil, though Deaf and Dumb, had like us, an idea of the past, the present, and the future, before he was placed under our tuition, and was at no loss for signs to express the differences. Did he mean to convey a present action? He made a sign prompted by nature . . . which consists in appealing to the eyes of the spectators to witness our current activity; but if the action did not take place in his sight, he laid his two hands flat upon the table, bearing upon it gently, as we are all apt to do on similar occasions: and these are the signs he learns again in our lessons, by which to indicate the present tense of a verb. Did he wish to signify that an action is past? He tossed his hand carelessly two or three times over his shoulder: these signs we adopt to characterize the past tenses of a verb. And lastly, when it was his intent to announce a future action, he projected his right hand: here again, we select his sign to represent the future tense of a verb.

Epée's disciple and successor, Abbé Sicard, pursued the master's course, conducting all instruction in Signed French, unaware that French Sign Language had its own grammar, albeit one quite different from French. "We all know the kinds of sentences in use among the Negro tribes," he wrote, "but those used by the deaf and dumb are even closer to nature, even more primitive." It mattered not a whit that Pierre Desloges had given a ringing defense of LSF in his book a decade earlier, showing how it served the needs of the deaf community of Paris, so that "No event in Paris, in France, or in the four corners of the world lies outside the scope of their discussions."

Gradually it became clear to disciples of Epée and Sicard, who had founded schools for deaf children throughout Europe and the Americas, that the effort to dialectize sign language was unsuccessful and that precious class time was lost in attempting to teach Signed English and Signed French. At the "mother school" in Paris, Abbé Sicard had learned from Epée's attempts that merely translating a French sentence into Signed French did not assist its understanding; therefore the meaning of each sentence was first explained in LSF. In the years after Sicard's death the intermediate step between French and LSF was dropped. Likewise, in the United States, the report of the New York Institution for the Deaf and Dumb in 1834 described methodical signs as "wholly discarded."

Writing from the first school for deaf children in America, founded in Hartford in 1817 by a deaf Frenchman, Laurent Clerc, and a hearing American, Thomas Hopkins Gallaudet, an instructor (later to become president of Columbia University) wrote: "The purpose of the school is not to teach signs but words and the labor thus spent in defining a [methodical] sign is the very labor, and no other, required to teach a word. . . . Truly the system of methodical signs is an unwieldy and cumbrous machine, and a dead weight upon the system of instruction in which it is recognized."*

By 1835, Signed English had been abandoned, not only in New York and Hartford, but in most schools for deaf children throughout the United States. Thus, one of the two strategies for annihilating the minority language had failed, not because the oral majority lacked prestige, power, and access to the schools, but for a linguistic reason: The structural principles of the two languages were so radically different that their bizarre superposition would not be transmitted from one generation to the next.

Although the failure of Signed French and Signed English was definitive, a hardy group of latter-day Sicards is trying again in the United States, Germany, and elsewhere. In historical perspective, we will not be misled by their stated goal—namely, to introduce a new and better way of teaching deaf children the national oral language.

When a single language is the national language of the great majority, the dominant language group can aspire to impose that language on all the people in an attempt to replace minority languages outright. In the period between the two world wars, so many European governments pursued this policy of replacement that it would appear to be almost an inevitable consequence of human ethnocentrism (often abetted by other motives), were it not for a few enlightened states that demonstrate true linguistic broad-mindedness. Heinz Kloss points out that successor states to the Turkish, Hapsburg, and Russian empires "ruthlessly pursued linguistic annihilation. A crucial method was, of course, to substitute the majority for minority languages in the schools. In 1918, there were 147 Lithuanian schools in Poland; in 1941 there were two. The number of German schools in Lithuania fell to one third in the same period. There were 2600 Ukrainian schools in East Galicia in 1918 and 400 in 1928."

In America, there were 26 institutions for the education of deaf children in 1867, and ASL was the language of instruction in all; by 1907, there were 139 schools for deaf children, and ASL was allowed in none. The French figures provide a comparable glimpse of ruthless linguistic imperialism: in 1845, 160 schools for deaf children, with LSF the accepted language; by the turn of the century, it was not allowed in a single French school.

The struggle to replace the sign languages of the Western world with majority languages began, significantly, after efforts at dialectization had failed, in the mid-nineteenth century. The decisive victory of replacement was gained, however, later in that century, beginning with a meeting of hearing instructors of deaf children that was hastily convened in Paris at the French Exposition of 1878. Only fifty-four persons attended, half of them instructors, and all but two of these from France. No deaf people were allowed to attend, although at the time a majority of the instructors in deaf education in France were themselves deaf. Nevertheless, the hearing group grandiosely proclaimed itself the First World Congress to Improve the Welfare of the Deaf and the Blind, affirmed that only oral instruction could fully restore deaf people to society, and chose Milan as the site of the second congress, to be held in 1880.

Despite its devastating impact on deaf children and adults for over a century, the Milan meeting was merely a brief rally conducted by hearing opponents of sign language. The congress amounted to two dozen hours, in which three or four audists reassured the rest of the rightness of their actions in the face of troubling difficulties. Nevertheless, the meeting at Milan was the single most critical event in driving the languages of deaf communities beneath the surface; I believe it is the single most important cause of the limited educational achievements of modern deaf men and women.

Writing from Milan, a British teacher raved: "The victory for the cause of pure speech was gained before [the] congress began." And the headmaster at the Royal School for Deaf Children in England reported that the congress "was mainly a partisan gathering. The machinery to register its decrees on the lines desired by its promoters had evidently been prepared beforehand and to me it seemed that the main feature was enthusiasm [for] '*orale pure*' rather than calm deliberation on the advantages and disadvantages of methods." The location chosen, the makeup of the organizing committee, the congress schedule and demonstrations, the composition of the membership, the officers of the meeting—all elements were artfully arranged to produce the desired effect.

Italians made up more than half of the 164 delegates, and there were 56 from France; the committed delegates from these two countries were seven eighths of the membership. In the opening address, the Italian host enjoined the delegates to "remember that living speech is the privilege of man, the sole and certain vehicle of thought, the gift of God, of which it has been truly said: 'Speech is the expression of the soul/As the soul is the expression of divine thought.' "

The congress of educators of deaf children, from which deaf educators were excluded (although one slipped in), elected a rabid enemy of sign language as its president, an Italian priest named Giulio Tarra. "The kingdom of speech," Tarra began in what would prove to be a two-day peroration, "the kingdom of speech is a realm whose queen tolerates no rivals. Speech is jealous and wishes to be the absolute mistress. Like the true mother of the child placed in judgment before Solomon, speech wishes it all for her own—instruction, school, deafmute—without sharing; otherwise, she renounces all. . . . I know that my pupil has only a few imperfect signs, the rudiments of an edifice that should not exist, a few crumbs of a bread that has no consistency and can never suffice for nourishing his soul."

The congress president eventually came to what he called his fundamental argument. "Oral speech is the sole power that can rekindle the light God breathed into man when, giving him a soul in a corporeal body, he gave him also a means of understanding, of conceiving, and of expressing himself. . . . While, on the one hand, mimic signs are not sufficient to express the fullness of thought, on the other they enhance and glorify fantasy and all the faculties of the sense of imagination. . . . The fantastic language of signs exalts the senses and foments the passions, whereas speech elevates the mind much more naturally, with calm, prudence and truth."

When a deaf-mute confesses an unjust act in sign, Tarra explained, the sensations accompanying the act are reawakened. For example, when the deaf person confesses in sign language that he has been angry, the detestable passion returns to the sinner, which certainly does not aid his moral reform. In speech, on the other hand, the penitent deaf-mute reflects on the evil he has committed, and there is nothing to excite the passion again. Tarra ended by defying anyone to define in sign language the soul, faith, hope, charity, justice, virtue, the angels, God. . . . "No shape, no image, no design," Tarra concluded, "can reproduce these ideas. Speech alone, divine itself, is the right way to speak of divine matters."

All but the Americans voted for resolutions affirming "the incontestable superiority of speech over sign" and the necessity of using spoken languages exclusively in the education of deaf children. In the closing moments of the congress, the French delegate cried from the podium, *"Vive la parole!"* "Long live speech!" has been the slogan of hearing educators of deaf children down to the present time. According to an American deaf leader, however, "The infamous Milan resolution paved the way for foisting upon deaf people everywhere a loathed method; hypocritical in its claims, unnatural in its application, mind-deadening and soul-killing in its ultimate results."

In the aftermath of Milan, the policy of annihilating signed languages by substituting spoken languages washed over Europe like a flood tide. Many people and schools were swept up in the advance of "oralism." There is no single explanation for such tides in human affairs. In *When the Mind Hears*, I discuss the confluence of nationalism, elitism, and commercialism that led to the Congress of Milan and its tragic legacy. For example, the ensuing demand for "English only" in American schools for ASL-using children coincided with, and was reinforced by, a similar demand made of schools here that used other minority languages, such as German. Americans were alarmed at the "rising tide" of immigration, which seemed to threaten the country's economy, mores, and "racial stock." The new immigrants could be discouraged from voting and educational and economic advancement by disenfranchising their native languages. Residential schools for deaf children meted out severe punishment for using ASL, and in federal boarding schools for Indians, children were beaten for using American Indian languages. It seems likely that the latest resurgence of the "English only" movement has been fueled by the Hispanic and Asian immigration of recent years.

The pronouncements of Milan also conformed with educators' desire for total control of their classrooms, which cannot be had if the pupils use a signed language and the teacher cannot. The teacher then becomes the linguistic outcast, the handicapped. Nor can he or she acquire the necessary skill in a year, or even two, any more than an Anglophone teacher can so rapidly prepare himself to teach in French. This understandable reluctance of hearing teachers to master a language radically different from their own continues to have the greatest weight in what are misrepresented as pedagogical decisions. There was a time when teachers of deaf children could not practice without a knowledge of their pupils' primary language. But the vast expansion of schools in Europe and America late in the last century created more professional positions than there were educators and administrators fluent in the sign language of their nation's deaf community. Increasingly, people with few ties to the deaf community dominated the education of deaf children.

Teachers who used manual languages were increasingly forced into retirement; whereas nearly half of all American teachers of deaf students had been deaf themselves, by the turn of the century only a handful were. Before the ravages of Milan, American deaf teachers had founded twenty-four schools for deaf children. Many more deaf teachers taught in these and scores of other schools, and some developed widely used teaching materials. Some published learned articles and appeared on the international deaf scene, shaping the future of their profession worldwide. Within a decade after Milan, however, the fraction of teachers who were deaf fell from one half to one quarter; by World War I, it was down to a fifth, and most of the fifth were in the South, teaching manual trades in just a few schools. Nowadays the fraction is about one tenth, and many of these deaf teachers are assigned by the hearing establishment to instruct multiply handicapped children.*

With the forced retirement of teachers who used manual languages, and the quarantine and then graduation of the older students who did so, signed language could be totally banished from the schools. Of course, deaf leaders protested. At the Convention of American Instructors of the Deaf, a decade after the Congress of Milan, a hearing principal affirmed: "A teacher in a pure oral school who understands the sign language is out of place. . . . He might demoralize the school in a very short time. Only insofar as he would suppress his inclination to use sign could he be useful." J. Schuyler

Long, Gallaudet graduate, superintendent of a deaf school, journalist, poet, and author of the first illustrated dictionary of ASL, rose to respond: "The Chinese women bind their babies' feet to make them small; the Flathead Indians bind their babies' heads to make them flat. And the people who prevent the sign language being used in the education of the deaf ... are denying the deaf their free mental growth through natural expression of their ideas, and are in the same class of criminals."

At the dawn of this century, the first president of the National Association of the Deaf, Robert McGregor, cried out against the oppression of manual language in these words:

> What heinous crime have the deaf been guilty of that their language should be proscribed? ... The utmost extreme to which tyranny can go when its mailed hand descends upon a conquered people is the proscription of their national language. By whom then are signs proscribed? By ... educators of the deaf whose boast is that they do not understand signs and do not want to ... by parents who do not understand the requisites to the happiness of their deaf children. ... Professing to have no object in view but the benefit of the deaf, [educators] exhibit an utter contempt for the opinions, the wishes, the desires of the deaf. And why should we not be consulted in a matter of such vital interest to us? This is a question no man has yet answered satisfactorily.

The deaf press labeled oralism the method of "violence, oppression, obscurantism, charlatanism, which only makes idiots of the poor deaf-mute children." A deaf leader urged the authorities to "stop tying the hands of the deaf, forbidding the colorful language which alone can restore them to moral life and the bosom of society." The international congresses of deaf people were established to resist the banishment of their language decreed by hearing educators in Milan. The first congress was held in Paris, on the centennial of Epée's death, under the presidency of one of the French deaf professors forced into retirement a few years earlier. Addressing that convention, the president of the American National Association of the Deaf declared: "Suppress the language of signs and the deaf man is excluded from all society, even that of his brothers in misfortune; he will be more isolated than ever." The congress of deaf leaders ended with quite a different set of resolutions for promoting the welfare of deaf people than those voted in Milan. It proclaimed manual language "the most suitable instrument for developing the intellect of the deaf" and closed with its own "Long live!"—"Long live the emancipation of the deaf!"

But the views of deaf people were ignored. In the final congress on the education of deaf children—held in Paris in 1900—which gave us our present legacy of English-based instruction, deaf teachers were again excluded by the hearing leadership. The president of the meeting, an otologist, wrote in a textbook on speech teaching: "The deaf-mute is by nature fickle and improvident, subject to idleness, drunkenness, and debauchery, easily duped and readily corrupted." Since deaf leaders had demanded that they participate in future congresses concerning their welfare and planned to participate in the Paris congress of 1900, the otologist president decided to separate the deaf from the hearing sessions, on the pretext that otherwise the sessions would be too long and translation between manual and spoken languages would produce confusion. The deaf leaders then proposed a compromise, a common meeting of all delegates at the end of the congress, to debate and vote on the resolutions. The presiding otologist rejected that as well. Then the deaf planners met to decide whether to acquiesce or attempt to block plans for the congress; they chose to acquiesce and convene a separate deaf section.

Right from the first session of the hearing section, Edward Minor Gallaudet and Alexander Graham Bell traded blows. Gallaudet was the son of Thomas Hopkins Gallaudet, the cofounder of deaf education in the United States, and Sophia Fowler Gallaudet, the foremost woman in American deaf society; the leader of deaf education in the United States, he was an ardent advocate of the "combined system"— ASL in the classroom and training in speech after class for those who could benefit (primarily late-deafened children). Alexander Graham Bell, the son of a distinguished elocutionist and a hard-of-hearing mother, husband of a late-deafened woman, was the leader of the oralist camp. Bell supported the exclusion of deaf delegates from the congress's deliberations: "Those who are themselves unable to speak," he contended, "are not the proper judges of the value of speech to the deaf." Gallaudet rose to attack the exclusion of those whose lives were vitally concerned. He called the Milan congress unrepresentative and its declarations a great error, yet "its decisions have been cited for twenty years as if they had the weight of a judgment of the Supreme Court." Now this congress, he said, is no more representative: Anyone with ten francs can vote. Milan decided nothing, for the controversy rages. He then moved a resolution calling for an open exchange of ideas with the deaf leaders. At this, the president declared—while giving no one else an opportunity to express an opinion, and without submitting the proposal to a vote— that the proposition was rejected by the congress, which was adjourned until the afternoon.

At the start of the next session, the French government delegate asked the congress to reaffirm that the right to vote was reserved for hearing delegates and any speaking deaf, "as it is inadmissible to grant the right to vote to people who cannot follow the discussions." Gallaudet asked permission to read his paper to a joint session of the two sections; the leaders of the deaf section supported this request, but the president refused. Gallaudet claimed that oralism had not lived up to its promises, and he raised the question of whose testimony should carry the most weight in determining whether this was true. That of the teachers? But they are partisan and too familiar with their own pupils' speech to make an accurate judgment. That of friends and acquaintances of the deaf? But they, too, adjust to the poor speech and gestures of the orally taught pupil. That of strangers? Their testimony is more important. But the greatest weight should be given to the views of the deaf themselves. You can imagine how those remarks were greeted by oralist teachers, who had repeatedly excluded the views of the deaf! But even harsher words were to come: Gallaudet raised the question whether oralist educators were defective morally. He stated that they were conspiring to deceive. It was hardly possible that these teachers were deceiving themselves about the poor fruits of oralism, so it must be that they intended to deceive everyone else.

Oralists and their opponents fought back and forth. The vice-president of Gallaudet College presented a resolution in behalf of the combined system. The director of a French oral school read the conclusions of the Milan congress and then presented a resolution of his own reaffirming pure oralism. When the question was called, the combined system received only seven votes, while nearly everyone else voted for the French resolution affirming the "incontestable superiority of speech over signs for restoring the deaf-mute to society and for giving him a more perfect knowledge of language."*

A deaf leader observed: "Government derives its power from the consent of the governed—but not when it comes to the affairs of the deaf." But deaf leaders did not have—do not have—the final word. To quote a major professional journal reporting on the Paris congress: "The oral method has been weighed in the balance . . . and it is not found wanting. Whereas Milan was a hope," it said, "Paris was a conclusion—a verdict after trial. The action of Paris will have the chief effect . . . [of] confirm[ing] the faith of those who practice . . . oral education of the deaf. . . . The question of methods is practically retired from the field of discussion."

Language in Another Mode

In the Bilingual Education Act of 1968, Americans institutionalized the premise that children are best educated, transitionally at least, in their most fluent language. The laws of most of the states soon came to require that schools with more than a certain percentage of children whose primary language is Navajo, or Chinese, or whatever, must offer a portion of their instruction in that language. In the fall of 1990, the federal government reaffirmed the merits of bilingual education when President George Bush signed a law "to encourage and support the use of Native American languages as languages of instruction." Yet American Sign Language, our nation's most prevalent indigenous language (estimates range from one-half million to two million users) and among its most prevalent minority languages, has no official recognition whatever in the federal government and no place in educating ASL-using children according to the states. Neither the laws that provide funding for bilingual education programs, nor the laws that require those programs in schools with large numbers of children who use a minority language, have been applied to ASL-using children. In Great Britain, the Linguistic Minorities Project, the Mother Tongue Project, and other initiatives point to a growing interest in the rewards of linguistic pluralism and the acknowledgment of minority languages. The discussion includes languages as diverse as Gujarati and Chinese, but never British Sign Language. One reason for this particularly severe oppression of ASL and other manual languages is the medicalization of cultural deafness. This is precisely the posture of the American government, where the same agencies that support research and training for the education of retarded people do likewise for deaf people, and the agencies that address the needs of minority language groups refuse to have anything to do with the million or so Americans who use some variety of ASL in everyday communication.

A further reason that signed languages have been subjected to more than the usual portion of suppression doled out to minority languages by dominant language groups is their unexpected mode, manual and visual. Once again, the extrapolative leap leads laymen and scholars alike into error. What would my communication be like, they seem to reason, if I were deprived of spoken language? I would be reduced to pointing to concrete things around me and to miming various actions—that is what manual language must be like. In a 1975 book on thought and language, for example, psychologist Judith Greene deplores "the crudity of sign language. . . . Even deaf and dumb humans who rely entirely on sign languages find it cumbersome to make complicated abstract statements because of a lack of subtle grammatical inflections." As we have seen, she is quite mistaken about the semantics and grammar of ASL.

Educators with passing familiarity with ASL have thought it primitive for a further reason. They have been misled by word-for-word transcriptions of signed utterances; the substitution yields a series of words that necessarily violates the rules of the reader's language and makes the source appear primitive and ungrammatical. For example, the American Sign Language for "A bear killed my father's geese; father shouldered his gun and went to look for it" is, word for word: GEESE, FATHER HIS, BEAR CATCH EAT; FATHER, GUN SHOULDER-ON, GO-LOOK-FOR BEAR. That this is no more evidence for primitiveness than the corresponding transcription from Latin—"Bear, father's geese my killed; gun shoulder leaned against and went so bear might search for"—should be obvious but is not, given the educators' bias against the very idea of manual language.

I think there is something to learn from turning the tables on the oral language snobs with this proposition: ASL is not only intrinsically as good as any oral language but better.

The argument goes like this: Our species, in common with all mammals, is much concerned with three-dimensional space. In fulfilling our needs, both biological and social, we move about in space. Commonly those movements are coordinated among the members of a pair or a group of people, and they relate to an arrangement of people or objects. Consequently, much of human communication is explicitly about spatial arrays. How do we get to the market from here? Where are you going to put the new couch? Where did you leave the car? Countless similar everyday questions and their answers require us to talk about space.

But so spatial an animal are we that we also choose to talk about nonspatial matters in spatial terms. Lists start at the top and end at the bottom. Political alignments range from right to left. The future is ahead of us, the past behind. Power relations extend from the high and mighty to the lowliest of us. Comparatives in general are expressed in spatial metaphor, above all other means. Space inheres in language more deeply, however, than in mere metaphor. A former doctoral student of mine found that English speakers asked to rate the similarity of English verbs are guided most of all by a spatial criterion—namely, whether the meaning of the verb involves translatory movement or fixed position. Thus, his subjects repeatedly rated "giving" closer to "pushing" than to "giving up," and "standing" closer to "waiting" than to "walking." Several linguists have presented the case that the meanings of many English words are fundamentally based on spatial concepts.

Let us see how adroit oral language really is, then, in this fundamental task of spatial description. How well does English convey arrangements and distances of people and things in three-dimensional space? Both literally and metaphorically, we will need to refer to left–right, in front–behind, and above–below. Suppose I am giving a lecture and I look into the audience at two adjacent people—say, Will and his wife. In English I might say, "Will is to the left of his wife," but in that case I can also say he is on his wife's right—that is, "Will is to the right of his wife." So I have been quite unclear. Which is it? Is Will to the left or the right of his wife? The answer is: both. Anna, who is seated behind them, disagrees with me; Will was never to the left of his wife. If you followed that and think that English is clear although complicated about left and right, try this one: Arrange Will, his wife, and Anna so that Will is to the left of his wife, his wife is to the left of Anna, and Will is to the right of Anna.

I have tried to illustrate that in English we must give different accounts of the same array, depending on two things: first, the speaker's point of view, and, second, whether the speaker is using verbal pointing or intrinsic reference. Verbal pointing, called deixis, requires the English listener to know where the speaker is. The intrinsic system requires an interpretation of the scene and an intrinsic orientation. It applies to people and houses, but it will not work for trees, tables, or heaps. To illustrate, let's go for a picnic. If I ask you to put the little picnic table in front of the tree, you can comply with the instruction by putting it anywhere on the planet Earth; I have been quite unclear.

There's a nearby dog track, and we take our seats at the start line. As they leave the gate, the only dog I can see is the dog closest to me, which is, of course, in front of the other dogs; but he may be behind them as well—especially if I bet on him. The rabbit that runs around the inside rail of the track is behind all the dogs up to the turn, even though it is always in front of all of them.

My dog loses, and the sky darkens. "The sun is behind the clouds," you say. When the sun comes out from behind the clouds, is it then in front of the clouds? Of course not! So the sun is always behind the clouds. Actually, the sun is only behind the clouds when there is no sun.

I have brought two balloons to the picnic and tied them to a branch so the red is above the green. You, however, are lying on your side on the grass, looking at the vault of heaven, and the red is to the left of the green—or to the right of the green, depending on which side you're lying on. Unless, of course, you can see the horizon, in which case the red is above the green. "My friend," I tell you, "there's a spider dangling above your head." You go to brush it away, but where to swing? Is it close to you or far? Is it near your cheek or near the top of your head? Who knows?

Will is to the left of his wife. The table is in front of the tree. The black dog is in front of the others. There's a spider above your head. All of these sentences are ambiguous, but they are like those we use all the time. Then we must be rather poor at communicating in English that most essential of human messages, spatial arrays. I decided to do an experiment.

I bought a dollhouse—my first—that came with a few pieces of plastic furniture and, most important, a picture on the box showing how to arrange the furniture in this two-story home. There was a sofa, a TV, a stereo, a picnic table and two chairs, and a barbecue. A graduate assistant and I asked pairs of English speakers to assist us, as follows: With the house set up and the furniture in a pile in front of it, one of the pair was to look at the box and tell the other where to place each item of furniture, in an effort to reproduce the arrangement shown in the photograph on the box. We asked the furniture mover not to talk, and we tape-recorded the speaker. Seven pieces of furniture to place in common ways: should be easy. Here is a typical transcript, influencies and all, from a native speaker of English.

Okay, we'll start with the table and chairs on the bottom floor. In front of the house, um, there's a patch of green, like a patio, and the round table goes in the—in the—uh—top corner of the pa—of the green square. Okay. And in front of the—at—in front of the table—um—between the ladder and the table—goes one of the red chairs. Okay. And across from that red chair, on the other side of the table, goes the second red chair. Okay. Now, the barbe—the barbecue goes on the strip of patio between the green square and the house. Um, um, over to the left, almost in the left corner. Not quite. Okay, now let's go upstairs. Oh, excuse me, we have to go back downstairs; I forgot the record player. Now we're in the house, and as you face the house, it's a—the—the right—your right corner; okay, that's where the record player will go. Against the wall, well, against the wall in the corner. Okay? Now let's go upstairs. Okay. Now, on the second floor—the floor's divided into a terrace and a bedroom, and just where the terrace and the bedroom are divided there's no—there's a frame but no wall there and the couch or the little red seat goes in that frame, at an angle, so it's mostly in the room but it seems to stick out onto the terrace just a little bit. Okay. And the television goes—okay, the floor in that room is separated by—there's a little ridge that sticks out of the floor, so the couch is on one side of the ridge—the television goes in the area that's separated with the other side of the ridge—and it's facing so that the person who is sitting on the couch can't see the TV screen—in other words, the TV screen is facing into the—is facing out of the house. Okay. Sort of facing the ladder. Okay. So we're done.

Now, because ASL is a spatial language, it can communicate arrangement and relative distance of things and people in quite a different way than English or, indeed, any oral language. This makes interpreting signed into spoken language and vice versa unique among translation tasks in that the interpreter must mediate between spatial and linear languages, utterly restructuring spatial discourse as he or she translates from the one language into the other. ASL, instead of conveying a spatial array by a linear chain of words, can map that spatial message right onto its surface form. Moreover, once ASL establishes a location for an object, it need not be reestablished in order to refer to it. When I asked pairs of signers to do my experiment, they were not only quicker at it than English speakers, they followed a different strategy: they created a verbal map of the dollhouse by naming fixed parts of the house and locating those parts in space. Then they named the movable items that had to be placed by their partner and positioned them in the verbal space they had just created. I don't really know how to translate their spatial sentences into a nonspatial language like English, but I have tried to do it using the words "here" and "there" to translate the locating of an object in a position relative to the others:

> Okay, take the round white table and put it outside, in front of the house, in the green area. The two chairs go next to the table. So the table's here and the chairs are one here and one here in front. Now, the cooking grill, you know, with the black hood that opens—the table's here, the grill goes here. The round table goes here, the chairs go here, the grill goes here. Now, the stereo—careful, it's heavy; find the living room wall with the bookshelves and the mirror and put it there in the corner, like this. Now, the TV—go upstairs, up the steps, enter where the roof begins, see where there's a dresser, pictures, and a lamp— put the TV there. Now, the chair, which folds open like a bed, it's red and white, take that upstairs. You see where the TV, the dressers, and the lamp are? Put it there. That's it.

So is speech, in the words of the Milan resolution, "incontestably superior to sign," or is it the other way around? My point is that no language is superior to any other, and none is beneath you if you look up to it. Languages have evolved within communities in a way responsive to the needs of those communities. ASL is attuned to the needs of the deaf community in the United States; English is not. And the effort to replace ASL with English lo these last hundred years will get a chapter all its own in the history of human ignominy.

PART FIVE

The Education of Deaf Children: Drowning in the Mainstream and the Sidestream

Mainstream : integr. into
public school

The Failure of Deaf Education

Today, more than a century after the Congress of Milan, the suppression of the languages of the world's deaf communities continues unabated, and in the crucial realm of education, that suppression is growing worse. The attempt to educate deaf children with teaching methods developed for hearing children continues to prove a failure, decade after decade. In a classroom where English, spoken or written, is the basic means of communication, deaf children are baffled and withdrawn, the more so as nine out of ten became deaf before they could learn English at home.* These children lack the knowledge of English and the skills of articulation and lip-reading required to succeed.

Consider the plight of, for example, a nine-year-old in an educational program for deaf children. The teacher is in the front of the room addressing the class, but the child is, typically, profoundly deaf; he can scarcely make out a single word by peering at the fleeting movements of her lips; even children with lesser hearing losses and hearing aids cannot understand the teacher. One study showed that, on finishing school, deaf students in Great Britain were no better at reading lips than the man in the street (despite the students' decade of training). Let the reader turn on the nightly television news without sound and see how little can be gleaned in this way. Now the child, undaunted, has something to say; he raises his hand, and if he is in one of the many countries where deaf children are required to speak in class, he strains to articulate clearly some words of the national language he has been taught. The tables have turned: the teacher cannot understand the child; two-thirds find their own deaf pupils hard to understand or utterly unintelligible.* Training in lip-reading and speech generally fails with children who have never heard speech, and most of the deaf children in school today have never heard speech. During the 1980s, I visited schools for deaf children on four continents; I did meet children who, with difficulty, could read my lips and whom, with difficulty, I (or my interpreter) could understand. In nearly every case they were children who had become deaf after learning spoken language or who were simply hard of hearing.

True, teachers in the United States do not solely speak English to their deaf pupils; they also write English. But English written down is still spoken English, just as a symphony written down is still a musical work. As I shall show, the deaf schoolchild is no closer to understanding the vowels and consonants on the blackboard than he was to understanding them on the teacher's lips; indeed, when we teach a hearing child to read and write, we call on his prior knowledge of speaking and understanding. The deaf child finds even the alphabetic principle puzzling: Why should ideas be designated by stringing out a small number of elements (vowels and consonants) in a row? When a noted deaf and blind American of the nineteenth century, Laura Bridgman, was corrected in her childhood for misspelling "cat," she asked why it mattered whether one spelled it "cta" or "act" or "tac."

As the child remains silent in the face of mutual incomprehension, the teacher may resort to accompanying her speech with some signs: not sentences of ASL, mind you—just some sign vocabulary she has learned. COW, she signs, then mouths some words impossible to lip-read, then signs something that looks like HORSE and RUN. Perhaps the story's about a farm, or a fair; someone did something to the cow and the horse; or one of them did something to the other. Someone ran—or one of the animals ran, or is running, or will run.

There are more important things in life than speaking the national language aloud or understanding it when it is spoken to you. Many millions of hearing and deaf people around the world do not speak the national language—they have their own minority language, which meets most of their needs. The tragedy is not that America's deaf children cannot speak or lip-read English; the tragedy is that their education is conducted exclusively in this English they do not know.

An educational disaster has thus resulted from using oral language, whether spoken or written, to instruct deaf children. Here is the result of a study of seventeen thousand deaf high school students in the United States: The average sixteen-year-old deaf student reads as poorly as an eight-year-old hearing child. Even in his best subject, arithmetic, he is four grades behind.* The same atrocious results were found in England: a study of nearly all deaf sixteen-year-olds found that despite ten years of strictly oral education, deaf students left school at sixteen years of age with a reading age of eight. Nor did these orally taught and trained deaf children have good oral skills, as I have reported. If we ask what fraction of deaf students at the end of their schooling can read complex subject matter, the answer is 4 percent—one in twenty-five. An estimated half of the British deaf population is unable to read at a functional level; deaf students there have one fifth the chance of hearing students to pass national achievement tests administered when students are fifteen or sixteen. Similarly, the average Japanese deaf student will go through life reading like a nine-year-old.

So it is around the world, wherever the education of deaf children is conducted exclusively in the national language. These abysmally low achievement levels are averages; roughly 50 percent of the children are even less educated. For example, 35 percent of deaf American high school leavers cannot read at second-grade level. Alas, these are real children, not merely statistics, and they are rapidly becoming illiterate adults. If it takes the reading ability of an average eleven-year-old hearing child to read a typical newspaper, then 75 percent of deaf school leavers cannot read a newspaper, and 85 percent of the profoundly deaf school leavers cannot do it.

We are living in an increasingly technological world. Nearly three fourths of all jobs now require technical training beyond a high school diploma. Projections for the year 2000—less than a decade from now—show that new jobs will require a work force with an average education of nearly fourteen years. That means that, on the average, the workers who fill these jobs must have some college education. Not to be the boss, mind you; just to bring home a paycheck.

Education is thus the key to the future of deaf people, but the education of deaf children in America as elsewhere is not now remotely capable of enabling deaf people to meet the challenges of that future. Since educational programs for deaf children have not succeeded in teaching them English and yet rely on English for all teaching, the programs long ago settled for instructing their deaf students in manual trades. The average deaf student now leaves school with few other qualifications and ends up in one of the rapidly vanishing unskilled or semiskilled occupations that are being replaced by jobs requiring higher levels of mathematics, language, and reasoning skills.* Moreover, the schools judge significant numbers of their deaf students unable to achieve even the modest goals they set for them, and they place these students in so-called living skills programs, a euphemism frequently for day care. In Great Britain, half of all deaf students leave school with no qualifications; two thirds are in unskilled or semiskilled employment. Many American teachers believe that a high school degree is the highest academic level most deaf children are capable of; to French teachers, even that seems unattainable; and Burundian teachers doubt that deaf children could profit from elementary school. The special-education system determines what the child is capable of; the child himself does not. Deaf youth are not only ill-prepared vocationally by audist education; they have also been deprived of the normal personal development and acculturation that would enable them to prosper in marriage, in the community, in recreation, in all the facets of a well-rounded life.

In 1986, the American Congress created a commission to look into the education of deaf children. After two years of fact-finding and testimony from deaf leaders, parents, scholars, and others, the commission concluded: "The present status of education for persons who are deaf in the United States is unsatisfactory. Unacceptably so." Alas, the same conclusion was reached by a similar national commission twenty-three years earlier. The audist educational establishment has successfully resisted significant change of its English-based methods and hearing-based values not merely over the last twenty-five years but for over a century.

In historical perspective, the audist program of forced assimilation of deaf people has progressed through five stages:

• *Oralism.* The first stage, as I have told, was the late-nineteenth-century movement to banish signed languages and deaf teachers from the residential schools in favor of spoken languages and hearing teachers. This was totally successful. Almost without exception, ASL is not to be seen today in the classrooms of American schools for deaf children, nor BSL in British schools, nor German Sign Language in German schools, and so forth. An American deaf college student who attended high school in the 1980s reports: "If we tried to sign, we would get our hands slapped."

With most deaf children in the schools deafened before the age of three, the effort to teach intelligible speech and lip-reading characteristically failed, and the child instructed orally was certain to be handicapped indeed. An increasing part of classroom time was devoted to the attempt at oralizing the children. Many schools became, in effect, speech clinics. Hearing educators of deaf pupils commonly were not trained in specific academic areas because none could be truly taught to the children under the oralist regime. The Scottish experience was representative: "Without the benefit of having sign language passed down through the generation grapevine," deaf leader A. Murray Holmes writes, "deaf school leavers were turning up at local deaf clubs unable to have proper conversation with their peers who were fluent signers. Because of [these students'] lack of life skills and behavioral problems, social workers for the deaf were finding it increasingly difficult to locate gainful employment for them."

In Japan, I was told by deaf leaders that the commitment of audist educators to oralism and to the suppression of Japanese Sign Language has been so prolonged and thorough that many deaf school leavers are frustrated in their desire to communicate with deaf adults, to participate in the life of the deaf community, to socialize and find a spouse. The head of the Osaka Deaf Club told me that its members came to the incredible conclusion that, for the first time in the history of the Japanese deaf community, older deaf people must offer classes in Japanese Sign Language for younger deaf people.

• *Day schools.* In the second stage of forced assimilation, day schools were established on a large scale at the beginning of this century, so deaf children could live at home in a majority-language environment. Classes were conducted in spoken English; the hope was that the deaf children would not learn the language of the deaf community and would not marry other deaf people, but nearly all, then as now, learned ASL, took a deaf spouse—whom they met in school, at the deaf club, or through friends—and entered the deaf community. Many of the day schools were actually small classes of deaf children located within an ordinary hearing school; thus the contemporary "mainstreaming" movement, integration of deaf children into hearing schools, already existed on a small scale around the turn of the century.

• *English dominance.* Next, the dominance of English (or French, German, etc.) was reinforced by encouraging its use in all forms of classroom communication: finger-spelling, lip-reading, written English, speech, speech accompanied by signs, signed English. This stage is dominated by the tidal wave of total communication programs that began in the 1970s. In theory, "total communication" means that the teacher uses every means of communication available to communicate with the deaf pupils: manual language, finger-spelling with the manual alphabet, writing, speech, pantomine, drawing—whatever. In practice, "total communication" merely means that the teacher may accompany his spoken English with some signs from American Sign Language, if he knows a few. While the teacher is speaking, he occasionally "shouts" a sign—that is, signs a prominent noun or verb if he knows it, in the wrong order and without using the complex grammar of ASL, which requires agreement in space, in number, in aspect, and so on. Because the teacher is speaking English while intermittently emitting these signs, he has the illusion of making sense, like a pilot in a simulator whose senses tell him he is landing a plane while, viewed from outside, he is headed nowhere.

Most American educational programs for deaf children report that they are using the method called total communication. The rest use spoken English in the classroom or one of the invented systems that, like Epée's methodical signs, code English on the hands.* Gallaudet University linguists Robert Johnson and Scott Liddell point out that teachers of hearing students never say that the method they use to teach science, history, or mathematics is "English"; however, "total communication" is usually the answer to questions of methodology in programs for deaf children. This is another indication that education is not the preoccupation of the classrooms for deaf children; English is. What is fundamentally an issue of cultural and linguistic oppression has been recast as a matter of methodology. Audist educators attempt the same sleight of hand when they characterize the centuries-old struggle between ASL and English as the "oral-manual controversy" or the "bitter methods dispute." The French refusal to allow Breton in the schools, or the British refusal to allow Gujarati, is not a methodological dispute, any more than the American rejection of ASL; it is a matter of culture, politics, and history.

As their poor results testify, schools that subscribe to total communication communicate very little to very few. Nearly fifteen years of total communication have not appreciably changed the discouraging profile of deaf academic achievement in America. The American initiative in total communication was taken up by numerous countries throughout the world, but with rare exceptions they made no place in the classroom for their indigenous signed language, and the practice failed to educate their deaf children. Deaf leaders who mistakenly thought total communication would rely less on the national oral language than the "pure" oralism of the first stage and would provide an entrée for manual language in the classroom were cruelly misled. It is simply impossible to use two languages simultaneously, so the hearing teacher subordinates the manual language to the spoken one, omitting the rich morphology of the signed language and scrambling the sign order, thus rendering the manual message ungrammatical and nearly unintelligible for most deaf children; speaking is also distorted and slowed by such bimodal performances. Nevertheless, the unfortunate teacher who has both English and ASL speakers but no interpreter in his classroom is obliged either to use this dreadfully awkward method or to say everything twice.

For more than a decade, deaf leaders in England, Germany, France, Italy, Japan, and many other nations that remained in the dark ages of oralism looked toward American total communication programs with envy. They now know better. I concede the possibility, however, that total communication may have been a necessary way station on the road from oralism to bilingual education of deaf children in America.

• *Mainstreaming.* In the fourth stage of forced assimilation the minority has been increasingly dispersed by placing deaf children in scattered local schools for hearing children. Although mainstreaming of deaf children was instituted on a large scale in France and in Germany during the last century and failed utterly in both cases, a renewed attempt began in the United States in 1977.* The mainstreaming movement is now taking place in Britain, on the European continent, and elsewhere.

• *Surgery.* Finally, a medical model increasingly guides the relations of hearing and deaf people in the majority's attempt to resolve the social issues by denying their existence. With the headline "Cochlear Implants—Oralism's 'Final Solution'?" *British Deaf News* assailed the 1985 International Congress on the Education of the Deaf for its preoccupation with cochlear implants. Cochlear implants are not the solution to a social issue; in common with other prostheses, they are a tool for living, one among many, appropriate for some and not others. That they are presented as a cure-all and are embraced by educators reveals once again the central program of forced assimilation and denial of a difference.

Though few deaf children are as yet implanted, most deaf children in America are now mainstreamed. Nearly three fourths of an estimated eighty thousand deaf schoolchildren in the United States now go to local schools with hearing children, and the specialized schools for deaf children they would have attended are closing or serving new populations, such as multiply handicapped children.*

The label "mainstreaming" embraces so wide a range of educational arrangements that, as with the label "total communication," people with divergent beliefs about deaf education can be gulled into endorsing it. In some urban schools, there are classes of deaf children, grouped by grade, without any contact with hearing children, or just the odd shared class in art or sports. Often these "self-contained" classes are only nominally within a public school—they are located in temporary trailers, separate buildings, remote corners of buildings, or in basements. In less densely populated areas, on the other hand, the deaf child may have no one with whom he can communicate; he is left to "make do" in the midst of a hearing class and in the occasional coaching session with a few deaf children of various ages and abilities. Most deaf children are in schools where there are only one or two other deaf children.

An ASL interpreter may be provided for the mainstreamed deaf child in some classes; but many of these interpreters are insufficiently skilled to cover the range of academic subjects required, and very few are board certified. Many communities can neither recruit nor afford qualified interpreters. Few schools in America would appoint a nurse, a counselor, or an audiologist without certification; standards are much lower when it comes to finding an ASL interpreter. Then, too, the child who depends on an interpreter relates very little, if at all, to the teacher. Moreover, he must keep his eyes glued on the interpreter for long stretches while classroom events suit his hearing classmates: maps are unfurled, slides are projected, tables of numbers are displayed, and all the while the teacher talks, the interpreter interprets, and the deaf child must never look away from the interpreter.

Immersed in a hearing, English-speaking environment, the deaf child frequently drowns in the mainstream.

"I have experienced both, mainstream and deaf school," eighth-grader Jesse Thomas testified to the National Council on Disabilities. He first explained, "I'm not disabled, just deaf," and then gave his reasons for opposing mainstreaming: "Learning through an interpreter is very hard; it's bad socially in the mainstream; you are always outnumbered; you don't feel like it's your school; you never know deaf adults; you don't belong; you don't feel comfortable as a deaf person." That's the gist of surveys of deaf college students who have attended mainstream high school or elementary school programs. Reports one study: "Almost every informant described their social life in terms of loneliness, rejection, and social isolation." In order to cope as best he can in a mainstream class, the deaf child hides his hearing aid, pretends he understands lessons when he does not, copies other pupils' work, rarely asks questions in class or volunteers to answer them, speaks as little as possible to hearing students, or even to other deaf students. Writes one child trying to pass in the mainstream: "I hate it if people know I am deaf."

Mainstreaming is a part of a wider movement in the United States that has removed large numbers of mentally and physically handicapped children and adults from custodial institutions. "Deinstitutionalization," as the movement was called, was accompanied by the promise of more normal life-styles for all and services in the community for those who needed them. There is a consensus that, overall, the promise was not fulfilled, not least perhaps because one motive for the change in policy was cost containment: It is less expensive to foist a deaf child on the local school, even with an allocation for special services, such as an itinerant special teacher or a resource room, than it is to provide education in a residential setting.

Deaf children were thus swept up in the movement to mainstream indiscriminately nearly all previously "institutionalized" children. The old custodial institutions were not only costly; they embraced many more mentally and physically handicapped children than needed to be there, and they fostered dependency and restricted freedom with no countervailing gain. This was not true of the residential schools for deaf children, however. Yes, the audist staffs of these "sidestream" schools frequently infantilized their charges, could not communicate with them, and were ineffective as teachers. Nonetheless, the residential school offered something of immense value: language—the ability to communicate with other human beings. For most deaf children, who came from hearing, languageless homes, this was a boon indeed, as was the community and the culture they found in the residential school. Although manual language was not used in class—although, indeed, it was often forbidden—still the school was a signing community, where the deaf student could get help after class with coursework, discuss local, national, and international events, obtain counseling, participate in student activities, develop friendships with other deaf students, emulate older students and deaf staff, and acquire self-respect as a deaf person.*

None of these advantages is available to the deaf child in an ordinary public school, where ASL, deaf adults, and a deaf community are absent. Moreover, in this setting the deaf child is hampered in learning the "indirect messages" of education: the implied and unintentionally taught beliefs, feelings, attitudes, and social skills. Since only one schoolchild in a thousand is deaf, most school districts have too few deaf children to establish an effective program with properly trained staff, a peer group of reasonable size at each age level, and extracurricular activities. The only plausible alternative to residential schools for deaf children, then, is regional programs, but children in those programs may spend almost as much time in the bus as in class, reducing the time they can devote to extracurricular activities, to homework, and to their families. Moreover, their deaf friends are likely to live out of reach.

Granted that the conditions in the local public school for the deaf child's social and emotional growth are quite poor. Is the child receiving a better education in the "three Rs" there? Not at all. The first report cards on mainstreamed deaf children show no improvement in their blighted English or mathematics attributable to mainstreaming, even though the first to be mainstreamed were the children with the best speech and hearing, and the academic qualifications of their teachers frequently surpass those in the residential schools. Indeed, there is some evidence that when achievement scores are corrected statistically for differences in the makeup of the deaf student bodies in residential and mainstream schools, the deaf child in the mainstream is at an academic disadvantage.*

The deaf children who do best in school, mainstream or residential, are—note it well—the fortunate 10 percent who learned ASL as a native language from their deaf parents, the core of this linguistic minority. These native speakers of ASL outperform their deaf classmates from hearing homes in most subjects, including reading and writing English—an achievement that is all the more remarkable when we reflect that they come from poorer homes, generally a disadvantage, and that the schools they attend, whether mainstream or residential, do not capitalize on their native language skills.* Deaf children arriving at school with a knowledge of ASL are also better adjusted, better socialized, and have more positive attitudes than their counterparts who have been deprived of effective communication.* Similar findings come from other lands. In Israel, deaf children of deaf parents were found more successful than those of hearing parents in reading comprehension, emotional development, self-image, and initiative to communicate; in Greece, they were found superior in expressive and receptive communication and in lip-reading; in Denmark, they communicated more effectively with peers.*

The superior performance of deaf children from deaf homes highlights the changes that most need to be made in the education of deaf children: namely, a return to manual language, deaf teachers, and deaf administrators directing residential schools—successful practices in the last century, when American deaf children studied all their subjects in their most fluent language, ASL. These changes have long been advocated by the deaf community itself. "How could we ever learn to cope as deaf people, without the shared experiences of other deaf people all around us?" asks a California deaf leader, assailing mainstreaming. "It guarantees the emergence of a deaf adult with serious doubts about himself. How can a child, probably with a reading problem and almost certainly intimidated by the sometimes hostile and generally distractive atmosphere of a mainstreamed classroom, learn comfortably through an interpreter (possibly one with minimal skills) and without direct contact with the teacher? It's puzzling to me that the parent will permit this." But parents are badly advised by the experts, who, in any event, ride roughshod over their wishes.

A further obstacle to revitalizing and expanding the residential schools and other specialized programs for deaf children is placed in the way by spokesmen for people with disabilities. Now that advocates for people with disabilities have gained their hard-won integration of mentally and physically handicapped children in the public schools, they fear that segregated schooling of deaf children, who belong to a language minority, would set a precedent for backsliding on mainstreaming of disabled children. That is why such advocates mounted a major campaign in 1990 to close the American School for the Deaf in Hartford, Connecticut. Deaf leaders from around the country, outraged at this assault on America's oldest residential school, which had spawned so many others, beat back the attack. Such discord between leaders of the deaf community and of the disability rights movement arises only because neither group has control of its destiny and must persuade a third group, the nondeaf, nondisabled experts, whose incomprehension each fears.

Advocates for children with disabilities are joined in their insistence on mainstreaming for all by those in the audist establishment who believe that education without assimilation is a failure and that assimilation can be achieved by brute force.* This is the counsel many hearing parents want to receive, as they prefer, understandably, to have their child live at home. According to the Commission on the Education of the Deaf, the intent of the law to have all handicapped children placed in the "least restrictive environment" was misinterpreted to mean mainstreaming in the local school for nearly all deaf children—precisely the most restrictive environment for those children, given the communicative and social barriers in the local school. The U.S. Supreme Court has ruled that when Congress passed the Education for All Handicapped Children Act in 1975, it recognized that "regular classrooms simply would not be a suitable setting for the education of many handicapped children" and it provided for alternative placements. The Code of Federal Regulations implementing the act also requires that educational placement be "appropriate," that potential harmful effects on the child must be considered, and that a child can be removed from "regular" classes when education cannot be achieved satisfactorily. One judge ruled in 1988 that "mainstreaming that interferes with the acquisition of fundamental language skills is foolishness mistaken for wisdom." But the federal and state departments of education and local school boards, frequently encouraged by the audist establishment, have largely ignored provisions of the act, of federal regulations, and of court rulings when full compliance favors placing a deaf child in a specialized program with other deaf children.

Like many mothers of bright ASL-using children, Jesse Thomas's mother appealed the local school board's insistence on mainstreaming Jesse; she agreed with her son's wish to go to the state residential school for deaf children. (Because she is hearing and could not provide a model of manual language for her son, Mrs. Thomas had made a point of placing Jesse in the company of deaf children and adults since his infancy.) The local experts claimed to know Jesse's best interests better than his mother did, however, and she lost her appeal. Teachers and administrators have their ways of keeping parents at bay, despite the law requiring that the parents participate in deciding the Individualized Educational Plan for their child. These ways include withholding information, presenting major issues as minor ones, limiting the topics on which parents may have a say, authoritatively identifying the source of problems as the child and not the school, and choosing the time, place, manner, and language in which the discussion is conducted. Although the professional's judgment may be based on class differences, on stereotypes, on invalid test results, or on an inability to communicate with the child, many parents are intimidated, the more so if they belong to an ethnic minority. Both parties believe that the parents need the professional more than the converse.

The experts present advice, which is really a demand for confirmation of their judgment; the parent is not invited to form a plan collaboratively but asked to accede to the audist's plan. Moreover, parents are encouraged to be compliant by their fear that protest will have harmful repercussions for their child. Determined and resourceful parents can sometimes outwit the establishment, however. Mrs. Thomas had heard of a county that sent its deaf children exclusively to oral programs. Informed that those programs would not accept pupils who used ASL, the Thomases moved to that very county. As they had hoped, the program administrators would not consider Jesse for admission and saw no alternative but to send him to the state residential school for deaf children.

When Susan Dutton, who is deaf, moved with her deaf son, Mark, to Harveys Lake, Pennsylvania, the boy was placed in a local school, in a special-needs class with children ranging in age from eight to eighteen. Mark was fluent in ASL, but neither the teacher nor the other students could sign. There was an "interpreter/aide" present, who had completed one class in sign language. When the school convened a meeting to formulate Mark's Individualized Educational Plan, Mrs. Dutton was not provided with an interpreter and was told that "despite my wishes, despite my right as a parent to decide what is best for my son, Mark would have to remain in the local school and be mainstreamed into fourth grade classes with hearing students two years younger than he." Since deaf peers, culture, and role models were utterly lacking in the mainstream and there was little effective communication, Mrs. Dutton refused to sign the IEP. A hearing was convened before the school assistant superintendent: "There was no interpreter present. There was no discussion. The assistant superintendent came into this meeting having already made his decision, and he communicated it to me via note writing. It was, of course, in support of mainstreaming." Mrs. Dutton consulted a lawyer, and nine nights of hearings ensued before a hearing officer employed by the Pennsylvania State Department of Education. The school district's lawyer argued that the mainstream was the least restrictive environment for Mark Dutton. Susan and Mark's lawyer and several scholars contended that the local school was the most restrictive environment for Mark's education since he could not understand his teachers and peers nor they him, and since the school could not nurture his linguistic and cultural development as a deaf person. The school district prevailed, but the Duttons appealed the hearing officer's decision, and it was overturned by a panel of two lawyers and an educator who affirmed that "communication is the essence of education" and that the hearing officer had misinterpreted the law. Susan and Mark were relieved to see their year-long struggle and expense finally end in success—until they learned that the school district had filed an appeal which as of this writing is before a federal court.

Confronted with the mainstreaming tragedy in Britain, members of the British National Union of the Deaf formally charged their government with a violation of the United Nations Convention on the Prevention and Punishment of the Crime of Genocide. That treaty prohibits inflicting mental harm on the children of an ethnic group, and it prohibits forcibly transferring them to another group. According to this deaf organization, mainstreaming will gravely injure "not only deaf children but deaf children's rightful language and culture." Their published *Charter of the Rights of the Deaf* asserts that "deaf schools are being effectively forced to close and therefore children of one ethnic/linguistic minority group, that is, deaf people, are being forcibly transferred to another group, that is, hearing people," in violation of the U.N. convention.

For nearly a century, parents of deaf children were told to place them in specialized programs that would teach them to speak and lip-read; at home, they were to drill their child in speech and never let him make a sign. Then, fifteen years ago, most parents were told that individual signs could be used at the same time as speech. Some were told that English expressed on the hands through real and invented signs held out the greatest hope for their child's mastery of English. Ten years ago, parents were told to place their deaf child in the local hearing school. Now they are increasingly told that an ear operation combined with oral drills and no sign is his best hope. If the local school cannot provide sufficient training in speech and hearing, they may need to enroll their child in specialized programs that teach him to speak and lip-read; at home, they are to drill their child in speech and never let him make a sign. So the advice comes full circle. The audists keep changing the rules because they have the power to do so as each version of the audist regime becomes a blatant failure. Moreover, the failure of a stage of forced assimilation, far from undermining the establishment and its normalizing principles, leads to an expansion of its regime. So, too, the prison system is offered as the remedy for its own ills and the failures of applied social science justify more research. The fundamental enterprise is never placed in question; instead, bio-power establishes as the question, how best to implement the fixed, accepted goals.

The deaf community, however, has held unswervingly to a single truth: deaf identity, hence deaf language and culture. "Methods are not acquired naturally like languages," writes deaf linguist MJ Bienvenu, "they are invented by individuals for specific purposes."

Deaf People Without a Deaf Community

Burundi provides an object lesson in what happens to deaf people when they are isolated in the mainstream, when they fail to gather together in schools, clubs, homes, and associations and to mutually instruct one another using their language. There are five types of instruction, according to the source of the instructive messages, that shape the child into an informed adult. There are the things we teach ourselves, those we learn from peers, parents, and community, and those we learn in school. Many children in the world do not receive the last kind of instruction, formal instruction, either because they simply do not have physical access to it or because—it amounts to the same thing—they do not have linguistic access to it since that instruction is conducted in a language they do not understand. A child without formal instruction frequently grows up to become an economically oppressed adult, but not one who is perceived as mentally retarded. Such a child still receives informal instruction from his friends, his parents and relatives, and his neighbors. With talent and luck, the child may become a leader in his community, hearing or deaf.

Consider, however, the plight of a deaf child of hearing parents who, like most, is alone in a "mainstream"—hearing—setting. Besides lacking access to formal instruction, that child lacks the opportunity to communicate with peers, and he cannot communicate with his parents or neighbors. That child grows into adulthood with self-instruction as his or her only resource. Such a person must inevitably be seen as mentally deficient and is assigned social roles accordingly.

In 1986, I traveled to Burundi to lay the groundwork for the formal education of deaf children in that country. En route, I visited schools for deaf children in Kenya, and there I met Assumpta Naniwe, a psychologist and the mother of a deaf boy, who had stopped in Nairobi on her way to her native Burundi; we agreed to join forces. We arrived in Bujumbura, the capital of Burundi, during the rainy season, so the view from my hotel, the Source of the Nile, was one of lush tropical vegetation reaching down to the banks of Lake Tanganyika. In order to meet deaf people, we sought out a Protestant mission in the outskirts of the city that provided some classes for deaf children. A class was in progress when we arrived, and, to my astonishment, the teacher was instructing the children using signs from American Sign Language accompanying his spoken French.

The teacher explained to me in French that he and a colleague had spent three months studying deaf education in Nigeria, under Dr. Andrew Foster. I had heard of Foster, the first African-American graduate of Gallaudet University in Washington, and of his years of labor in Africa establishing small church-run classes for deaf children. It was Foster, deaf himself, who had taught the Burundi teachers a little ASL, at least some vocabulary, so that they could teach signs to the deaf children and thus communicate with them. The one-room chapel that served as a school for four classes could accommodate only two classes at a time (a burlap curtain was hung down the middle), so each of them met for half a day. The youngest children, seven to eight, studied math and written French, I was told, although the government had criticized the school for not first teaching written Kirundi, the national language, as in the regular schools. In later grades, natural and physical sciences were added, and in the last, history and geography.

I had brought a videocamera and recorded a geography class; the children knew the locations and names of neighboring states and finger-spelled them rapidly. I asked to meet a child who was clearly following every move and whose hand was often raised first; this was ten-year-old Claudine Umuvyeyi, from a family with five children—two teenage brothers, an older sister, and a younger brother—four of them deaf.

Claudine and I conversed using signs from ASL in French word order, as did her teachers. I asked Claudine if we could visit her family and film their signing; she offered to take us there directly, and we set out on foot. At Claudine's home, Assumpta explained to Mme Umuvyeyi, in Kirundi, the reason for our visit. Claudine's mother looked to be in her forties. Like many Burundians of Tutsi origin, she was rather tall and thin. Her skin was quite dark and contrasted with the brightly colored floral print of her dress. She seemed to me shy and deferential and looked away from me much of the time, as did many of the women I met in Burundi. Mme

Umuvyeyi told us that her fifth child was losing his hearing, yet he, like the other children when their deafness was discovered, had not been seriously ill. She had noticed with her first child that by the age of two, she still was not speaking as other children would, so she tested her daughter's hearing with various kinds of noises and came to the sad and unexpected conclusion (her husband and all relatives were hearing) that her child was deaf. Her second child spoke fluently by age two but shortly thereafter stopped responding to sound, and gradually his speech disappeared. The mother was despairing.

In time, however, and especially with the advent of two more deaf children, a manual system of communication grew up in the home. Mme Umuvyeyi could understand all that her children said to her in this language—their complaints, their requests, their reports—and they understood all she said to them. So in the end she had adjusted to the situation, although the father, who had never learned the "home sign," never did adjust.

At my request, Mme Umuvyeyi told her daughter to go and see if the beans she had put up to cook were tender. Claudine left immediately and returned a moment later, her hands flying. "They're not ready yet," her mother translated. I had brought a set of drawings with me (a cat on a chair, a dog jumping through a hoop), and I asked one of the teenage brothers to describe my pictures to the other in their home sign language, which he did readily. With Claudine interpreting from ASL to home sign, I asked the brothers about their friends. They were mostly deaf people from "around." Perhaps a dozen. The friends had picked up the family sign language, though of course they were not as fluent as their hosts. I urged the deaf brothers to consider forming a deaf club, and I described what one was like in America.

The brothers had a question to put to me (through Claudine): What trades did deaf people practice in America? I listed a few, then I added that some deaf people went to university and into professions; their eyes were filled with wonder. They themselves worked as assistants to a tailor in the city. "Who exploits them," added the father, who had meanwhile returned home from his job as a clerk in a government office. I complimented him on his family: two employed sons, his youngest daughter in school, his oldest, Christine, employed at a shelter for the handicapped. "Five deaf children," he said. "Some days I really wonder: Why me?" He paused. "What is to become of them? Will Christine be able to marry? Claudine should go on in school, but there are no more classes." I had to acknowledge that it might be some years before she could continue in an official government school for deaf children.

Burundians take justifiable pride in their national university. I sought out the rector, to whom I made the following proposal. In order for formal education of deaf children to begin in Burundi, teachers would have to be trained. The Faculty of Psychology and Sciences of Education already offered many of the necessary courses. If the rector would designate a graduate of the faculty and arrange for the candidate's transportation to Boston, Northeastern University would provide a fellowship to train that person in methods of educating deaf children. The fellow could then return to the faculty to provide the additional courses needed by teachers of the deaf. The rector agreed.

The next day I met with various government officials, who endorsed our undertaking, and before long the university had chosen a candidate for me to interview: a tall, engaging high school principal of twenty-seven, Adolphe Sururu, who was highly recommended by the dean of the Faculty of Psychology, from which he had graduated with distinction. I soon came to know the intelligence and commitment of this fine young man, and we filled out his application to Northeastern University together. We were launched on a great adventure, one that could well enhance the lives of hearing and deaf people in our two countries and beyond.

At the start of this enterprise, we were anxious to know what the "soil" was like in which deaf education in Burundi would take root. Using the incidence of childhood deafness in Kenya as a guide, we estimated that there were some four thousand deaf children of school age in the Burundi population. Since most families are dispersed over the countryside, where they eke out a subsistence by tilling their small plots of land, and since most travel is done on foot, we doubted that we would find a deaf community with a manual language in widespread use. Lacking that resource, it was hard to see how deaf children of hearing parents could obtain much instruction.

My Burundian colleague Assumpta Naniwe set out to meet some of these children and their parents and neighbors; not surprisingly, she found that each family had developed its own idiosyncratic gestures and "home sign"; except for those that had a child at one of the two church-sponsored schools, the families seemed to have no sign language in common, so Assumpta interviewed the parents at length in Kirundi, while unobtrusively recording the conversation on tape.

In this society virtually without communication for many deaf people, Assumpta's twelve interviews with parents of deaf children reveal wildly inaccurate conceptions of deaf people and of their possible social roles. As a common result of those misconceptions, both parent and child suffer greatly and behave badly. Two representative interviews (translated and abridged) illustrate the debasement of the deaf child in the absence of manual language and the profoundly enabling consequences of introducing it. The first interview took place in the thatched hut of a woman with a deaf daughter whom we will call Jeanne, but who is called Deafie by her parents and neighbors. Jeanne was in her early thirties at the time of the recording and had numerous hearing brothers and sisters.

"When you see a deaf person walking down the street," Jeanne's mother told Assumpta, "you think he is perfectly normal, someone like everyone else, but in fact he has no intelligence whatever. You have to feed him, supply all his wants, dress him; in fact, you have to do everything for him." Assumpta asked her if she really meant to say that deaf people have *no* intelligence. "Alas, yes," she replied. "Do you think I consider my deaf daughter to be like all my other children? A child whom you can't rely on, who relies on other people for everything? Now she is in her thirties, and the other women her age have three or four or even five children, and she—what is she? She's always trailing around behind me, she never got married, she can never get married. But you know, it's not that she doesn't want to. I've done everything on earth to stop her running after men." Here the mother laughed out of embarrassment. Assumpta learned later from a relative that the mother had obliged her daughter, against her will, to have three abortions. "You know, men only think about having a good time [with her]; none of them considered marrying her. You understand, Deafie doesn't know what it means to have children out of wedlock, so it's I who must think of these things for her."

"Why not explain the birds and the bees to her?" Assumpta asked.

"How am I supposed to talk to someone who doesn't speak?" the mother replied. "Tell me how I'm supposed to explain all that to someone who seems to live in another world? It's hard enough as it is with someone normal, those who have a language as we do, to whom you can say, this is not good, this is very bad, this is good, and who manage anyway to get into trouble. So when it comes to a creature without ears, without intelligence . . .

"I gave her little tasks," Jeanne's mother continued, "like cooking, sweeping, getting water from the well. You could never rely on her, but since I had other children I could ask them to keep an eye on her. After her younger sisters got married, she realized that she would never leave our home. She explains in her own particular gestures that everyone has found a husband, has had children, but she, she will always remain at home. All I have is problems with her; bringing up a child who can never turn out good, who can never fit in—that's truly a waste of time."

Assumpta asked why she thought her daughter didn't "fit in." "Who can befriend a deaf woman?" the mother replied. "People see her, take pity on her, and that's it. She's her mother's baby, and as long as I live I will take care of her, and when I'm no longer around, the family will look after her, but I'm quite concerned about her future."

The second interview is with the mother of a boy named Vincent, the oldest child among four; he is thirteen and attends the third grade of a church-related school for deaf children. His situation is quite different from Jeanne's, although he, too, is the only deaf person in his family. It is striking, for example, that his mother begins the interview by talking about competence rather than incompetence.

"I myself feel that every deaf person should have some kind of work he can do, a profession, and I'm sure that even if he is deaf he can do his work well. For example, that child there," she said, pointing to her deaf son, "took it in his head once to sell peanuts, and I let him do it because once he gets an idea in his head, Vincent doesn't let anyone tell him otherwise. I was afraid because I thought he'd never succeed in doing it. But he stuck to it, and he makes a lot of money with it. If other people understood that he can do as they do, if people would give him work, Vincent could do all right in life."

Assumpta asked who stood in the way of Vincent's doing as hearing people do. "Everyone," his mother answered, "starting with me. It's not because I don't love him; it's because I'm afraid of what can happen to him. Look, when you can't communicate with him, it's hard to know exactly what you're supposed to do. When Vincent wants to sell things, I'm afraid. I'm worried that he won't know how to count his money, that some robbers will come along and cheat him of everything he's got or attack him and steal all his money. There are lots of things that can eat away at the heart of a mother who knows her child's problems. Whereas other people, they simply underestimate him, they take him for an idiot. Even though he's a good worker, as I've told you, I'm sure that when the day comes for him to find a job as a mason, no one will bother with him because everyone thinks he is incompetent."

"Even though you tell me that he has a nice little peanut business?" Assumpta countered. On the tape, you can hear Vincent's mother laugh heartily. "Well, this deaf little fellow knows his business well and he knows what he wants. For, as I have already told you, when he decides to do something he does it, or if he can't, he has fits of anger that everyone in the family dreads. Actually, he is known in these parts as a brawler, and I think no one dares touch him for fear of being flattened. I think that's why his little business is working out okay. Everyone's afraid of him."

"So you don't think people will cheat him, after all?" Assumpta asked. "Cheat him! Don't worry about it," Vincent's mother replied. "Ever since he started school, he can count. He knows the difference between a hundred-franc note and a thousand-franc note. He's quite familiar with the value of money. It was from that moment that he began to do business. It's three years now that he has been going to school, and I have the impression that he's learned a lot. Don't ask me what, because I can't read, I don't understand a word of all that they write, but I notice that he has changed his ways a lot. He's learned to read, to count, to speak with gestures. I don't understand those gestures, but when he's with his schoolmates, they communicate with their eyes, their arms, their mouths. It's quite intriguing, but no one else understands them. When you come down to it, that's the only situation in which I see Vincent really come alive—he makes fun, tells stories, you can hear him laugh, whereas with the rest of us, and his sisters and brothers, all you hear are slaps echoing."

Clearly, Vincent will have a better life than the deaf woman "Deafie" from the generation before him. Vincent has found people with whom he can communicate; Vincent's manual language is allowing him to learn such basics as buying and selling with money.

Burundi is a country where, because of geography and history, most deaf people apparently send very few messages and receive even fewer. It is also a country where most deaf people are called not by their names but rather by a common designation, *nyamuragi*— "deafie," or, closer, "dumbo"; "deaf" in Kirundi is related to the word for "mentally retarded."

The interviews with the parents of deaf children make clear that when hearing people cannot communicate with deaf people, they conclude that deaf people are mentally retarded, and they assign deaf people social roles and even perceived traits consistent with that belief. Then the epithet that deaf people bear, *nyamuragi*, the modest social roles they are allowed, the demeaning traits they are perceived to have, all reinforce the belief in their mental inferiority. Naturally, this society has not had arrangements for schooling its deaf children.

The parents of deaf children in Burundi for the most part see their own children as, fundamentally, stupid. Speaking of her teenage daughter, Imelda's mother explained that "a deaf child doesn't know anything; you have to attend to her all the time." The mother of a sixteen-year-old deaf boy, Pierre, said, "You know deaf people are not intelligent, they always do as they like, and they don't understand the consequences of their actions." Spès's mother says of the day she realized her daughter was deaf: "It was the saddest day of my life. In vain people told me a child's a child, accept her as God gave her to you—I couldn't do it. I was thinking of her future and wondering how she could survive, deaf as she was." She had heard of schools for deaf children, "but I do wonder what one could possibly teach them. Because they don't have enough intelligence." Assumpta asked the mother of a deaf boy to imagine for a moment a society made up only of deaf people. She replied: "Deaf people together? Are you serious? What language could they speak? They couldn't live together; their intelligence is very limited."

Most of the parents have established some rudimentary communication with their deaf children, but it is so limited that they cannot gauge their intelligence, not to say instruct them as they do their hearing children. And though in some cases they see their deaf child communicate fluently in sign with other deaf children, still they do not see the possibility of taking that route themselves. Vincent's mother, for example, said that the only situation in which he comes alive is with his signing schoolmates, yet she apparently does not entertain the possibility of learning the signs herself. This is not the result of bad professional advice or of wrongful practices in the schools. Imelda has begun to go to the mission school. Now things are better, her mother reports, because they are teaching her some signs. "I don't know them, but ever since she goes to the school, her friends come to see her—and you've got to see them together! They make all these gestures, they laugh like we do—it's quite a show! They understand each other like you and me."

Pierre also goes to school now. "When he is with his schoolmates, he becomes a different child," his father reports. "They have their signs that they learn at school; sometimes he teaches me these signs, but I forget them quickly. His brothers and sisters, however, know signs a bit. They talk to each other and tell each other things. Sometimes I hear them laughing and when I go to see what's happening, I find it's Deafie who makes them laugh." Didier, fourteen, has three brothers and sisters, to whom he has taught some signs. His father recounts: "Now things are much better. They teach signs at the school; for example, to say 'father' [he shows the sign], to say 'tree' [he shows the sign], and for each thing there's a sign. It's really quite interesting. As he's an alert boy who gets along well with everyone, he comes home and shows us everything that he has learned. Now his brothers and sisters know all these signs, and for everyday communication, there's no longer any problem."

Here is how Jeanne's mother describes communication with her daughter. "Ever since we have lived together, we understand each other with certain gestures. For example, to say that her sisters are married [she makes a gesture]; to say that they have children [she portrays a mother breast-feeding her child]. She uses little gestures with me that I understand, that her sisters and brothers understand. For example, her father has a beard, so to speak about him she makes a gesture that refers to the beard. So in this way, even if you have trouble saying what you mean, you can sometimes guess what she means. We don't have conversations, because that's impossible with a deaf person, but when I want her to go fetch water, I can take the jug that she always uses, show it to her, and point my finger in the direction of the well, and she knows that I need some water. She may go or she may refuse to go, depending on her mood."

Thus the heartbroken parents find some solace in their children's signed conversations with deaf friends and in their own ability to direct their children with gestures. Yet they do not see that deaf people have presented them with the key to their child's future success—namely, signed language; in other words, an affirmation of deafness rather than its rejection.

If Burundi is backward in raising deaf children, then so is the United States, for it is hard to see how most American mothers and fathers do better in these matters. American parents, misled by the experts, make little or no use of the rich opportunities provided by America's large deaf community, its long heritage and its rich language. They see no lesson implicit in the fluent manual communication of deaf adults. They commonly allow their child to go without substantial communication for the first six years of life. Then they tolerate or encourage an educational plan that isolates their deaf child further. In this way America's deaf children are commonly deprived of parental, community, and, finally, formal instruction through a breakdown of communication.

In the weeks after my visit to Burundi, the eager deaf pupil I had first met and whose family I had visited, Claudine Umuvyeyi, was frequently on my mind. Claudine and children like her, it seemed to me, were not only part of the problem I had undertaken to alleviate; they must be part of the solution. Deaf adults and their manual language must be at the service of the schools for deaf children in Burundi, yet how could this be achieved when there have been no schools to educate those deaf adults? How could deaf education lift itself by its own bootstraps? I was moved to write a letter to Claudine's mother, asking her to allow her daughter to come to America for several years so she could join the deaf community here, continue her education, and then become the first deaf teacher of deaf people in Burundi.

"It is difficult, I know, to imagine a deaf adult as a teacher in Burundi," I wrote to Claudine's mother. "But that is just what I ask you to imagine, for there can be no successful education of deaf people in Burundi without Claudine and deaf people like her as teachers. There is abundant evidence in America that hearing people as a group cannot single-handedly, without the involvement of deaf people, educate deaf children successfully."

How can I decry the conduct of deaf education in America and then ask that Claudine come here to be educated? For one thing, the education that I criticize is certainly better than none at all. Moreover, it will provide Claudine with credentials as well as knowledge and skills that she will need to get a professional job in her country. And although deaf education has for decades largely failed to educate deaf children, it has at least brought deaf people together so that they could learn from one another—about school, culture, sports, and love, about life. True, nowadays educators in America willfully ignorant of the language of deaf people have increasingly isolated deaf children from each other and have cast a majority into neighborhood schools where only English is spoken. But I would see to it that Claudine was not placed in such a program. The American deaf community can offer her a fully developed language; richly textured, profound communication; friendship and solidarity; and a new vision of the possible lives for her deaf countrymen. As, in the early nineteenth century, American Sign Language developed from French Sign Language, thanks to Laurent Clerc, so, perhaps, a Burundian Sign Language will develop from ASL. And as, in the last century, deaf education using ASL in residential schools was fundamental to the development of the American deaf community, so might deaf education in Burundi serve a like purpose.

"My reading of the lessons of deaf history in Europe and America," I wrote in my letter to Mme Umuvyeyi, "leads me to believe that deaf people must be given the power of self-determination as only a few decades ago Burundi people affirmed their own self-determination. Hearing people can work alongside deaf colleagues, provided that they learn their language, that they are endlessly vigilant against the disease of paternalism, and that they can persuade their deaf colleagues to hold them to account.

"What many Americans, hearing and deaf, yearn for but have not been able to achieve is a relationship of equals in which different is simply different, neither better nor worse. If Burundians achieve this, deaf and hearing adults together, in mutual respect, will conceive and operate the first school for deaf children and teach in its classes. This is how deaf education began more than one hundred and fifty years ago in my country, before it drifted off course: a deaf man from France, Laurent Clerc, came here and opened the first school, in Hartford, with a hearing colleague. Who will be the first Burundian called to this noble mission, the role of Laurent Clerc, Apostle of the Deaf? If you and your husband believe it might be your daughter Claudine, then let us join forces to find a way to enable her to continue her education."

Claudine's parents responded to my letter, saying that they and their daughter wanted very much for her to continue her education; the United Nations agreed to provide funds for her first years in high school in America; and, as I have told, Claudine enrolled at the Model Secondary School of Gallaudet University; she will graduate in 1992.

There is reason to be optimistic about the prospects for deaf children in Burundi, but reason to be pessimistic indeed about their prospects in the United States. In Burundi, Adolphe Sururu, after two years training in the United States during which the deaf community taught him ASL and much more besides, has returned to open the first official school for deaf children, which provides instruction using manual communication. A signing community is coalescing around the school, hearing teachers are learning to communicate manually, and Claudine will soon join their ranks. Moreover, hearing people willing to sacrifice communication do not yet have a stranglehold on deaf education in Burundi, since it is so new.

In the "first world," on the other hand, that stranglehold is a century old and tightening. The breakdown of communication perseveres in Europe and grows worse in America as deaf children are placed in growing numbers in hearing schools. Our educational programs for deaf children continue to graduate poorly educated students in large numbers. And cochlear implant surgery has become a significant menace, as it threatens to delay effective manual communication while offering the child born deaf or deafened early no substantial oral communication in return.

The Parents' Ordeal

I have described briefly the history of the struggle between language minorities that use manual languages and the oral language majorities that surround them. I propose to illustrate how this history of struggle shapes the lives of deaf children and their parents by considering an archetypal family, Mr. and Mrs. Rue, hypothetical hearing parents of a deaf child, Sammy. As each challenge arises, the Rues will make the wrong decision, guided by a witch's brew of emotions, including love, guilt, and fear, and misguided by the experts.

The Rues' ordeal begins the day they discover their son Sam is deaf. Perhaps it happens in the way Thomas and James Spradley describe in their account of life with a deaf child, *Deaf Like Me*. Thomas and his wife, Louise, had been at a clamorous parade with their three-month-old daughter, Lynn: "Only a few seconds had passed," the father wrote, "when it occurred to me that Lynn might be terrified by the pealing dissonance that sent a current of excitement through the crowd. When I saw that she lay awake, quiet, undisturbed, gazing up into the elm tree as if no one were present, I relaxed. Then some instinct made me look closer. She did not flinch or turn; there was not the slightest movement or reaction to suggest that she even heard these sounds that vibrated in the air with such force. . . . I had the strangest feeling in the pit of my stomach, like something dreadful was about to happen and I couldn't stop it. I thought she might be *deaf*."

Since the Rues are typical hearing parents, they react to their discovery with profound emotional shock. As they know nothing of deaf people and the deaf community, their minds are prey to the worst fears—their child will never have a happy, healthy life. At first, disbelief spares them mercifully from fully confronting this needless fear; but then a series of visits to "experts"—the pediatrician, the otologist, the audiologist—confirms Sammy's profound hearing loss. There is no room for disbelief, but the experts offer the Rues the next best thing—denial. Sammy can be made normal again with enough effort, time, and expense. He will learn to lip-read, to hear people with his eyes rather than his ears, and to speak, but this will require extensive training; Sammy will not acquire spoken language automatically, as a hearing child would.

The months pass; Sammy's parents live with frustration, anger, impotence, sorrow, guilt. Unwittingly, they, not their child, have become the problem. They do not realize that there is a deaf community in America with some million members, most of whom view being deaf simply as a way of being, not as a calamity or even, indeed, a disability, and that there are parents of deaf children who treat their arrival as a joy and not a tragedy. Thomas Gallaudet put the choice confronting the Rues in words to this effect: You can welcome the birth of your deaf child as a source of great joy and instruction. At first you wonder at him, sympathize with him, do all you can to make him happy, rejoice to see that the infant seems more and more to appreciate what you do. He is constantly struggling to make his wishes known by various expressions of his face, by the signs and gestures that his own spontaneous feelings lead him to employ. If you have not experienced it, you cannot imagine the joy in witnessing the child's growing originality and skill in doing this, his graphic panto-mime, his evident pleasure when he is understood, his rapid progress in this singular language, the development of his intellect, your plea-sure (and that of the other children) in learning signs from him, in your newfound power to express to him increasingly subtle ideas and desires. . . . Or will the advent of your deaf child be a tragedy? Will you quail before the onus of learning a new language? Will you pretend that there is nothing for you to learn, that you can raise him as you raised your other children?

Unhappily, the Rues take no pleasure in Sammy's developing "pan-tomime." Far from trying to learn it, they see it as pathetic gesturing, and they have been told, moreover, to ignore it, as Sammy will have little incentive to use his voice if he can use his hands. And now the true tragedy begins, for Sammy becomes a virtual "bubble-child"; like those seriously immunodeficient children who must be raised in complete isolation, literally within a glass "bubble," lest they contract a fatal infection, he is surrounded by a barrier—in his case, a communicative barrier. The world goes on around him, but he can rarely anticipate events or understand their significance once they occur. Even more rarely can he shape those events. His parents cannot communicate with him orally, and following the advice of experts, they will not communicate with him manually, so few messages indeed pass between parent and child, and those that do are generally about present concrete objects.

Thomas Spradley describes the struggle simply to tell his daughter not to wait on the corner for the school bus since it was Saturday. Lynn had eaten her breakfast and rushed blithely out the front door as on a weekday. There she stood on the corner for over a half hour, stamping her feet impatiently, waiting for the bus to come. "Shall I go bring her in?" her father asked her mother. "No," she answered. "Let's wait; she may have to learn this by herself." Finally, Lynn came back in and curled up in a chair in front of the television.

At the urging of the professionals she has consulted, Mrs. Rue enrolls Sammy in an oral day school. The director tells her that unless Sammy proves to be mentally retarded, he will learn to speak and lip-read—provided that she never lets him use sign language and that she spends several hours a day practicing speech with her son at home. Mrs. Rue is led around the school, and truly, the deaf children there speak; they answer questions and they read aloud; Mrs. Rue sees with her own eyes that they are not "deaf and dumb."

Alas, parents, scholars, teachers, have been misled in such circumstances since the beginnings of oral education of deaf children. There are three great traps; they concern the pupil, the audience, and the material. Every large school has a few outstanding pupils who can be trotted out for inspection. But how representative is the star deaf pupil? At what age did he lose his hearing? There is a world of difference between instilling a knowledge of oral language in one who is deaf and slowing the deterioration of oral skills in someone who once spoke, perhaps even on arriving at school. Is the pupil only hard of hearing, can he hear speech addressed directly to him in a loud voice? Does the star pupil communicate only with a familiar audience—the teacher, perhaps, or another pupil? It generally happens that deaf pupils come to understand the teacher better than they understand anyone else, and the teacher returns the compliment. Is the material rehearsed? Oral teachers often have a few pupils prepared with common utterances for use with visitors: "Where do you come from?" and the like. Furthermore, if the question or the text is familiar to the visitor, it can easily appear more intelligible to him than it really is. Visitors are often unwitting accomplices to this charade when they ask to hear the Pledge of Allegiance or the Lord's Prayer, or when they follow by eye the pupil's reading from some text.

Knowing none of this, the Rues do not presume to ask how deaf the children are whom they have heard speak, or when they became deaf; nor do they try to engage the pupils in conversation. Sammy soon finds himself in an oral class. What is it like? Here is the description given by one deaf author:

> The first steps were to make me shape my mouth so, place my tongue such and such a way, and then make a sound by studying the movements of my teacher's mouth and by passing my hands over his throat or nose. If the letter F was to be pronounced, I was to place my upper teeth on my lower lip and then to blow at a scrap of paper lying on the back of my hand. If the letter were a V, I had to add a sound. The letters M, B, and P looked so much alike when formed by the lips that I was confused in knowing which of the three letters my teacher was asking me to articulate. The R, Ng, K, etc., were so modestly concealed within the throat, that I thought I should dive into my teacher's mouth and locate them. This entire process or method is both tedious and discouraging. I might also add that it was a bit disgusting when the teacher had partaken of onions. . . . To be fair, I must concede a high motive and perfect honesty of purpose to *some* of the oralists. But insofar as results are concerned, one may as well concede the same [honesty of purpose] to Thomas Torquemada of the infamous Inquisition, or to the witch hunters and burners of heretics. So deep-rooted is the prejudice against the sign language among some classes, that it approaches a form of persecution.

The months, the years, pass, but Sammy makes little progress in speech and lip-reading. To quote the conclusions of an early study by Alfred Binet and Theodore Simon: "The [orally taught] deaf-mute cannot carry on a conversation with a stranger, nor even with his relatives; and for his immediate wants, he can communicate only by a combination of methods, in which the gesture constantly supplements the word." Sammy does not understand anyone except his mother and his teacher, and then only if they address him in a good light, full face, slowly, and on everyday matters. They can scarcely understand him, however, and strangers do not understand him at all. I imagine Mr. Rue protesting in the words of another father of a deaf child, one of the founders of the first school for oral education in America. "Probably there are persons here today," he said at the school's public exercises, "who will go away disappointed. They will be able to understand but a part, perhaps a small part, of what the pupils shall say; and there will be lurking in their inmost thoughts the query whether this institution hasn't undertaken the impossible, and whether a large amount of time, labor and money isn't half-wasted here. But a wooden leg is a pitiful semblance of bone, nerve and muscle. . . . A glass eye is utterly useless for vision. . . . The poorest articulation pays in the increased self-respect and happiness of the pupil."

This is of course a parent's fantasy, though no doubt well-meaning. Sammy's sham speech, if ever he could learn it, would no more make him like hearing people than blackface makes a black person. The father who communicates so fluently with the world around him announces that "the poorest articulation pays in self-respect." The quest for this kind of self-respect will exact a terrible price from Sammy. If he barely can communicate orally and is not allowed to communicate manually, he cannot communicate at all. Can self-denial ever be the way to self-respect?

Not only is Sammy not becoming a hearing person; he is not becoming an educated deaf person either. He cannot grasp messages about history or arithmetic or geography from a few evanescent movements of his teacher's lips, and moreover, those messages are not there in the first place. For oral education of deaf children, in its desperate drive to win the deaf child to the community of English users, drives out all other instruction. As a leading textbook in deaf education puts it: "Because teachers of the deaf have been expected to be teachers of language and speech, even class time designed for academic subjects has often been devoted entirely to speech and language remediation. Since most teachers of the deaf have not been trained in specific academic areas, the tendency to sacrifice content is intensified."

Sammy's parents are told that they must be part of the language and speech remediation, that his achievements will be their own, and his failings theirs as well. Relieved that she can finally do something about her feeling of guilt, Sammy's mother enrolls in a correspondence course on speech training of deaf children and drills her son an hour a day. The work is long and tedious, her son rebellious, and progress difficult to discern. Numerous studies have shown that hearing parents of deaf children tend to be more manipulative, more tense and antagonistic, than deaf parents (or hearing parents of hearing children). The deaf children of hearing parents are, in turn, less compliant, less attentive, and less responsive.

Time passes. Sammy enters his teens, but he cannot read and write; in fact, he never will with any fluency. I have already recounted the sad statistics. Despairing of Sammy's lack of progress, Mrs. Rue goes to see the director of the oral school. Sammy has been "picking up signs" from deaf acquaintances, she reports. So perhaps he would do better in one of the total communication programs, where all means of communication—voice, signs, finger-spelling, gesture—are employed. The director urges her to think carefully: Does she really want to embrace sign language, surrender her son to the world of the deaf, where he will marry a deaf woman and take up manual labor? Mrs. Rue has heard about mainstreaming. Why not enter Sammy in the regular public school, she asks. He could do no worse, he would be among English-speaking children, and a great deal of money would be saved. Absurd, the director replies. If he cannot succeed in a specialized school with highly trained teachers, how is he to manage on the deaf bench in his neighborhood school?

Sammy is living a melancholy adolescence. He cannot use the telephone, but he has no TTY—a teletypewriter for deaf people—for he has no one to call. He cannot be hearing and his society will not let him be deaf, so he falls between both cultures and both languages, English and ASL. In his book on bilingualism, François Grosjean reminds us of the similar predicament of adolescent children of North African parents in contemporary France: born in France, but often speaking only marginal French, they are rejected by French society, they are poorly educated, and they are destined for lives of manual labor. Too Frenchified, however, to be truly North African, they are rejected by Arab society as well. So, too, the second generation of Turkish laborers in Germany, euphemistically called *Gästarbeiter* (guest workers), relate that they are losing their own identity while unable to take on a German identity because of linguistic and social barriers.

Nearly fifteen years have passed since the Rues' traumatic discovery that Sammy is deaf, and yet they have never met a deaf adult. At last they meet a deaf couple, who, let us say, have a deaf daughter, Lucy, Sammy's age. Lucy is fortunate to have deaf parents who, although less educated and less prosperous than the Rues, have passed on their manual language to their daughter and raised her much as any parents would raise their child, with love, discipline, instruction—in short, with communication, using ASL. As I have told, Lucy's prospects in education and personal development are much better than Sammy's because of this.

If Mrs. Rue is typical, however, her encounter with the deaf couple merely confirms her prior beliefs. They were unable to communicate with her, she reflects, for ASL is not the language of society at large. And, as she had been warned, ASL appeared a highly emotional language of grunts, grimaces, and gestures, not a true language at all.

The Rues do not see what an opportunity has been presented to them by their meeting with the deaf couple. They were disquieted by their new acquaintances' signing, but even more disturbed by the fact that they *were* a couple. Although deaf, they had married and had given birth to a deaf child. How selfish that was, to people the earth with deaf children! Thanks to his oral education, Sammy at least would marry a hearing woman, who could help him through life and give him a hearing child.

The Rues are quite mistaken, however. In the first place, 90 percent of deaf children have hearing parents. That is Sammy's crucial problem: He has to learn to be culturally deaf from other people—and that despite his parents. In the second place, 90 percent of children born to deaf parents are hearing, and many of these will leave the deaf community as adults. Third, Sammy will in all likelihood marry a deaf woman in any event; 90 percent of deaf unions involve two deaf spouses, no matter the type of schooling they have received. The reasons for deaf intermarriage are not hard to find: facile communication, shared experience, the friends of the one more readily become the friends of the other. Deaf people know, too, that for these reasons, marriages with two deaf partners are less subject to divorce. And as I have told, marriage within the culture is valued positively by the culture.

Suppose Sammy and Lucy married and had a deaf child. Is there anything to regret? Deafness does not entail a crime, disgrace, physical suffering. Educated deaf people, like their hearing counterparts, manage their affairs judiciously, raise their children well, become useful and respectable members of the community.

When he is old enough, Sammy drops out of high school and takes a job in a machine shop. Mrs. Rue has never expected anything else: only two deaf children in a hundred go to college, and for many decades most attended one of only two schools: Gallaudet University in Washington, D.C., and the National Technical Institute for the Deaf in Rochester, New York. Nowadays an additional dozen schools have sizable programs for deaf students. Hundreds of other colleges in the United States have been unwilling, for the most part, to hire or train interpreters so that deaf students can participate in classes taught in English.

One evening, Sammy comes home from work with a hearing man who knows ASL, and he explains to his mother through the interpreter that he has been offered a transfer to his company's plant in a large city where there is a sizable deaf community. Mrs. Rue wants to protest, but the shock of pleading with her son through an interpreter reminds her of the gulf that separates them, that has always separated them, reminds her that this has never really been his home. Soon Sammy moves away.

If only the Rues had been encouraged to place communication above prejudice, to embrace manual language, recognizing that oral language could not reach their child. If only they had made their home bilingual, accepting that their son was a member of a language minority. If only they had come to know some members of the deaf community, studied their language, observed how they conducted their lives, listened to their counsel and not to that of the audists. If only they had seen to it that their son was taught in his most fluent language. If only they had tried, as Sammy grew into the deaf community, to grow with him. Jesse Thomas's mother did much of this and recounts: "My life has proven richer and more rewarding, my relationship to my son perhaps even closer, than if Jesse had been born hearing."

Most of us are not aware of the cultural premises that guide our lives; we are ethnocentric and naturally so, for social life would be impossible if every action required our reflection. We have an unconscious mental model of our culture that makes most of our choices for us, leaving us free to grapple with the ones that remain. Our ideas about wealth, family, sexuality, and disability, for example, all seem more or less given and appropriate. We know abstractly and vaguely that other people live in other ways; but we do not know the premises beneath those differences; we do not see the linkages among the differences; and we cannot make the empathic leap and see the world from another vantage point. Not seeing that there is a range of choices of how to live, we do not realize we have made such choices; and since we do not realize we have made choices, in some sense we have not, since to choose is to perform an act of conscious volition. The fundamental choices have been made for us—by our parents and, even more, by history.

In these circumstances, the study of another culture can be a revelation; it can liberate and empower us by helping us to imagine other premises and other ways of life. Liberated by cultural perspective, we are more able to fashion our own lives and to "connect" with the lives of others. These are some of the rewards that the good fortune of having a deaf son placed within the reach of the Rues but that audism held beyond their grasp.

Many Americans can recall their initial shock when they realized fully for the first time that other people were conducting their lives in an entirely different language. Perhaps that shock reflects a kind of egocentrism that it is in our mutual interest to overcome; for the growth of social consciousness, like that of the child, is largely a series of triumphs over egocentrism. As I am not less but more when I recognize the heliocentric movement of the planets and the biological continuity of the species, so I am not less but more when I recognize that there are other languages, manual and oral, on a par with my own. That recognition opens the way to collaboration with people who speak another language and can teach it to me. When Thomas Gallaudet went to France to learn how to educate deaf children, he turned to Laurent Clerc, the leading deaf professor at the Paris school, and said, "Teach me." They came to America together. "We spent the voyage," Clerc later wrote, "in useful employment. I taught Mr. Gallaudet the method of signs, and he taught me the English language." All Mr. and Mrs. Rue's misfortunes can be traced to one completely understandable error: they trusted those whom society had taught them to trust, the audist establishment; therefore, they saw deaf people as defective, closed their minds to them, did not seek their counsel. Victor Hugo put the moral well: "What matters deafness of the ear," he wrote, "when the mind hears. The true deafness, the incurable deafness, is deafness of the mind."

PART SIX

Bilingual Education and Deaf Power

For Progress, a Return to Deaf-Centered Education

Early in the last century, American deaf children studied all their subjects in their most fluent language, ASL. As the first generation of pupils completed their primary education, the need arose for high school classes so they could continue that education. Several schools established such programs, which included courses in English, history, geography, astronomy, mathematics, and foreign languages. Many deaf students completing the high school classes, in turn, sought to continue their education and to enter the professions, especially the profession of teaching deaf children. Thus the need arose for a college that used their primary language, ASL, as well as their secondary language, English, and Gallaudet College was born in 1864. Its lower division was a high school. Candidates for the upper division, far from reading at third- or fourth-grade level, were examined in English, Latin, history, geography, physiology, philosophy, and mathematics through quadratic equations. Graduates in the first class were journalists, translators, inventors, editors, and teachers, among other professions.

In the century since the Milan congress, as I have told, much of this progress has been undone. Now there is an audist establishment; now educational practices are largely ineffective; now deaf people and their language are locked out of deaf education. The single most important reform, from which many more will follow, is to get deaf adults—teachers, administrators, and parents—involved once again in the education of deaf children. This is the right course for us to follow, not only out of a sense of fairness, or out of respect for human dignity and democratic principles, but especially because the present social policies serve neither deaf people nor hearing people well. Deaf adults can provide a language model for young deaf children from hearing homes; it is vital that deaf children do not remain languageless for years on end, for this is to undermine their intellectual and social development. Hearing parents who study ASL and acquire some degree of fluency can foster that development.* Without deaf adults, however, the implicit message the parents send to their child is that this is a world in which deaf people have no place. Only deaf adults can provide the best language model, can convey a sense of the hearing world from a deaf perspective, can teach the child how to deal with that world while remaining a proud, informed deaf person.

Speaking practically, this means that deaf and hearing adults need each other and must be willing to take steps toward each other, frequently against their instincts, in the interest of deaf children. Only if deaf organizations and individuals are willing to share a measure of deaf culture and language with these outsiders, only if preschools and hearing homes will seek out deaf adults and open their doors to them, can this necessary collaboration take place.

Reason dictates that deaf adults would be particularly effective in the classroom: Most would be fluent in the primary language of the pupils; they share a common set of experiences with their pupils and could provide them with examples of what it is to be a highly educated deaf adult; they can readily teach deaf history and culture; and having survived the special-education system, they know just how disabling it can be and how to minimize those effects. Furthermore, deaf teachers, because they are visual people, who gather and express information primarily in the visual modality, would tend to conceptualize their lessons in a visual way, which would match most closely the pupils' best strategies for processing information.

A few years ago, UNESCO called in consultants on deaf education from around the globe to advise it on the different approaches to the education of deaf children. The UNESCO report concludes that deaf adults have an important role to play "in the development and education of deaf children" and finds that the interaction of deaf adults with the parents, the deaf children, and the teachers also "enriches the socialization of the deaf child." If deaf adults were once again substantially involved in the education of deaf children, there would be role models for those children, manual language would be reintroduced, spoken language skills would take their appropriate priority, literacy would improve, schools would no longer be speech clinics but be educational institutions. We need to recognize the deaf community for what it is and approach deaf education from the perspective of the education of language minorities, rather than exclusively from the perspective of education of the handicapped.

For over a quarter century, the U.S. Congress has steadfastly pursued the reform of education to accommodate children whose primary language is not English. It has succeeded in budging the local schools, using a carrot and a stick. The carrot is the Bilingual Education Act, which provides funding for a wide variety of programs promoting the use of minority languages in the schools. The stick is composed of civil rights statutes, which impose an affirmative duty on the schools to afford children who speak a minority language an equal educational opportunity by lowering the English-language barrier to their education.

The Bilingual Education Act affirms that many children in America have only limited proficiency in English because they have a distinct cultural heritage and that the federal government has an obligation to assist children from language minorities in acquiring equal access to education and in mastering English. The act goes on to affirm that children learn primarily by using their native language and cultural heritage and that bilingual education is thus appropriate for many American children.

According to the Code of Federal Regulations, the test for whether a child comes under the act is whether he or she normally speaks English. For the purposes of the act, it does not matter what language the child's parents speak. What matters for the success of the educational enterprise, and therefore for the application of the law, is the language the child speaks. According to the code, if the child normally speaks a language other than English, then his native language is not English, and if the child has limited proficiency in English, then he or she can benefit from the programs funded by the act.

Some of the activities that are currently funded by the act to benefit children in various language minorities include model bilingual/bicultural programs; teacher training; programs to develop accurate tests; fellowships for bilingual teachers; and special resource centers that have bilingual materials.

Bilingual/bicultural instruction includes many components: academic subjects taught transitionally at least in the pupil's primary language; English taught as a second language (ESL); the history, culture, and language arts of the student's minority-language group; American culture and history. The goal of many bilingual programs is to teach the student English so that he or she can ultimately be educated exclusively in English, while assuring that the student does not fall behind in other studies. This objective is met by: fostering a healthy self-image in the learner; developing his cognitive powers; creating a bridge to the learner's existing linguistic and cultural knowledge; and developing the student's reading and expressive skills in English.

While the Congress provided the carrot to motivate the schools to serve their bilingual children, the Supreme Court provided the stick. In a historic ruling that greatly promoted bilingual education, the Court decided in *Lau* v. *Nichols* that the Civil Rights Act of 1964 (Title VI) requires local school authorities receiving federal financial assistance to provide special instruction to students from language minorities. The Court wrote: "We know that those children who do not understand English are certain to find their classroom experience wholly incomprehensible and in no way meaningful [if the language of instruction is exclusively English]."

Ten years after the Civil Rights Act, Congress passed the Equal Educational Opportunity Act, which explicitly requires local authorities to take "appropriate action to overcome language barriers that impede equal participation in the instructional program." Speaking in behalf of this legislation, President Nixon said: "This Act would further establish an educational bill of rights for Mexican-Americans, Puerto Ricans, Indians and others who start their education under language handicaps to make certain that they, too, will have equal opportunity."

The Court ruled in another test case concerning children with limited English proficiency, *Rios* v. *Read*, that the Civil Rights Act and the Equal Educational Opportunity Act and other laws "mandate teaching such children subject matter in their native tongue (when required) by competent teachers . . . and [strongly suggest] the requirement of a bicultural [component] as a psychological support to the subject matter instruction." The Court found that the school district was not in compliance merely by providing students with intensive training in English while they fell behind in subjects that required a knowledge of English. The Court ordered school officials to add three features to their bilingual education program: to educate teachers about the special cultural background of children from language minorities; to train all instructors in the teaching of English as a second language; and to actively seek and employ instructors of the same minority group as the students.

The carrot and the stick are based on a simple idea. We Americans want our children to be educated and in command of English. We recognize that to achieve this goal, if their most fluent language is not English, their schooling must be conducted in their most fluent language, until they have achieved a sufficient command of English. This is true for children who can hear the teacher, and it is true for children who cannot hear the teacher. More than twenty states have legislation promoting some kind of bilingual education, and in 1985 there were three hundred bilingual programs in New York City alone. The UNESCO report on deaf education states as a principle that "We must recognize the legitimacy of the signed languages as linguistic systems and they should be accorded the same status as other languages . . . it is no longer admissible to overlook them or to fail to encourage their integration into deaf education." The European Parliament made a similar proclamation in 1987. Yet bilingual education of ASL-using children is virtually unheard of in the United States. Courts have ruled that language barriers addressed by the Equal Educational Opportunities Act need not involve a foreign language but may involve an indigenous American language (*Guadalupe* v. *Tempe Elementary School District*) or an English dialect departing significantly from standard American English (*Martin Luther King Elementary School Children* v. *Michigan Board of Education*). Thus it seems reasonable to believe that the protection of language minorities provided by these statutes and related cases should and does extend to children who belong to the ASL-speaking minority. These children are thus discriminated against in monolingual English schools, and the remedy is a bilingual/bicultural program; such a program brings them together, it instructs them in a language they understand, and it affirms the value of their unique heritage. Legal advocates for the deaf community have been remiss in failing to work with parents of ASL-using children to demand in court the same access to education for their children as that accorded Spanish-speaking children, for example. This demand for equal treatment under the law has been grievously delayed because most parents of deaf children, unlike Hispanic-American parents, for example, do not share their child's unique linguistic and cultural heritage and do not realize how much the affirmation of that heritage has to offer to their child's development.

Times change. We can't blame educators or administrators for not having known all along that ASL is a full-fledged language, before the fact was discovered and confirmed in the 1970s and '80s. But we can blame any who rigidly adhere to old and unsuccessful practices now that the evidence is in and scholars, educators, and community leaders alike are calling for change. The Commission on the Education of the Deaf states: "We urge that outmoded educational policy be brought into line with recent scientific discoveries in linguistics and psychology. It has been shown repeatedly that children whose primary language is ASL, like those who speak other minority languages, such as Spanish or Navajo, are at a severe educational disadvantage in a system that disbars, denigrates and denies their primary language. It is reasonable to believe that the same educational remedies provided by the Congress and the courts for the speakers of all minority languages will benefit ASL-speaking children. In any case it is the law." The Department of Education has yet to implement this recommendation, however.

There is a substantial scientific literature comparing monolingual and bilingual education for children whose primary language is not English. The most comprehensive review of that literature to date finds a consistent advantage favoring bilingual education on "tests of reading, listening, language skills, mathematics, social studies, total achievement, and attitudes toward school and self." An independent review added that the greater the incorporation of the minority student's language and culture in the school curriculum, the greater his success in that curriculum. In his 1986 book summarizing research on bilingualism, psychologist Kenji Hakuta concludes that bilinguals also have an advantage over monolinguals in cognitive flexibility; a Canadian expert on bilingualism, Wallace Lambert, reached the same conclusion about a decade earlier: bilinguals are more sensitive to semantic relations among words than monolinguals; they are better at analyzing sentence structure and discovering rules generally; they are more able to reorganize perceptual situations; they are more creative in solving problems.

The potential advantages of extending bilingual/bicultural programs to ASL-using children are similar to those for other language-minority children. There would be an infusion of new ideas and methods for teaching this minority, including new strategies for teaching them English; enhanced communication between teacher and pupil; improved English literacy; improved academic achievement scores; improved emotional adjustment; decreased need for counseling services; increased class size without reduction in individualized attention; decreased dropout rates; decreased underemployment on school leaving; an increase in bilingual fluency of classroom teachers; teaching careers opened to adult minority-language users. Some educators of deaf children, rather attached to their current practices, ask for proof of the merits of bilingual education for ASL-using children. They did not ask for proof before endorsing total communication, nor did they ask for proof before embracing mainstreaming. When some schools acquired significant numbers of, for example, Vietnamese-speaking children and applied for federal funds to train teachers and develop materials for bilingual education, there was no demand for proof that current practices with two dozen other languages would succeed with this one. Nevertheless, we should acknowledge that most ASL-using children have little or no familiarity with *any* oral language and many spent the first years of their lives languageless. The results of properly conducted research on bilingual education of ASL-using children surely would be welcome. Meanwhile, we have proof that current practices in the education of deaf children are failing, and we have a familiar line of reasoning, grounded in linguistics and psychology, that leads us in a direction demanded by the minority concerned.

Bilingual education has its outspoken critics. They charge that programs that are supposed to make the transition to English persist in using Spanish (for example); that instruction using Spanish is time lost for familiarizing the student with English; that many bilingual programs show no advantage over the mainstream in academic achievement; and that Hispanic children would pick up English rapidly in an all-English school. Hakuta rebuts each of these claims: Surveys show bilingual programs are mainly transitional; there is evidence that skills learned in one language—for example, reading— transfer to the other; bilingual programs vary in quality and in the extent to which they really implement bilingual/bicultural education; and it is not clear that children from language minorities pick up English in a flash, especially the kind of English used in the classroom. These rebuttals, Hakuta notes, usually lead the critic to voice some words of respect for scholars and research, an affirmation of the importance of English in the United States—and renewed criticism of bilingual education.

Let's be candid: The source of the strong feelings on this issue lies deeper than disputes over educational policy. Hakuta's observation that research findings frequently fail to persuade the critic of bilingual education is one piece of evidence; another is that critic's first charge: Some programs actually perpetuate the child's linguistic and cultural heritage. Bilingual education has become symbolic of a larger issue that divides us as a nation: the commitment of some Americans, and the hostility of others, to cultural pluralism.

But we need not be divided when it comes to educating ASL-using children. While it is true that many immigrant children become bilingual on their own without special programs and that others rapidly become English monolinguals, take a husband or wife born in America who speaks only English, and assimilate into mainstream American society, this informal acquisition of a second language cannot and does not happen with deaf children, for the elementary reason that nearly all cannot hear sufficiently well to acquire English. Consequently, ASL becomes and remains their primary language, and they marry other people whose primary language is ASL; most do not and cannot disappear into the mainstream English-speaking society. Thus, although the education of deaf children is predicated nowadays on a denial that the deaf community is a linguistic minority, the fact is that the deaf community is the one language group that can never be totally assimilated and whose language can never be totally eradicated. Vocal opponents of bilingual education do not, of course, have deaf people in mind when they advocate sink-or-swim immersion in English-speaking society.

It is not hard for such opponents of bilingual education in general to see why an exception must be made for children who cannot hear. Indeed, even transitional bilingual education, which aims at replacing the child's primary language with English, is unrealistic for most deaf children; a more appropriate goal is maintenance bilingualism, in which a command of written English (and spoken English for the rare few) is built to stand alongside a command of ASL, each to be used with its appropriate audience and occasions.

While the necessity of bilingual education for ASL-using children is evident, the need for a bicultural component in their education may be less clear. Yet deaf studies as an obligatory part of the curriculum has much to offer the deaf child. In learning about historic deaf figures, the El Mudos and Laurent Clercs of our world, the deaf child gains ideas of possible lives that he can lead and finds a basis for self-esteem in a society that insists he is inferior. Possessing knowledge about one's heritage is part of being a well-informed adult, and such knowledge provides a useful framework, as well, for organizing other knowledge. Thus, the deaf student who learns about Laurent Clerc's life as he traveled about New England in the early 1800s, seeking charity for the first school for deaf children, will learn, too, about early American government, medicine, agriculture, and religious values. Further, a knowledge of the forces that shaped the deaf community as it is today will give the deaf student insight into the mechanisms of oppression that will influence his life as they have his forebears' lives—mechanisms that he may otherwise use, in turn, to oppress minorities within and beyond the deaf community. Finally, profound thought, aesthetic values, the universals of the human experience, can be taught by examining any of numerous literatures, but allowing the deaf child to learn these through deaf literature expressed in ASL and in English gives them an extra measure of immediacy, clarity, and emotive power. Deaf studies need not be at the expense of social studies, natural science, and the rest of the curriculum. On the contrary, all learning is facilitated when it takes place in a setting that is validating for a child, and all learning is hampered when the school is an alien place.

These academic gains will not be had merely by changing the fundamental orientation of deaf education from education of the handicapped to minority education. That is the first step. But there must also be a phase of development in which new materials and methods are conceived, tried out, and modified. Teachers must be trained in new ways and new subjects, and means must be found for greatly increasing the numbers of teachers and administrators drawn from the deaf minority.

Like other children who use a minority language, ASL-using children are not a homogeneous group with respect to language use, social class, race, and many other educationally important factors. In an ideal world, Chinese American students in bilingual education programs might have a teacher who not only spoke a Chinese language but who spoke *their* Chinese language. After all, Mandarin Chinese and Cantonese, for example, are quite different languages. Likewise, there are many American children whose most fluent language is that of their Sicilian parents but whose Italian-speaking teacher uses the Italian spoken in the Tuscany region. The term "ASL-using," like "Chinese-using" or "Italian-using," covers quite a range of linguistic performances, so all communication problems are not solved when the teacher addresses the child with whatever mastery he has achieved in ASL. The problem of incomprehension may be substantially reduced, however, and the advantages still accrue from the affirmation of the child's language and identity.

For the purposes of education, we should consider that most of the children in deaf-education programs in America today are ASL-using in this sense. They do not all speak the same dialect or register; they have not all mastered the language to the same degree. ASL is not the mother tongue of most of them—if by mother tongue we mean "acquired naturally from one's parents"; neither is English. But the one language that is accessible and thus holds out the greatest common hope for a comprehensible and meaningful education is ASL. And ASL is the birthright of America's deaf children as they are future members of the American deaf community. English is also their birthright and for some so is Spanish, Chinese, or another minority language. We need not worry about the school's readiness to present and espouse mainstream culture and values. What we need to ensure is that its curriculum reflects minority cultures and values that are validating for the minority deaf child who is doubly oppressed. In many educational programs for deaf children, what is called for is a multilingual/multicultural curriculum that capitalizes on the knowledge and sense of self that the deaf child brings to the school.

The Danish sociolinguist Tove Skutnabb-Kangas, one of the world's leading authorities on bilingual education, has reviewed the many published studies assessing educational programs for children who do not speak the majority language and has identified the properties of a successful program:

- *The linguistic goal is bilingualism and not dominance of the minority language or the majority language.* This is not true of current education for ASL-using children, where only English is taught and used.
- *The social goal is positive for the group and not to keep it in a powerless, subordinate position.* This is not true for ASL-using children, who are primarily prepared for unskilled and semiskilled labor.
- *A choice exists among educational programs using the various languages.* This is not true for ASL-using children.
- *Teachers are bilingual and well-trained.* This is not true in programs for ASL-using children. "Especially with small children," Skutnabb-Kangas writes, "it is close to criminal psychological torture to use monolingual teachers who do not understand what the child has to say in its mother tongue."
- *Bilingual materials are available.* This is not true for ASL-using children.
- *The cultural content of the materials is appropriate for the students.* This is not true for ASL-using children.

- *The teacher is not authoritarian but supportive and promotes a low level of anxiety.* According to my deaf informants, teachers are more often authoritarian than supportive; it is difficult to be supportive for a child if you cannot communicate fluently with him.
- *The students have high internal motivation; they are not forced to use the majority language.* This is not true for ASL-using children, who are generally obliged to use only the majority language.
- *The students have high self-confidence: they know they have a fair chance to succeed, and the teacher reinforces this with high expectations.* This is not true for ASL-using children; they commonly have low self-esteem in a system that does not esteem them, and they are realistic about their poor chances for success. The teachers of these children have low expectations of most of them.
- *The students' linguistic development in their primary language is promoted. They learn language registers, art forms, reading and writing, etc., in their primary language.* This is not true for ASL-using children.
- *There is enough relevant, cognitively demanding subject matter provided to promote common underlying proficiency for all languages.* This is not true for ASL-using children.
- *There is adequate emphasis on linguistic development in the majority language.* This is true for ASL-using children.
- *The samples of the majority language studied in class are appropriate to the students' proficiency.* This is frequently not true for ASL-using children.
- *There is an opportunity to practice the majority language in peer group contexts.* This is true but limited for ASL-using children.
- *There is exposure to the majority language used by native speakers in linguistically demanding formal contexts.* This is frequently not true for ASL-using children.

As we see, most educational programs for deaf children would receive very low scores indeed on this checklist.

The relation between language and power seems to be at the root of the poor English literacy and academic achievement of deaf children. For many in the audist establishment, the present state of affairs may be quite acceptable. How else can we explain the failure of most programs for ASL-using children to provide more than one or two of these fifteen features of a successful program? How else can we explain the lack of discussion of the most important fact about deaf education today—its failure in educating deaf children, the very reason for its existence? Neither the professional meetings nor the professional journals are centrally concerned with diagnosing the reasons for the failure, proposing remedial steps, or evaluating progress. The focus of the seventeenth International Congress on the Education of the Deaf in 1986 (the third was the infamous Congress of Milan in 1880) was not the failure of deaf education but, as I have told, the promise of cochlear implants. The profession of deaf education apparently believes that the best hope for deaf education is to provide it miraculously with hearing children.

Why is there a conspiracy of silence about the failure of deaf education? Whatever our profession, it is, of course, more agreeable to parade our few successes than to study our many failures. In this particular case, moreover, successful education is not entirely in the interest of the educators. If most deaf children acquired critical thought and a command of written language once again, as they apparently did in the last century, they would once again enter the teaching profession in large numbers, reform that profession, and make obsolete the present hearing teachers' training, so endangering the employment of many. Moreover, the present deaf illiteracy has been acceptable to deaf education for nearly a century because the low achievement of deaf children corresponds to their teachers' low opinion of their potential for achievement, of their intellect, of their maturity. Believing their deaf students to be intellectually handicapped, hearing teachers handicap them.

Most deaf students are illiterate, further, because their own extensive language skills are not acknowledged in the school; they are demeaned or denied. Nothing is said in school about the manifold forms that deaf literacy takes in manual language: the narrative traditions, the poetry, the handshape games, the pantomime, and so on. Although English-using children study English nearly every year of their schooling, ASL-using children are never permitted to study their language, to gain an awareness of its grammar, its art forms, and its manifold possibilities.

Most deaf students are illiterate in the national language because the systematic denial of their primary, manual language shuts out the most effective strategy for teaching them a second language in school. Modern methods of teaching foreign languages in the classroom are based on a contrastive analysis of the student's first language and the structure of the language he is striving to learn. There are fundamentally two sources for students' errors in learning a second language: structural principles in the student's first language that he wrongly extends to the second (the Frenchman who says "My brother is engineer") and principles of the second language that he applies too broadly ("What a nice weather!"). And yet, although French is a source of interference and errors for the Frenchman learning English, it also facilitates his learning because of its structural similarities with English: Many French words have cognates in English; verb conjugation is organized in similar ways, and so on. The student of English whose primary language is, say, Japanese is not so fortunate; and the ASL user can expect even less facilitation, since his language exists in another mode and uses the possibilities presented by space and vision. What is needed, therefore, is a systematic mapping of the discrepancies between ASL and English (in marking time, in describing space, in word order, and so on), as well as a systematic exploration of the errors that arise when the ASL speaker extrapolates the model of English he has constructed in the course of acquisition. With this analysis in hand, an ordered sequence of instruction can be set down, which will lead the ASL-using student from what is naturally easy for him to what is difficult, and which will build a metalinguistic awareness at the same time: Languages have different ways of achieving similar ends.

Most deaf students are illiterate because the teachers conceive of language as a set of exercises on the one hand or an aesthetic and moral norm on the other, but rarely as a reflection and reinforcement of cultural patterns, including group loyalty, problem solving, recreation, perception of space and time.

Most deaf students are illiterate because they are taught English fundamentally as mentally retarded children are. The written language they see is neither high-level nor newspaper-level but imbecile-level, reduced language. And as with mentally retarded hearing children, the language used for teaching English is English itself, precisely the language deaf students do not know and are trying to learn; no account is taken of the language in which most deaf students are fluent: their manual language. Educators of deaf children have not developed materials or teaching strategies that address the basic differences between deaf and hearing children in the ways they go about reading.

When a hearing child learns to read, he relies on his knowledge of the spoken language; written text is not an entirely new communication system but an unfamiliar version of a familiar one. Fundamental to the prior knowledge that he uses is his knowledge of the sound system of his language, the vowels and consonants of English and their allowable sequences. Here is some evidence: Poor readers are as skilled as good ones in detecting most sounds in noise but inferior to good ones when it comes to detecting speech sounds in noise. Likewise, poor readers are as skilled as good ones in remembering unfamiliar faces or nonsense designs but worse at remembering words. Poor readers are worse than good readers in breaking up words into their component sounds. Good readers have trouble remembering lists of consonants if some of them rhyme, as this increases the similarity of the items when they are remembered in terms of sound or articulation, but poor readers are less bothered by the rhyming. Evidence such as this has led many cognitive scientists to conclude that when hearing children read, they use their knowledge of the sound system of their language. Poor readers also have difficulty with syntax, but this may be a by-product of strain on sentence processing because of their difficulties with the sound system of their language.

A related but distinct picture of the reading process emerges from studies of deaf students. When deaf college students whose primary language was ASL were given lists of visually dissimilar printed words to recall, the lists that rhymed proved the most difficult; lists of (nonrhyming) visually similar words and also lists of words whose sign translations are visually similar proved easier to recall. Thus, these relatively skilled readers, who knew ASL, appeared to use knowledge of the vowels and consonants of English and their allowable sequences in reading and remembering the lists of words. Deaf college students asked to think of words that rhyme with a given word can frequently do it, but they come up with words that look alike in lip-reading. They also know how to pronounce invented words like *flaim*. In sum, it is possible for deaf readers to use knowledge of word formation in reading, and such use is characteristic of good readers. What is relevant is not how well the deaf student can speak but rather how well he has mastered the elements and regularities of English words; deaf students' oral proficiency does not correlate with their reading achievement.*

There are many ways in principle in which the profoundly deaf child could learn about the elements of English words and their regularities: from articulation, to the extent that he has such skills; from lip-reading; from finger-spelling; from a distillation of experience with the writing system—that is, by learning the regularities in the sequences of letters. When deaf children and adults are asked to write something down, they frequently finger-spell the word to themselves, producing a hand configuration for the letter before beginning to write it. All in all, it appears that the best deaf readers use some such strategy to represent spoken words; readers with intermediate levels of skill call on their knowledge of signs; and the poorest readers are unable to use any of these strategies. What we need, then, are new teaching strategies that explore both avenues—ways of bringing into relief for the deaf student the regularities in the construction of English words, and ways of associating his prior repertoire of signs with their English translations.

Thus, deaf students continue to be illiterate in English, Japanese, and other national languages because this state of affairs is often acceptable to the schools; the children's prior language skills are demeaned and not utilized; the relations between language and culture are ignored; English is taught in English, Japanese in Japanese, which the students can't hear and don't know; and teaching techniques are appropriate for hearing students but not deaf students.

Illiteracy is a national problem, in America as in many other lands, that is not peculiar to deaf students. However, deaf students are particularly harmed by the schools' failure to teach them to read. How are deaf students to acquire knowledge? Not directly from the teacher, because the schools also fail to communicate with deaf students in their primary, manual language. Not from their parents, since communication is too rudimentary except for the privileged few with deaf parents or hearing parents who have studied ASL. Not from older deaf students, unless mainstreaming, which increasingly disperses students, is reversed. Not from deaf adults, since most deaf students have little contact with deaf adults. Reading—textbooks, newspapers, captioned programs—is a lifeline to knowledge for the deaf student more than for any other student. Thus, the schools' failure to teach literacy to deaf students is a disaster indeed; academic achievement is necessarily depressed in all subject matters, and the acquisition of knowledge may be hampered lifelong.

Educational programs for deaf children seem to reflect more the needs of the hearing teachers than they do those of the deaf students they are trying to serve. We come back to Padden and Humphries's observation that culturally deaf people and culturally hearing people have different "centers." In teacher-centered education, the difficulties of the student who does not speak the teacher's language fluently are imputed to the student, to his parents, to his entire minority group, or to all of these. In student-centered education, the learner's own knowledge of language and culture is a starting point. When the student is in trouble in school, the explanations tend to be quite different. His troubles are imputed to the extra work involved in learning through two languages; to racism and discrimination; and to all the factors that hinder monolingual students.

Is deaf education in America really hearing-teacher-centered?

Whose language is used to deliver instruction? The hearing teacher's.

Whose language is the student required to use in class? The hearing teacher's.

Do the role models provided in school—the teaching staff, the principal, the distinguished visitors, the historical and contemporary figures studied in class—do these role models reflect the possible lives of the deaf children, or do they reflect the hearing teacher's possible lives? The hearing teacher's.

Whose values determine the learning agenda? The relative weights assigned to educational goals? The activities carried out in class—storytelling or essay writing, acting plays or reading plays? Whose are the goals and subgoals? The hearing teacher's.

Whose themes are the themes of the classroom? Do they include student-centered themes like ASL, deaf friendships, sex, family, money, work, food, sports, growing up, drugs, cars, and so on? School has little to say about these themes, and what it has to say isn't in the language the children speak. No, the themes are generally the hearing teacher's.

Whose outlook on life dominates the class? Whose conception of success? Whose idea of good social relations? Or of humor? Or of personal space? Or of community responsibility? Whose worldview is presented as the only possible personally relevant worldview? The hearing teacher's.

If deaf education has evolved across the decades into a structure that is centered on the hearing teacher, it is no accident. This arrangement minimizes what the teacher has to learn; the burden is not the teacher's to study the language of the students, nor to become familiar with their cultural and historical context. Moreover, students submerged in an alien language environment are submissive rather than autonomous; they recognize that their world and language have no place in the school and correctly assume that they are not valued.

Then, too, education centered on the hearing teacher is consistent with the premise on which the teacher frequently entered special education in the first place. That premise was not one of mutuality. On the contrary, it presupposed that the teacher had a language and the deaf student little or none. It presupposed that the only culture relevant for the student is the teacher's culture. So, too, the last to yield to decolonization are the *colons*; they refuse to give up their status; thus they learn at great cost of human suffering that their status is a liability.

Isn't it time to try another way? To move deaf education toward the deaf student? To build on the native gifts and acquired knowledge of the pupils, and foremost their language? To adopt student-centered education is not to abandon all that the teacher represents. Student and teacher share many values and experiences, and the teacher, after all, represents the majority in power. The students need to learn much of what is on the teacher's agenda. But the successful teacher will acknowledge and use what the deaf pupil brings to the learning process and will identify the teacher-centered agenda for what it is. For example, teacher and students can study complex written English as they can study ASL narration, and they can examine the entrée that each communicative form provides. Likewise, reading texts and reading life—the pupil's life—can be integrated.

Building on the student's entering skills, affirming the learner's own identity, providing role models with whom he or she can identify, addressing the real issues of the student's life—this is all good psychology and good educational practice. Three principles in particular from cognitive science encourage the belief that student-centered deaf education will be more successful than its precursors. The process of decoding a message, of taking an utterance and discovering the speaker's intention, is normally unconscious. Speakers telling stories in English or in ASL go at the rate of forty propositions a minute, so there's scarcely time to be consciously thinking about vocabulary, and word order, and word endings, and so on. The child who is forced to bring these unconscious grammatical processes to consciousness because the message is clothed in a language he does not know well is in serious trouble. Even if he knows all the facts of the language, he cannot do the analysis quickly, and he must allocate much of his intellectual capacity simply to reconstructing the message. Less is available for considering the message itself, for relating it to other ideas, and for formulating a response. Student-centered education uses the child's most fluent language and removes this handicap.

The second principle of cognitive science that favors a student-centered approach to deaf education is that message processing is "top-down" as well as "bottom-up." Sound waves, movements of the lips, printed words, or signs play only a small role in leading us to understand a sentence. The meaning of each word and its grammatical class are likewise not the basis of comprehension. In interpreting a sentence, in arriving at its sense, we rely unconsciously, and thus much more than we realize, on our knowledge of life, knowledge that is not specific to the particular language in which the sentence is communicated, knowledge that comes from general acculturation. Would a person commit an action like the one I understood? Can it even be done in principle? Would the subject of the sentence be likely to do it? Acculturation is also the key to composing good sentences; children who know a lot about life have a lot to talk about, and they know which words and structures tend to come together. Thus, student-centered education conducted in the child's most fluent language is actually fostering his literacy in English even without a single word of English spoken. Of course, English must also be taught explicitly, with the aid of the child's most fluent language.

A third relevant observation from cognitive science is that cognitive skills transfer from one language setting to the next. The largest study of bilingual education to date in the United States found that the majority of Hispanic children who were taught to read Spanish before learning to read English learned later to read English quite well. The children who had difficulty learning to read English were not those who spoke Spanish at home but those who had poor language and prereading skills whether the home language was English or Spanish. And if those children did not get assistance in their native Spanish, they did not do well in later years. The *best* readers of English, on the other hand, were the children with the best skills in Spanish. A Canadian study of children from various language minorities—e.g., Russian—who were learning French came to a similar but broader conclusion: Those children who could read and write in their minority language outperformed nonliterate children on all measures of French achievement, not just reading French. There was evidence, furthermore, that the results were not due simply to the children's spoken fluency in their minority language; what mattered for success was their literacy in their native language.

Now apply these findings to ASL-using children. They suggest that instruction using the deaf child's most fluent language would actually improve his or her performance in English—just the premise of student-centered deaf education. I submit that ASL literacy and English literacy have much in common, and that by developing and using the deaf student's ASL literacy we can advance that student significantly along the road to English literacy. A Greek study found evidence of precisely this association between the two kinds of language skills: Those deaf children who were the best at expressing themselves in Greek Sign Language were the best at writing Greek compositions.

English texts differ from English talk in many ways. If we aim to teach English literacy, we must not focus exclusively, as we tend to do, on the mere fact that English texts are written down. If that were all there was to it, if English texts were simply a record of everyday conversational speech, many more hearing people would be literate, as all engage in everyday conversation. In fact, we rarely if ever encounter a text that is merely a written version of an intimate conversation, and a person who could read only such texts would not be considered literate. On the contrary, written texts are generally quite different from spoken conversation in structure, vocabulary, tone, and values. Written text is more complex, coherent, integrated, decontextualized, and emotionally detached than face-to-face communication. Thus, a hearing student learning to be literate in English confronts a different kind of discourse than the one with which he is familiar; his problem of decoding English print is only a small part of the overall task of uncovering the multiple messages of this secondary kind of discourse.

I propose that literacy is above all the ability to process such secondary discourses. So deaf children are frequently illiterate in English not only because of an imperfect command of English grammar and vocabulary but also because their primary discourse is so different from, and conflicts with, the particular secondary discourse taught in the school—that is, essay-text literacy. Essay texts are explicit, complete, clear, closed, self-sufficient. But face-to-face communication, which the student knows well in his primary, manual language, is frequently not explicit but suggestive; not complete but fragmentary; unclear in itself but made clear by its connections with context, hence neither closed nor self-sufficient.

In expository prose, linguist James Gee observes, the important relations are between sentence and sentence, not between a speaker and a listener. Thus, the reader must actively research structure and make connections within and between sentences; underlying propositions must be figured out and their logical implications developed. It is these logical relations that are important, rather than the audience or the rhetorical situation. Indeed, there is only an imaginary audience in expository prose, and an invisible, abstract author, who is under few clear rhetorical constraints.

Considering all the differences between their primary discourse, talk, and the secondary discourse that is written expository prose, it is no surprise that minority children in America often have difficulty in mastering expository prose and becoming literate. But many of the members of these minorities have other secondary discourses. Fluent users of ASL can often engage in such secondary discourses as tall tales, folk speech, naming practices, jokes, wordplay, pantomime, and poetry.

I hypothesize that when any one secondary discourse is mastered, further secondary discourses are easier to acquire. That is why the Hispanic-American children who could read Spanish well are also those who did best in reading English expository prose. And the children most fluent in ASL seem to have an advantage in mastering English prose over those with less mastery of ASL. In this sense, then, ASL literacy and English literacy are indeed related. If the hypothesis is correct, if learning an easier secondary discourse facilitates learning a harder one, then we should be interested in fostering ASL literacy and in building on such skills in order to develop English literacy as well.

Gallaudet University linguists Liddell and Johnson and anthropologist Carol Erting have published a controversial paper, "Unlocking the Curriculum," advocating bilingual education of deaf children and setting down some principles. Deaf children should learn ASL early from deaf adults. This, their most fluent language, should be used as the primary language for instruction. English should be taught as a second language, using ASL and written texts for instruction. No child should be asked to understand speech and learn through speech at the same time. Mainstreaming is ill-advised because, for one thing, instruction is likely to be based on English. Deaf education must incorporate deaf culture and interactions with deaf adults.

Isn't it time to try "unlocking the curriculum" by centering deaf education on the deaf child rather than on the hearing teacher? The teacher or school principal who is ready to do so faces challenges but also great rewards. There are new lesson plans to be formulated; new instructional materials to be developed. Teachers must have the opportunity and the incentive to work toward bilingualism. New roles have to be defined in the school so that deaf adults can play their necessary part. Deaf adults can help their hearing colleagues to learn their pupils' most fluent language and come to know their culture. In the process, the hearing teacher may bring his own culture to consciousness as never before. This can be emotionally and intellectually expanding. Deaf adults can provide language and role models for the children. And deaf adults can play a special role for hearing parents: They can provide practical advice born of their personal knowledge of deaf people, language, and culture; they can give information about community services; and they are a living example to the parents of how their child may one day be a knowledgeable adult and a contributing member of society. When hearing parents arrange for their deaf children, before starting school, to come to know deaf adults—for example, by visiting those adults and welcoming their visits, and by placing their children in day care programs with deaf staff—they are hastening the day when their child can engage in real communication, and they are building the basis for later bilingual/ bicultural education. This partnership of teachers, deaf adults, and parents promises great rewards for each party and, most of all, for the children. The potential reward for the school, which must inspire and organize the partnership, is nothing less than the joy of seeing today's youth finally equipped for tomorrow's challenges.

The Politics of Deaf Education

The great progress of various minorities in the West—for example, of African-Americans and Hispanic-Americans in the United States —has led deaf adults to realize that rights are won by struggle. Two courses are open to deaf leaders: to work for reforms within the present audist system, or to challenge that system. When following the first course, deaf people pay a price, for they implicitly subscribe to the hostile definition of the deaf experience as infirmity. For example, they may lobby the Congress to pass the Americans with Disabilities Act, with its provisions for deaf people; while the deaf leaders know they are not disabled, their actions lend credence to the belief that they are and weaken their demands for access to funding under the Bilingual Education Act. When the Congress, in response to deaf activism, proposed a national research institute addressed to the concerns of deaf people, deaf leaders lobbied for this initiative, even though the institute would be placed within the establishment of the National Institutes of Health and would affirm in its title (Deafness and Other Communication Disorders) the very principle that the activism was aimed at negating. Moreover, deaf leaders were subscribing to a policy in which organizations *for* deaf people (run almost exclusively by hearing people) get large allocations from the government, while organizations *of* deaf people do not.

In order to participate in the conduct of their own affairs, deaf people have had to participate as disabled. Audists have placed deaf people in this double bind. One means of ensuring that an oppressed group internalizes its managed identity is to make rewards contingent on embracing that identity. In a society in which families are given money or tax relief for each child, women are presented with a double bind. In a society that exempts gays from the military service on psychiatric grounds, gays are presented with a double bind. Why not enjoy the perquisite if it is legally yours, in a society that has, in any event, oppressed you and owes you much? Yet each such act victimizes the beneficiary and his or her group.

If the audist establishment continues to lock out deaf people themselves, to silence their narrative and prevent their collaboration, we must expect deaf adults to take the course that has typically been followed by other frustrated language minorities. "You may be forced to raise the level of your protest," I told the 1986 meeting of the National Association of the Deaf: newspaper interviews; leafleting campaigns; demonstrations at the statehouse; student sit-ins. Indeed, British deaf leaders, determined to break the century-old silence over the exclusion of deaf people, culture, and language from deaf education, demonstrated, picketed, and leafleted during the 1985 International Congress on the Education of the Deaf in Manchester, and held their own "alternative congress" concurrently. There has been growing deaf protest in Europe and America ever since.

The most significant event in contemporary deaf history, the Gallaudet Revolution, was the fruit of this kind of deaf activism. March 6 to 13, 1988, was the week that the world heard from Gallaudet.

During this week, American deaf people rose up and took control of the premier deaf institution in the world. The revolution breathed pride into young deaf children and into deaf adults. It exposed hearing parents of deaf children, many for the first time, to successful deaf professional people. It added impetus to the development of bilingual and bicultural educational programs for ASL-using children. I was privileged to hold the Powrie Doctor Chair of Deaf Studies at Gallaudet University during the spring of 1988 and was therefore on the campus when the revolution broke out. Here is how it happened.

On Sunday, March 6, word spread on campus that the governing board of Gallaudet, seventeen hearing and four deaf persons, had made their selection of the university's new president from among the three final candidates. Two of those candidates were deaf. One was the dean of the largest faculty at Gallaudet, the college of arts and sciences; I. King Jordan had a Ph.D. in psychology and was a widely admired administrator and scholar. The other deaf candidate was the director of the Louisiana School for the Deaf, a child of deaf parents and a leader in the American deaf community, Dr. Harvey Corson. The one hearing candidate, Dr. Elisabeth Zinser, was known to the chairman of the board and some of its members from her candidacy during a presidential search some years earlier. She knew very little of the deaf community and their language. Her training was in the helping professions—nursing and educational psychology—and she was an administrator at the University of North Carolina, Greensboro.

In the weeks leading up to this day, several deaf leaders from around the country had converged on Washington and led rallies on campus advocating the selection of a deaf president for the first time in the history of the university, since its establishment by Abraham Lincoln in 1864. From the choice of finalists presented to the board of trustees by the faculty and staff, there was reason to believe that the university had indeed been sensitized to this aspiration of the deaf community. A small crowd of students and some employees gathered on campus to hear the news of the board's decision. The board proclaimed that Dr. Zinser was the new president. I watched the crowd react with shock, anger, disbelief, and tears. Posters and news releases were burned, and speeches were made in ASL. The crowd swelled.

A large group of students and their supporters—including many faculty, staff members, and alumni—took to the streets and marched, without a permit, to the hotel where the board was staying. The police tried to stop the march with bullhorns, but of course, the students did not respond to the warnings. Unable to communicate with the largely deaf crowd, the police blocked off the avenue and escorted the marchers to the hotel.

At the hotel, the chairman of the board, wife of a millionaire furniture manufacturer, agreed to talk with a group of three student representatives. She told them that the board had not picked a deaf candidate because (as the newspapers reported it) "deaf people are incapable of functioning in a hearing world." The remark added fuel to a volatile situation. The chairman later claimed that her interpreter had misconstrued her statement. From the hotel the students marched to the Capitol building and then, still with police escort, back to campus.

Hundreds of Gallaudet employees returning to work on Monday found all the entrances to the campus blocked. The students had parked their cars in front of the campus gates and let the air out of their tires. They refused to admit top-level administrators, so the university was forced to close down. The students issued four demands that the board would have to satisfy before they would reopen the campus: first, the board must withdraw Dr. Zinser's appointment as president and replace her with a deaf president; second, the chairman of the board must resign; third, the deaf membership of the board must increase to 51 percent; fourth, there must be no reprisals against the student protesters.

The board agreed to meet in the morning with a delegation to discuss the demands, and then to meet in the afternoon with the campus community at the field house. A large crowd, gathered at the field house in the afternoon, heard from the student delegation that the board had refused all their demands. The chairman of the board was there to "talk sense into the students." Inside the field house, someone tripped the fire alarms. "It's hard to talk above the noise," the chairman told the students through an interpreter. They responded in ASL: "What noise?" The crowd stormed out of the building and marched a second time on the Capitol.

The next day, the students organized a "Deaf President Now" rally that filled the stands of the football stadium. They burned effigies of the chairman and Dr. Zinser. "Deaf President Now! Deaf President Now!" became the protest chant. After many speeches, the crowd marched around the campus and then dispersed.

The Deaf President Now Council was formed to coordinate developments, make plans, and oversee the protest. The third day ended with the lines of battle drawn up.

On Wednesday, March 9, unable to get on campus, the university's administrators set up office in a downtown building. Dr. Zinser was flown into Washington at once (four months early) to attend a much publicized press conference, where she announced, "I am in charge!" thus becoming the first president of Gallaudet to try and run the university from off campus. At the press conference, deaf candidate I. King Jordan stated that as dean of Gallaudet's college of arts and sciences, he felt it was best to support the board's decision.

While the chairman and Dr. Zinser were holding the press conference, a group of students, alumni, faculty, staff, and members of the deaf community were meeting with several congressmen. The group explained to the legislators the seriousness of the situation, pointed out that it was a national issue, not just a campus matter, and declared that the students would never back down.

Later in the day, these congressmen met with Dr. Zinser and warned her that the prolonged upheaval could hurt the university's funding by the government. The staff of the university voted overwhelmingly to support the students' four demands. The faculty did likewise, although they had originally ranked Dr. Zinser above the two deaf candidates in their recommendation to the trustees.

The national media—television crews, newspaper and radio reporters—swarmed over the campus. The Deaf President Now Council set up a communications center and a team of interpreters for the reporters. That evening deaf student leader Greg Hlibok appeared on the nationally televised news program "Night Line," along with Elisabeth Zinser and deaf film star Marlee Matlin. It was probably the most watched event in all of Western deaf history. The consensus on the Gallaudet campus: Hlibok held his ground well against Zinser.

The heavy media coverage attracted much support to the students' cause. Letters, telegrams, and phone calls poured in. Rallies were held at deaf schools all over the United States. Members of the American Postal Workers union and their wives joined the student barricades at the campus. A linen company donated forty bedsheets for banners. A law firm provided their services free. Twenty thousand dollars in contributions came from Americans who cared all over the United States.

Late the next evening, Thursday, Dr. Zinser announced that she was resigning. Greg Hlibok wrote her a letter wishing her success in her future endeavors and calling her "an innocent victim and unfortunate target of our collective anger." He was generous in victory, but much of the nation wondered why it had taken someone from outside the audist establishment so long to understand the justness of the deaf community's demands; perhaps her training in managing the sick and the infirm had prevented her from recognizing her role in cultural oppression of deaf people. Word of Elisabeth Zinser's resignation spread quickly. Early-morning arrivals on campus Friday were therefore surprised to see students still guarding the gates. "Haven't you heard the news? Dr. Zinser has resigned," said one. "Yes, we know," replied the students guarding the gates, "but we still have three and a half demands to go!"

Friday's march to the Capitol attracted three thousand participants from all over the nation, including busloads of deaf students and their parents. The march began with a huge banner, which proclaimed, "We still have a dream!" The banner was lent by an African-American museum. People along the parade route cheered and waved. Cars and trucks honked their horns in support. Government workers stopped their office labors and leaned out windows to cheer the students on.

At the Capitol, congressmen stood in line to address the rally. The students' determination and behavior in the struggle won their praise and admiration. Said one senator: "You have succeeded in educating the world about deafness, the concerns of deaf people, and the simple truth that we all need and are entitled to dignity and respect." Candidates for the presidency of the United States, George Bush, Michael Dukakis, and Jesse Jackson, sent the students letters of support. Said Jackson: "The problem is not that the students do not hear; the problem is that the hearing world does not listen."

On Saturday, hundreds of students and their supporters gathered on campus for a "Board Buster Day." There were lectures, a picnic, free food, strategy meetings. Meanwhile, members of the board of governors were returning to Washington from their homes around the United States to pick a replacement for Dr. Zinser and to discuss the remaining student demands.

Sunday, March 13, 1988, was a historic day for deaf people. It was also a day of anticipation and waiting. A call finally came through to campus from a deaf member of the board, meeting downtown. The seventh president of Gallaudet, and its first deaf president, would be

Dr. I. King Jordan. The chairman of the board had resigned. The board would be reconstituted with a deaf majority, and there would be no reprisals against the protesters. The board had agreed to all the students' demands. There was a huge celebration on campus, and then the students went home for spring holidays.

After the Revolution

The Gallaudet Revolution was the high point of contemporary deaf history. Unfortunately, journalists and the nation's political leaders, who with rare exceptions enthusiastically supported the Gallaudet students' demands, generally missed the point. They conveniently categorized the uprising as a legitimate demand for the rights and dignity of disabled people, thus evading the necessity of rethinking and revising the conceptual and social framework in which hearing people relate to deaf people. That is how the absurdity came about that the Congress, impressed by the national lovefest with the deaf students, endorsed their demands and then created a national institute of health to address them, when the revolutionary principle of their demands was that the deaf community, like the African-American community, had a right to minority leadership; health was irrelevant.

Of all the different issues that concern the deaf community, none illustrates better the operation of oppression and none is more vital to deaf people themselves than deaf education. The hearing people in charge of special education are in a position to mystify others—that is, to mask social reality—in behalf of their own interests. I have told how teachers of deaf children continually make judgments about the capabilities of the pupils they teach, judgments often based on social rather than educational criteria. Deaf children, condemned to vegetate ten years in an environment in which learning is not possible for them, are said to have a so-called learning disorder. This is mystification of the role of the teacher and the school in the educational failure. Its logic proceeds as follows: Demonstrable lesions of the brain can cause academic underachievement; therefore, deaf underachievement must be due to some undetectable lesion of the brain—as if the audist practices of the teacher and policies of the school could not themselves be the primary reason for academic under-achievement.

All over the world, powerful social groups categorize and classify weaker social groups and treat them unequally. The rationalizations differ, but benevolent humanitarianism is a common one. The audist establishment wants at the same time the denial of deafness—mainstreaming, oral education, hearing aids, cochlear implants—and its maintenance; without the deafness market, there is no audist establishment. No one believes any longer in the image of the colonizer as a self-sacrificing purveyor of civilization. We are aware of colonialism's economic motivations and the dehumanization of the colonized and the colonizer. Yet we still accept the image of the self-sacrificing speech teacher or educator of the deaf. This explanation denies and masks the vested interests of hearing teachers, administrators, and other professionals. Deaf history is replete with teachers purportedly acting for humanitarian reasons only but in fact motivated as well by personal goals. Abbé de l'Epée wanted to convert the heathen deaf children. The first great oralist, Jacob Pereire, labored to leave a legacy for his children. The founder of British deaf education, Thomas Braidwood, sought to create a lucrative family empire and monopoly on deaf education. Thomas Gallaudet had failed in four attempts at a career and needed one.

Interests that particularly affected the early period of deaf education were the economic interests of industrial society; the emphasis was on training in trades, where, in much of the world, it remains today. Government is asked to fund a large audist establishment not as a right of deaf children—that is, fundamentally for humanitarian reasons—but as a good capital investment. It was not benevolent humanitarianism that resisted a deaf president for Gallaudet University, nor benevolent humanitarianism that dictated its policy prohibiting ASL in the classroom; it is not benevolent humanitarianism that requires Gallaudet students to study audiology but does not require them to study deaf history or culture; and it is not benevolent humanitarianism that has largely excluded deaf people from the profession of teaching deaf people; it is, instead, audist self-interest.

Before the Gallaudet Revolution, it was possible for the deaf community and hearing people of goodwill to accept uncritically the explanations that people with power gave for their actions. This is not to deny that compassion and humanitarianism sometimes played a role in determining those actions. Many thought about deaf education, however, without making allowance for conflict. Deaf leaders who examined deaf education considered the "special needs" of deaf children in special education but failed to consider the needs and interests of the teachers and others with power who have shaped deaf education into the audist form it now has.

Then came the Gallaudet Revolution, laying bare the conflicts among various interests in deaf education. It was deaf studies, the scholarship of the cultural renaissance, that made the Gallaudet Revolution possible, for outrage requires a standard of just treatment. Once deaf leaders came to understand fully, thanks to deaf studies, that they were members of a language and cultural minority in America, they saw hearing paternalism no longer as benevolent concern for their welfare but as brazen and intolerable discrimination against them. Now, after the Gallaudet Revolution, prerevolutionary oppressed forms of thinking are no longer possible. Deaf studies knows now that it must examine critically the roles assigned to teachers, parents, pupils, and professionals. What are those roles and the stereotypes that have dictated them? Pupils are associated in deaf education with negative attributes: incapacity, inability, and powerlessness. Parents are viewed as incompetent. Teachers are trained only to combat the supposed special limitations of the pupils, as the system perceives them, and not to actually instruct in academic subjects. Teachers and professionals tend to come from socially dominant groups. Professionals are outside and above the working-class clientele that accepts the mystique of their superior abilities and rational decisions.

Deaf studies also now knows that this critical analysis of roles must be conducted within a wider social, historical, and political perspective on deaf education. American deaf leaders are aware as never before that they must engage in a struggle for power if they wish to see the lot of the deaf community improve in vital areas where hearing people have staked out a conflicting interest. In short, the field of deaf studies in America has grown up and lost its taste for fairy tales.

The Gallaudet Revolution added momentum to demands for reform pressed by deaf leaders around the world. French deaf leaders and their hearing allies had begun actively militating for reform two decades earlier, when a summer institute at Gallaudet brought them face-to-face with hearing and deaf linguists investigating ASL, with politically active deaf groups such as Deafpride, and with the American civil rights movement. On return to France, these leaders worked to repossess French deaf history, to investigate *La Langue des Signes Française*, and to initiate the first bilingual courses for deaf children. During this period the Paris-based International Visual Theater, with a deaf director and an all-deaf cast, presented avant-garde plays in LSF on themes in deaf culture. The high visibility of the theater group inspired respect for LSF among both deaf and hearing audiences and led to the first classes in which members of the deaf community taught LSF to parents and professional people. When, in 1985, hearing teachers at the residential school in Poitiers, joined by deaf adults, staged a hunger strike to demand the inclusion of LSF and deaf teachers, they brought the sorry state of deaf education to national attention.

A call to deaf people and their friends a year later to rally at the Bastille in behalf of official recognition of LSF resulted in a media event in which three to five thousand people, including legislators and parents, marched through the city to the offices of the prime minister. The march not only enlightened millions of Frenchmen but also breathed pride, vigor, and a sense of power into the deaf community of France. The reform of deaf education has also been fueled by a hard-hitting and insightful "underground newspaper," focused on the deaf community and its language and called *Coup d'Oeil* (At a Glance). A nationwide association of hearing and deaf people committed to the bilingual education of deaf children, Deux Langues pour Une Education (Two Languages, One Education), which had its own magazine, *Vivre Ensemble* (Living Together), conducted summer institutes where parents, professionals, and deaf leaders gathered and created bilingual classes for deaf children in several cities. This gave rise, in turn, to regional groups engaged in applied research and development related to LSF—for example, the Association les Iris in Toulouse.

Several major books on French Sign Language and the French deaf community, as well as a spendid journal of French deaf history, the *Cahiers de l'Histoire des Sourds*, have appeared since the 1970s. As part of the bicentennial of the French Revolution, a magnificent panorama of French deaf history was prepared and placed on display in the Sorbonne.* An international conference on signed languages held in Poitiers in July 1990 drew inspiration from the Gallaudet Revolution and was in many respects a political gathering to chart a course for reform. This was followed in the fall of 1991 by a major Franco-American conference on "Deaf People in Society," where the

Americans learned from early French initiatives—for example, in bicultural and bilingual education of deaf children—and where the French had much to ponder in the scholarly distinction of the nearly all-deaf American delegation. Shortly before the conference the French legislature passed a law affirming the right of parents to choose between an education for their deaf children conducted exclusively in French and one conducted in both French and LSF; shortly after, some two thousand deaf people took to the Paris streets to demand implementation of the law. I confidently predict major changes in French deaf education in the next few years as deaf adults win their rightful part, and that of their language, in the schools for deaf children.

In Great Britain, deaf people, working together with hearing people, have been broadcasting national and regional television programs aimed at the deaf community and featuring deaf leaders. They have produced two full-length films for television based on my history of deaf communities: the first, aired in 1987, called *Pictures in the Mind*; the second, to be shown in 1992, *The Count of Solar*. The BBC's magazine program for deaf people, "See Hear!," began over a decade ago; "Listening Eye," a current affairs program, first appeared on Channel 4 in 1984. Deaf and hearing Britons have published books on the British deaf community, its language, history, and leaders. Durham and Bristol universities prepare deaf people to teach British Sign Language. The London Deaf Video Project and Deaf Owl make programs for television. The group Deaf Comedians is another expression of the cultural upsurge. And Britons have established the International Sign Linguistics Association and its journal, *Signpost*.

In Canada deaf leaders, spurred by the Gallaudet Revolution, staged rallies that brought their concerns to the attention of the Canadian government. I remember vividly one march in sleet and rain in which it was my bone-chilling privilege to participate; we drew comfort from our numbers and the thought that our ordeal was a persuasive sign to the legislators of our determination. This kind of deaf activism has led to official recognition of ASL in three provinces and a farsighted plan for reforming deaf education in Ontario; that province has appointed a deaf scholar, Dr. Clifford Carbin, to direct bilingual/bicultural programs for deaf children, and it also elected a deaf member of Parliament, Gary Malkowski. School doors have been opening to deaf teachers, bilingual/bicultural educational programs for deaf children are under development, and there are strong prospects that ASL shortly will be declared an official language of instruction for deaf children.

In Germany deaf and hearing people collaborate in research on German Sign Language in the Zentrum für Deutsche Gebärdensprache at the University of Hamburg. Innovative educational programs using German Sign Language with deaf children are under way, and the Gesellschaft für Gebärdensprache (Society for Sign Language) publishes a trailblazing journal, *Das Zeichen,* as well as books and videotapes concerning deaf communities and signed languages. There are new programs for training interpreters in Germany, Austria, and Switzerland, and a center for sign language research in Basel. An International Congress on Sign Language Research and Application convened by the Hamburg center in 1990 helped fuel the reform movement in Germany. German audists then mounted a campaign against German Sign Language, writing letters to government officials denying it had the status of a language. So ill informed is German government about the deaf community in its society that scholars felt it necessary to rebut audist claims with a petition affirming that German Sign Language is a natural language with a crucial role to play in the lives of deaf children and adults and reminding the government that the European Parliament had voted unanimously for member states to recognize their deaf communities as linguistic minorities.

The president of the Moscow Deaf Club, Igor Abramov, informs me that deaf people in his country were greatly encouraged by news of the Gallaudet Revolution, which appeared in *Pravda* and spurred them on in their efforts to break free from the government ministries that have so long exercised control over their lives.

Sweden must be singled out for particular notice, for its deaf leadership has been the most successful and its government's policies toward the deaf community the most enlightened in the world. In 1981, as a result of the activism of the Swedish national association of the deaf, the association of parents of deaf children, and linguists at the University of Stockholm, bilingual and bicultural education was instituted as the official policy in the nation's schools for deaf children. The knowledge that deaf people have concerning their language and culture is now widely respected and seen as essential to the successful education and psychological development of deaf children. The schools have been hiring deaf teachers and other deaf staff members in large numbers, though the effects of banning them for many decades cannot be quickly undone: After ten years, the fraction of the faculty that is deaf now ranges in various schools from a fifth to two thirds. Swedish is taught as a second language, using the children's Swedish Sign Language as the vehicle for this instruction, and there are courses in the history, language, and culture of the Swedish deaf community.

On a visit to the oldest such school in Sweden, founded by a contemporary of Abbé Sicard, I was startled and moved to see the genuine exchange of ideas between teacher and pupils in a fifth-grade discussion of a Swedish poem. (I was accompanied by an interpreter, but you can tell when two people are genuinely engaged in their conversation even if you do not know exactly what they are saying.) The hearing teachers I met told me that they valued their deaf colleagues not only as a source of instruction in the language and culture of the deaf community but also as models of quite novel ways of teaching various subjects. One teacher gave me the example of a deaf colleague's spatial approach to teaching algebra, which proved more successful than the method, based more on notation, that she had been using. I was told, however, that many teachers found the burden of learning Swedish Sign Language onerous and the radical change in the politics of deaf education disorienting and disturbing, initially at least.

"No one in Sweden today advocates mainstreaming of prelingually deaf children," a Swedish educator writes. Because education of deaf children in Sweden uses their signed language but most such children have hearing parents who cannot teach them that language, and many regions are sparsely populated, with few deaf adults, a major outreach program is bringing Swedish Sign Language and deaf adults into the lives of such families. There are special preschools, deaf home visitors, and short-term live-in arrangements, and the nation's deaf clubs host Swedish Sign Language classes and parents' meetings. The success of the present system in Sweden, according to Swedish deaf leader Lars Wallin, is the product of collaboration between the Swedish deaf association, the association of parents of deaf children, and scholars who have investigated Swedish Sign Language and its community of users. Working together, they have put a stop to depriving deaf children of language, they have forged bilingual education, and they have blocked mainstreaming.

Progress toward bilingual education has also been taking place as a matter of national policy in Uruguay and Venezuela, as well as in

Denmark, although in the latter case without a clear government mandate. In America, there are bilingual education programs for ASL-using children in Santa Monica and Fremont, California, in Framingham, Massachusetts, in Philadelphia, Pennsylvania, and in Indianapolis, Indiana; and the list grows longer as the months pass.

Progress is impeded in the United States, however, by the gulf that has separated the National Association of the Deaf and the American Society for Deaf Children (the leading organization of parents), a gulf promoted by the actions of the audist establishment. Audists here contend that parents can never or will never learn manual language—but they do en masse in Sweden and in scattered instances throughout the U.S. and other lands. Audists here contend that parents will never accept their child residing away from home—but they do en masse in Sweden and they did at one time in the U.S. If only organizations representing the deaf community and parents would work in concert here, and elsewhere in the world, as they have in Sweden—what vast progress would be made for deaf children!

Deaf adults around the world are playing a growing role in research on their manual languages, in international congresses and publications concerned with the grammar and use of manual languages, in training interpreters and putting through legislation requiring them, in teaching signed languages to college students and parents of deaf children, in developing teaching materials, in counseling other deaf adults and conducting job training—and in many other areas. However, no matter how much research there is on manual language, no matter how many hearing people learn signed languages and interpreters are trained, no matter how many resolutions are passed by national and international bodies, no matter how self-aware deaf communities have become, the stark and terrifying fact remains that in most countries current educational and medical practices with deaf children are leading more than ever before to a devastating impoverishment of their lives individually and communally.

Because they brought about an abrupt redistribution of power and a heightened awareness of power relations between audists and deaf people, not only on the Gallaudet campus but throughout the nation and beyond, the events of those eight days in March 1988 were, politically speaking, a revolution. But they have yet to bring a revolution in a deeper sense, the sense in which one speaks of the Darwinian revolution or the Freudian revolution: a profound reorganization of thought, in which old categories are demolished, new ones created, and people, artifacts, and events redistributed and reinterpreted. It is *that* revolution that the leaders of the uprising, all deaf children of deaf parents, were seeking in the councils of war that I witnessed. The aim, in my view (they must speak for themselves), was a reconceptualization of deaf people, especially by hearing people but also by many deaf people themselves, in terms of language, culture, and shared experience.

The Gallaudet Revolution has yet to fulfill its promise. If it succeeds in crystallizing a new structure of thought about deaf people, then it will have achieved something of value enduring long beyond the lives of those who participated in it. If deaf children grow up in a world in which there is a conceptualization of deaf people different from the one that dominates now, there will be different kinds of deaf people, and different kinds of hearing people who interact with them regularly. The deaf children will see themselves in another light right from the beginning; so will their peers, parents, and teachers, who will relate to them accordingly, and the children will grow into another kind of deaf person, potentially prouder, stronger, better educated, bringing a unique contribution to the knowledge of humankind and the ordering of society.

When oppressed peoples have taken control of their destiny in the former colonies, frequently by the use of force, the dreams that seemed to justify the struggle and sacrifice were often not realized. Political repression and economic hardship continued under the new local authorities. That development cannot be divorced from the history of oppression under the colonial authority, but neither can it be totally explained or justified by it. What are the dangers of reforming the professions serving the deaf community so that deaf people play a preponderant role? To try and formulate these dangers and to reflect on them is the first step in guarding against them.

Perhaps the first danger to consider is unrealistic expectations. Literacy, for example, is an unsurmountable challenge for some hearing children, and it will probably remain so for some deaf children as well. A second concern must be that the new leaders will repeat the sins of their forebears. Where the audist establishment was ethnocentric, the new leadership could prove so too. For example, in reaction to the long years of oppression of ASL, English teaching might get less attention than it deserves in some of the new bilingual programs, just as, according to critics, it is slighted in some bilingual education for Spanish-speaking children. Where the audist establishment locked out deaf people, the new leaders may lock out some hearing people and shortsightedly give a large measure of solidarity to some deaf people who do not warrant it. It may be difficult for the new leaders to engage in and allow self-criticism, which may seem like betrayal after the long struggle.

Another area of potential concern lies in how the new leadership deals with deaf children and adults who are acculturated to the hearing community. This group has accused the deaf community in the past of using their numbers to win concessions but not really seeking to address their specific needs. Hearing parents must be concerned, too, that their deaf child, welcomed into a "new family" with which he shares language, history, and culture, is not led to loosen the bonds to his hearing family.

If we are prepared to respect deaf leaders, then we must accept that deaf people have the same right to make mistakes that hearing people have. Indeed, deaf leadership may have a greater right, since hearing people so often preempted their chances to try managing things for themselves. It seems to me that the wisest course is for deaf leaders to have internal control combined with external accountability. Services for deaf people should be organized so that they themselves have a preponderant voice in shaping the future of the deaf community while, at the same time, deaf and hearing managers are accountable to other concerned groups, the deaf community, hard-of-hearing people, hearing parents, and, ultimately, the nation at large.

We are very far from placing deaf destiny in the hands of deaf people, however. The concerns I have mentioned and others like them pertain to a world we are still far from realizing. The truest friends of deaf people, those with the deepest commitment to effective education of deaf children, will work together with deaf individuals and organizations to forge a hearing and deaf partnership in deaf education. For that partnership to be forged, both parties must bring their cultural frames into consciousness, construct a mutual understanding of those frames, and make an empathic leap, trying to position themselves at each other's "center."

PART SEVEN

Bio-Power Versus the Deaf Child

12 pt
on final

Oralism's Ultimate Recourse

The challenge presented by the cultural renaissance of the deaf community, the continued failure of special education, and the Gallaudet Revolution is to stop thinking of culturally deaf people as hearing people who have lost their hearing and to start thinking of them as members of a linguistic minority, as hale as the rest of us, as wise and as foolish, and equally entitled to self-determination. Far from facing this challenge, however, rethinking our premises and reforming our policies, we permit the disastrous mainstreaming of deaf children to proceed apace, and now the Food and Drug Administration has authorized the most extreme measures of cultural denial, the most aggressive medical reaffirmation of the infirmity model of the deaf community in all of deaf history. If true reform is to come, it will be because the deaf community and society at large have brought sufficient pressure to bear on those who are interposed between our two groups, namely, the audist establishment.

The desperate plight of deaf people portrayed by sham psychometrics, the design and failure of special education, which that portrayal is invoked to justify, and the desperate "cure" undertaken with highly experimental surgical implants are interrelated and interlegitimating programs of the audist establishment. "An essential component of the technologies of normalization," writes Foucault interpreter Paul Rabinow, "is the key role they play in the systematic creation, classification, and control of 'anomalies' in the social body. Their *raison d'etre* comes from two claims of their promoters: first, that certain technologies serve to isolate anomalies; and second, that one can then normalize anomalies through corrective or therapeutic procedures, determined by other related technologies. In both cases, the technologies of normalization are purportedly impartial techniques for dealing with dangerous social deviations." The connections among measurement practices, special education, and ear surgery are not only intellectual and abstract, they are also administrative and operational. If cultural deafness were not medicalized by psychometrics and audiology, there would be no special education but simply bilingual education for children whose primary language is ASL. There is no need for special education of deaf children as the term is now construed, any more than there is a need for special education of Native American children or Hispanic-American children. Of course, each group needs teachers with special credentials—a knowledge of cultural mores, language, and history. In this sense, all language minorities require a special education. If the members of the deaf community were characterized in cultural terms and bilingual education was largely successful, parents would be less motivated to subject their deaf children to surgery of little value and unassessed long-term risk.

When the U.S. Food and Drug Administration approved the Cochlear Corporation's request to market its cochlear prosthesis for surgical implantation in deaf children over the age of two, essentially one group of doctors gave another group of doctors permission to operate on a new population of patients. The Ear, Nose and Throat Devices Panel of the FDA, which ruled on the fate of innumerable deaf children and adults in the decades to come, consists entirely of hearing people: five ear doctors, an audiologist, a representative of implant manufacturing, and a "consumer representative"—not a deaf person, mind you, or the parent of a deaf child, but a hearing educator of deaf children, a member of the audist establishment. The choice seems bizarre until it is understood as one more reflection of the intimate relations in audism between measurement, education, and medicine. In America there is no place for deaf people where decisions about deaf lives are being made.

The cochlear implant teams thus authorized to conduct surgery generally consist of a surgeon, several audiologists and speech/language pathologists, and special educators. The teams have, in turn, resuscitated outmoded oralist practices—drills in pronunciation and lip-reading, instruction using spoken language only. The few oralist educational programs that had remained in the United States, serving largely children who once heard and spoke English, are experiencing a rebirth: Their ranks are growing anew with children who have been implanted; some of these were deafened late in childhood, others at birth or in early childhood. Cochlear implant teams are seeking the maximum commitment to postsurgical training in listening and speaking. They ask a profound commitment of the parents, who are to be trained in the elements of speech therapy and then apply them in daily sessions with their deaf child at home. One mother of an implanted child recounts: "I was so into the therapy training, I even went when I was in early labor [with my next child]."

The implant teams equally ask a commitment to oral practices by the school and consider it a counterindication for implant surgery if the school will not use speech with the child and provide speech and listening therapy. Some implant teams send team members out to the schools to ensure oralist practices, and they seek to influence directly or indirectly the formulation of the child's Individualized Educational Plan to include extensive training in listening, speech, and lip-reading—at the expense, inevitably, of time devoted to academic subjects. Parents are frequently led to supplement this oral training given at home and at school with further training delivered several times weekly by private therapists.

There is no evidence that these oralist practices at home, at school, and in the clinic are effective, any more than there was evidence of their effectiveness in the era before they were abandoned in the schools in favor of total communication.* They are not undertaken because they are of proven value. They are sought by the implant teams because childhood implantation and oral education are expressions of the same underlying system of values—namely, audism.

The three-pronged endeavor takes control of the body of the child psychometrically, educationally, and surgically. Those who orient the parents to the service their child supposedly requires and those who provide the services are in league: Audiologists are commonly sympathetic to oral-education programs; otologists to audiologists and speech therapists. Deaf people must be kept away from orienting roles. Michel Foucault was right when he said that in such social struggles, bodies are the battlefield. Cochlear implantation requires that the child be defined as several sets of numbers and then categorized accordingly. The audiologist makes measures and labels the child, say, "profoundly hearing-impaired"; the psychologist makes measures—we have seen some of the problems here—and assigns labels that are taken to reflect how intelligent the child is, how well-adjusted, how modest his expectations are for the benefits of the implant. What is needed is a full measurement "profile" of the child, and only those children with the right "profile" will be accepted by the implant team.

Cochlear implantation also dictates the child's communicative relations with his parents and others and shapes his home environment; it influences the school to commit itself to nonacademic goals and specific methods in striving to reach them; and it implants experimental electronic devices in the child's skull that continually affect his sensory milieu, his relations with those around him, and his image of himself. The intervention is comprehensive and long-term. The National Institutes of Health Consensus Conference on Cochlear Implants said it clearly: "Children with implants still must be regarded as hearing-impaired [and] will continue to require educational, audiological, and speech and language support services for long periods of time." This is bio-power: massive intervention in the life of the child in an attempt to impose the majority's language, culture, and values.

Substantial amounts of money are involved. The psychologists or others administering the psychometric tests must be paid. The audiologists who measure the remaining hearing, if any, must be paid. The radiologists who make x-rays of the inner ear to guide the surgeon must be paid. The surgeon, the anesthesiologist, and the hospital must be paid. The manufacturer of the implant device must be paid. The audiologist who tunes the device after it is implanted must be paid. The speech and hearing therapist who gives the child training at the hospital must be paid. The psychologist who counsels the parents and possibly the patient must be paid. The special educator who evaluates the school, monitors its oral training, and often trains the teachers must be paid. The school's speech therapist must be paid, and the private therapist must be paid. There are no hard figures available, but cost estimates run between $30,000 and $50,000 during the first year. The parents pay some, insurance pays some, local taxpayers pay some; and since many of the roughly four hundred children implanted in the U.S. have been research subjects, the National Institute on Deafness and Other Communication Disorders (fruit of the Gallaudet Revolution) also pays some.

An embarrassment for the medical model of cultural deafness heretofore was that this "pathology" had no medical treatment. With cochlear implants, however, the medical specialty of otology has been expanding its traditional clientele beyond adventitiously deafened hearing people who seek treatment, for whom an infirmity model is appropriate, to include members of the deaf community, for whom it is not. There are various measures of the success of medicalization, but one that is understandably important to the health professions is whether the medicalized group seeks their services. By this measure, there is no prospect of medicalizing the million or so deaf adults in America's deaf community—they reject the claim that they have a medical problem. This apparently came as a surprise and a great disappointment to the early manufacturers of cochlear implants, who envisioned selling some three hundred thousand devices (sales of four and a half billion dollars) in the United States alone. There is, however, the possibility of medicalizing culturally deaf people before they become adults, while they are still children. Why? Because of the remarkable fact that most members of this cultural and linguistic minority have hearing parents who do not transmit and will not share the linguistic and cultural identity of their deaf children. The children themselves are too young to refuse treatment or to dispute the infirmity model of their difference. Their hearing parents, frequently beset by guilt, grief, and anxiety, and largely ignorant of the deaf community, commonly accept the infirmity model uncritically, and consequently turn for help to the related social institutions, such as medicine, audiology, and special education.

As a reasoned position, the medicalization of cultural deafness faces several difficulties; here are five.

• Adults with this putative medical problem insist they do not have a medical problem.

• The putatively handicapped population has a common language and social organization; their shared culture puts us more in mind of, say, Hispanic-Americans than of, for example, blind Americans. History provides many examples of more dominant cultural groups labeling less dominant cultural groups as defective, but no example of an entire linguistic and cultural minority that is truly infirm.

• The otologists and audiologists who apply the infirmity model to culturally deaf people are often unaware of the language and mores of those whose way of being and behaving they consider infirm.

• There is no medical treatment that will improve the quality of life of the putatively infirm population as a whole.

• Some of the professions collaborating in the medicalization of this population have a financial and social stake in designating cultural deafness as a medical/handicap problem.

Although these considerations weigh against the infirmity model of cultural deafness, many hearing professional people hold tenaciously to that model. Surgical implantation of deaf children with cochlear prostheses has grown in just a few years from a closely regulated research procedure for a few children to an open market for the many; when the FDA approved implants for deaf children, it stated that there are more than one hundred centers offering surgeon/audiologist teams who implant the device in the United States alone.

Cochlear implants can be a useful prosthesis for some hearing people who have lost their hearing. According to the 1988 Institutes of Health Consensus Conference, a suitable candidate for an implant is usually a healthy, postlingually deafened adult with a profound hearing loss, whose performance in lip-reading is not enhanced by a hearing aid. By requiring that the implant recipient be healthy, this policy ensures that the adult makes the decision to have an implant calmly, after mature reflection, long after the medical crisis that led to deafening. By requiring that the recipient be postlingually deafened—that is, deafened after having acquired oral language—the consensus greatly increases the chances that the patient will profit from the implant, for it takes a knowledge of how the language sounds (and usually skill at lip-reading as well) to associate the unfamiliar sounds coming from the implant with the words intended and spoken by the speaker.

Why, then, are growing numbers of culturally deaf children, who do not meet several of these criteria, receiving implants? It is, of course, because the cultural differences of the deaf community—different language, different mores—have been medicalized. The active agent in the medicalization of cultural deafness is the audist establishment, but it cannot succeed without the consent of the "patients," who reject it, or their surrogates, the parents of deaf children, who embrace it. The medicalization of cultural deafness not only "makes sense" to uninformed hearing parents; it also holds out a false hope—that their child will not embrace a minority language and culture, which they find alien.

The medicalization of deviance is part of a larger social phenomenon that Ivan Illich has called "the medicalization of life": The purview of medicine has come to include contraception, fertility, pregnancy, childbirth, child development, hyperactivity in children, reading difficulty, learning problems, drug addiction, criminality, child abuse, physical disability, exercise, hygiene, sleeplessness, diet, breast and nose size, wrinkles, baldness, obesity, shortness, cultural deafness—the list seems never to end. Not all medical intervention in social issues is bad; sometimes it serves us well and derives great prestige from doing so. That is just why we have to be wary of its abuse. Children are particularly vulnerable to medicalization: They are considered not responsible, they are not politically organized, and experts have greater authority over their bodies than they do over the bodies of adults. The medicalization of childhood deviance is fueled by the great prestige of medicine in our society; by the willingness of insurers to pay for treatment if it is rendered by a doctor; and by the efforts of interested parties in disguising social issues as private troubles. The locus of the educational problem of deaf children is not in the child. The forces at work have to do with language, power, and social groups. When the audist establishment affirms that the locus of the problem is in the individual deaf child, it asks that we seek to change the victim rather than the society that has victimized him.

Likewise, in the medical treatment of overactive children, doctors and parents, urged on by teachers, administer drugs to the individual child instead of addressing the relevant social forces in the family and the school.* By locating the source of the problem in the individual—the source of poor educational achievement in biological deficit, the source of criminality in psychiatric disorder, the source of deaf underemployment in cochlear malfunction—medical discourse mystifies; it screens the social origins of these problems. It also provides a reassuring aura of professional competence to solve them. Medicalization is the tranquilizer we take to put our social problems out of mind. Deaf children and the deaf community in America today pose social challenges to the audist establishment, which it refuses to acknowledge and accommodate.

Illnesses are socially constructed. The construction is constrained certainly by physiology; it is also constrained by the ecology of the culture in which the illness occurs and by the nature of medical discourse and medical institutions in that culture. "How Short Is Too Short?" asked the *New York Times Magazine* in June 1991. Doctors working for Genentech, Inc., which manufactures an experimental human growth hormone costing each "patient" $20,000 a year, answer: shorter than 97 percent of the population. "Until growth hormone came along," an ethicist quoted by the *Times* points out, "no one called normal shortness a disease. It's become a disease only because a manipulation has become available, and because doctors and insurance companies, in order to rationalize their actions, have had to perceive it as one." Despite the synthetic hormone's side effects and its high cost, its sales amounted to $157 million in 1990, up more than 40 percent from two years earlier. Ninety thousand children born annually are below the 97 percent cutoff, which corresponds to a potential annual market of $8 billion to $10 billion. Best of all for Genentech, this "disease" can never be eradicated, for no matter what the height of our population, there will always be a shortest 3 percent. According to Genentech doctors, however, treating these children is not a minor matter of cosmetics: statistics show that our society is "heightist," and short people do not get a fair deal.

Whether one holds baldness to be a genetic disease, medical ethicists point out, "depends on one's judgment of the importance to a proper human form of a full head of hair. . . . If disease and health are to be identified as unsuccessful and successful adaptations, one must specify the reference environment . . . , the goals of the adaptation . . . , and whether one is regarding the species or the individual."

What one society considers a disease, another may not. Many societies in which alcohol or tobacco are widely and heavily consumed, in which eyeglasses are a commonplace, where teeth are normally lost with aging, where plumpness is favored over slimness, or where minor hookworm infestation is widespread would reject the claim that most of their population was suffering from diseases such as alcoholism, nicotine addiction, presbyopia, periodontal disease, obesity, or parasitic infection. To attribute sickness is to imply the existence of another state, which is more desirable. Thus, if a physical condition is widespread enough in a community and does not interfere substantially with the community achieving its goals, it will be seen as an illness only by outsiders with a different cultural frame of reference and different goals.

In prerevolutionary China, upper-class women whose feet were bound and who walked with difficulty and pain were not considered diseased or infirm. In northern Iran, "heart distress" is a common illness; patients complain of their hearts pounding, quivering, or feeling squeezed or pressed. People are also aware that the heart is associated with affective life, with feelings of sadness, anxiety, and being trapped. "Heart distress" occurs most often among adult women, especially those in the lower classes. It is associated with feelings of weakness, weak nerves, general malaise. The physicians who have studied it have concluded that it is a "culturally specific illness." In Sri Lanka, mental illnesses are commonly thought to be supernaturally caused and to be easily cured. Although Western psychiatrists faced with a patient who is withdrawn, lethargic, and excessively laconic may diagnose depression, these are seldom thought of as symptoms of an illness in Sri Lanka. A 1981 study found that the proportion of individuals labeled schizophrenic who had no further episodes of illness after the first one ranged from 58 percent in Nigeria, 51 percent in India, and 40 percent in Sri Lanka to 7 percent in the U.S.S.R. and 6 percent in Denmark. Mothers in many nations—India, for example—see pregnancy as normal and not requiring medical intervention. In the West, alcoholism has gone from a crime to an illness. Masturbation was considered a disease in the nineteenth century, the cause of epilepsy, blindness and deafness, vertigo, headache, and many other disorders; clitoridectomy and castration were among the treatments. Homosexuality was demedicalized in the 1970s, but "lack of sexual desire" has followed the opposite course. As Harvard psychiatrist Nancy Waxler has put it: "What kind of illness an individual is believed to have is not a cut and dried affair dependent simply on a physician's diagnosis. Instead, illness labels are created in social negotiations."

The physicians who have conducted research on cochlear implants with young children, and those on the Ear, Nose and Throat Devices Panel who have approved the marketing of these devices, have been guided apparently by an unreflective naturalism—what is natural is to hear, see, reproduce, behave oneself, work; nature gone awry is to be remedied by natural science applied. This framework is more suited to laboratory animals than to human children who have a language, a culture, and a cultural history within which any medical intervention takes place and which determine the final value of that intervention. Frequently the doctor does not consider the consequences of his intervention beyond the organ of the body concerned, because there are latent assumptions: Fertility is better than infertility; "normal" weight and height are best; a little hearing is better than none. But those assumptions can be wrong for any individual, and the risk that they are wrong increases with the distance between the doctor's culture and the patient's. In other cultural frames, these seemingly self-evident goods do not appear meritorious in themselves. In particular, enhanced hearing is not a good within the cultural framework of the deaf community. Fluency in ASL, however, is an evident good.

Heroic Treatments in Historical Perspective

Desperate and useless medical measures to address what we hearing people see as the desperate plight of culturally deaf children have a long history. The otologist who succeeded Jean-Marc Itard as resident physician of the Paris school for deaf children captured the audist medical view well, writing in 1853: "The deaf believe that they are our equals in all respects. We should be generous and not destroy that illusion. But whatever they believe, deafness is an infirmity and we should repair it whether the person who has it is disturbed by it or not." It was necessary for Dr. Prosper Ménière to make this outrageous affirmation precisely because deaf people were not disturbed by being deaf. On the contrary, in the last century, as in this one, culturally deaf people thought deaf was a perfectly good way to be, as good as hearing, perhaps better.

Itard undertook the most extravagant medical procedures with culturally deaf children once his many years of trying to teach them oral skills had utterly failed. He started by applying electricity to the ears of some pupils, since an Italian surgeon had recently found that a frog's leg would contract if touched with charged metal. Itard thought there was some analogy between the paralysis of the hearing organ and the paralysis of a limb. He also placed leeches on the necks of some of the pupils at the school founded by Abbé de l'Epée and directed at that time by his successor, Abbé Sicard, in the hope that local bleeding would help somehow. Six students had their eardrums pierced, but the operation was painful and fruitless, and Itard desisted. Not soon enough for one student, who died following this treatment. At first, however, his ears discharged some foreign matter and he reportedly recovered some hearing and with it some speech, which led Itard to think the deaf ear might be blocked up rather than paralyzed.

It was said that the postmaster at Versailles had cured his own hearing loss by inserting a probe in his Eustachian tube, which leads from the throat to the ear, and "flushing out the lymphatic excrement." The method had been widely tried by physicians and abandoned as impracticable and ineffective. Itard made improvements to the probe and then subjected to the treatment one hundred twenty pupils, almost every last one in the school (two dozen would not be subdued). Nothing at all was accomplished.

Following this failure, Itard dispensed a secret brew into the ears of every pupil in the school who was not born deaf, a few drops a day for two weeks—without effect. With other students he tried a regime of daily purgatives; still others had their ears covered with a bandage soaked in a blistering agent. Within a few days, the ear lost all its skin, oozed pus, and was excruciatingly painful. When it scabbed, Itard reapplied the bandage and the wound reopened. Then the cycle was repeated, with caustic soda spread on the skin behind the ear. All of this was to no avail. Still Itard remained relentless in his search for a cure. He tried fracturing the skull of a few pupils, striking the area just behind the ear with a hammer. With a dozen pupils he applied a white-hot metal button behind the ear, which led to pus and a scab in about a week. Yet another of his treatments was to thread a string through a pupil's neck with a seton needle, which caused a suppurating wound that supposedly allowed feculent humors to dry up. It was all a miserable failure. "Medicine does not work on the dead," Itard finally concluded, "and as far as I am concerned the ear is dead in the deaf-mute. There is nothing for science to do about it."

Early in the next century the medicalization of cultural deafness was promoted by the eugenics movement, which sought to "improve" the race by selective breeding. If the members of the deaf community indeed suffered from an infirmity, as the medicalization of cultural deafness would have it, and if deafness ran in families, as it clearly did at times, then it stood to reason for many audists that deaf people should be discouraged from reproducing. The most renowned and influential audist in this period was Alexander Graham Bell, and he devoted his great wealth, fame, and prestige to these measures. When the Breeders' Association created a section on eugenics "to emphasize the value of superior blood and the menace to society of inferior blood," Bell agreed to serve. In 1920, he published a warning that Americans were committing race suicide, for "Children of foreign born parents are increasing at a much greater rate than the children of native born parents." As selective immigration laws had been only partially successful, he argued, restriction on marriage or childbearing might be necessary: "It is now felt that the interests of the race demand that the best should marry and have large families and that any restrictions on reproduction should apply to the worst rather than the best." He was opposed, however, to laws forbidding marriage of deaf people and other undesirables (as he called them). "This would not produce the desired improvement," he wrote, "for even were we to go to the extreme length of killing off the undesirables altogether, so that they could not propagate their kind . . . it would diminish the production of the undesirables without increasing the production of the desirables."

Bell specifically engaged the issue of eugenics and the deaf population beginning in the 1880s, shortly after the Congress of Milan. Sign language and the residential schools were creating a deaf community, he warned, in which deaf people intermarried and reproduced, a situation fraught with danger to the rest of the society. He sounded the alarm in a *Memoir upon the Formation of a Deaf Variety of the Human Race*, presented to the National Academy of Sciences. Since there are familial patterns of deafness, he wrote, "It is to be feared that the intermarriage of such persons would be attended by calamitous results to their offspring." Congenitally deaf people without deaf relatives also run a risk in marrying, as do people deafened adventitiously who have deaf relatives. If these persons marry, Bell reasoned, and some of their children marry congenitally deaf people, and then some of theirs do, and so on, the proportion of deaf children born of such marriages will increase from generation to generation until nearly all their children will be born deaf. These families "would then constitute a variety of the human race in which deafness would be the rule rather than the exception."

In his recommendations, Bell considered repressive and preventive measures. Under the first heading, a law prohibiting deaf adults from marriage might merely promote deaf children born out of wedlock. A law prohibiting only congenitally deaf adults from marrying "would go a long way towards checking the evil," but it is difficult to prove whether a person was born deaf or not. "Legislation forbidding the intermarriage of persons belonging to families containing more than one deaf-mute would be more practical. This would cover the intermarriage of hearing parents belonging to such families." But more data are needed before we can justify the passage of such an act, he said.

Thus, for the present, Bell found that preventive measures must suffice. "We commence our efforts on behalf of the deaf-mute by changing his social environment." Residential schools should be closed and the deaf educated in small day schools. Coeducation with hearing children would be the ideal, "but this is not practicable to any great extent." Sign language and deaf teachers should be banished, speech encouraged by hearing teachers. As an audist par excellence, Bell believed speech to be the highest possible value for deaf people. When the Conference of Principals of Schools for the Deaf placed on its agenda the question "What is the importance of speech to the deaf?" Bell was flabbergasted: "I am astonished. I am pained. To ask the value of speech? It is like asking the value of life! . . . What is the object of the education of the deaf and dumb if it is not to set them in communication with the world?" This belief persists in the audist establishments of many nations, and the desperate educational plight of deaf children in those nations makes them particularly vulnerable to heroic medicine. For example, British experts on deaf education wrote in 1982: "Developing deaf pupils' ability to communicate, preferably in an oral way, is the central goal of deaf education"; and, in 1986, "Language development must be the central facet of their educational programme."

Bell's memoir on the formation of a deaf variety of the human race received wide newspaper coverage. There was much consternation among deaf people contemplating marriage, and numerous letters to the press, as well as journal articles, vigorously repudiated Bell's views. Whatever his intention, his actions led many to believe that there would be, or already were, laws prohibiting the marriage of deaf couples. Proposals to segregate congenitally deaf adults were made, as were counterproposals to allow them freedom as long as they did not reproduce. News of Bell's memoir spread rapidly among parents of deaf children, "their family physicians, and among surgeons generally throughout the world," a pastor to the deaf community has written, "and suggested to them a senseless and cruel procedure—the sterilization of children born deaf." This observer had come to know many deaf couples who were childless and unhappy as a result of having been sterilized in infancy; he laid the blame on Bell.

A 1912 report from Bell's eugenics section of the Breeders' Association cites his census of blind and deaf persons and lists "socially unfit" classes, including deaf people, whose supply should, if possible, "be eliminated from the human stock." The model eugenic law called for the sterilization of feebleminded, insane, criminalistic ("including the delinquent and the wayward"), epileptic, inebriate, diseased, blind, deaf, deformed, and dependent people ("including orphans, ne'er-do-wells, the homeless, tramps, and paupers"). By the time of World War I, sixteen states had sterilization laws in force. By 1940, thirty states had such laws, providing for compulsory sterilization of confirmed criminals, moral degenerates, prostitutes, "and other diseased and degenerate persons." Physicians were actively involved in this eugenics movement. We are shocked at the extremity of the measures that our society was willing to take; but our surprise at some of the classes of people to be sterilized teaches an even more important lesson. What "common sense" and medical science plainly show to be an illness in one culture and epoch are plainly considered not to be so in another place and time.

Bell presupposed, first, that familial deafness is a defect to be avoided; and, second, that society's interest in avoiding that defect outweighed deaf people's interest in compatible marriage choice and childbearing. For someone who believed that Italians were adulterating American racial stock, it was inconceivable that deaf people were not. Indeed, so hermetic was Bell's egocentricity that he was sure the outrage of deaf people and their friends at his proposals must reflect some misunderstanding, and he welcomed an invitation to address deaf students personally at Gallaudet College. "It is the duty of every good man and every good woman," Bell told them, "to remember that children follow marriage, and I am sure there is no one among the deaf who desires to have his affliction handed down to his children. . . . I therefore hold before you as the ideal marriage, a marriage with a hearing person." This amounted to urging the students to forgo marriage altogether, for nearly all the hearing people they knew who understood them and their kind had deaf relatives, and Bell enjoined the students from those marriages as well, since such marriages were as likely to transmit deafness as the students' preferred pairing with another deaf person.

The Risks and Limitations of Childhood Cochlear Implants

Among the biological means aimed at regulating and, ultimately, eliminating deaf culture, language, and community, cochlear implants have historical antecedents, then, in medical experimentation on deaf children and reproductive regulation of deaf adults.

The child who receives a cochlear implant runs the usual medical risks associated with general anesthesia and surgery. According to one report, about one child in thirty who is implanted develops complications such as pain, infection, drainage, or slow healing of his wound; displacement or misplacement of the electrode; and damage to his facial nerve during the surgery; another study reports complications as often as one patient in seven implanted with the standard Nucleus-22 device; the FDA's "Summary of Safety and Effectiveness Data" cites the alarming figure of one child in six with adverse reactions and complications. Usually, the surgeon can resolve these problems—frequently at the cost of more surgical intervention. Even if there are no complications associated with the initial implantation, however, the child may have surgery again one day, since the internal parts of the implant could break down and since improvements in the design of implants over the next sixty or seventy years of his life could require changing the internal coil or electrodes. As a pioneering otosurgeon in this field put it: "Once a child is implanted, he is an implant patient for life." However, the deeply inserted wire electrodes that the FDA has approved may be difficult to remove without serious structural damage. Furthermore, the effects of damaging the ear through insertion, as well as the effects of long-term electrical stimulation, are unknown. There are children who have had electrodes removed because of device failure or improvements in design and who were then reimplanted. The surgeons of some of them say their patients have never recovered their prior level of perceptual ability; but other surgeons claim explanting and reimplanting poses no problem. In any case, it is clear that a cochlear implant is not a hearing aid; hearing aids go into the ear canal without any difficulty, and their insertion does not cause structural damage, although their prolonged use may. They may be cast aside permanently (many deaf youngsters put them aside when they become adolescent), or they may be replaced.

Moreover, the cochlear implant approved for children by the FDA has many more external parts than the typical hearing aid and is much more visible. The child wears, first, an earpiece that resembles a hearing aid; it contains a microphone that picks up the sound. Then there are two wires running from the earpiece; one ends in a transmitter that contains a small magnet, which holds it in place over the coil the surgeon implanted under the skin behind the ear. The second wire hangs loosely down to chest or waist level, where it connects with the third external part—an electronic circuit in a box about the size of a pack of cigarettes. This speech processor, strapped to the child's chest, or placed on a belt or in a pocket with older children, selects the parts of the sound wave generally most useful for understanding speech and sends them over the wire to the earpiece and on to the transmitting coil. The coil in turn sends electromagnetic waves across the skin, which are detected by the internal coil, and the signal is sent along the wire to the appropriate electrodes in the inner ear.

The implant has twenty-two electrodes spaced at intervals along the wire the surgeon has placed in the inner ear; when an electrode receives pulses, it creates an electromagnetic field that stimulates nerve cells located near it in the core of the cochlea. Those cells excite other cells, and so on up to the auditory region of the brain, where the pattern of nerve firing is interpreted as a pattern of sound. In a person with normal hearing, there are some 35,000 nerve cells in the core of the cochlea. Research in progress indicates that the more cells remain, the more the implant can aid the patient in understanding speech; however, persons with hereditary deafness, the most common cause, seem to have particularly low numbers of nerve cells in the cochlea.

Apart from hereditary factors, the most common cause of deafness in the child's first years is meningitis, a viral disease. The physiology of children deafened by this disease, like those with hereditary deafness, potentially poses a special problem for implantation. On the one hand, a sequel to the disease is bony growth in the inner ear over the next half year; that growth will impede the insertion of an electrode, and the operated child then incurs the risk of little perceptual benefit from the implant. "I wish parents would realize that the clock is ticking," said a leading otologist, urging prompt surgery in these cases before the bony growth occurs. On the other hand, parents are still grieving and are confused by conflicting advice concerning ASL and English and school placement; the child is alarmed by his inability to communicate, and it is difficult to conduct the necessary tests. Time is needed to counsel the parents, train the child in lip-reading, assess the recovery of hearing that occurs in some cases, and see what benefits a hearing aid provides. Hasty surgery may yield little auditory gain; the child may even hear less with the implant than he would have without the surgery and with hearing aids instead.

It would be a mistake to think that someone who has received an implant can hear again as he did before deafening. After all, the complex mechanism of the ear "designed" to convert sound waves into nerve impulses has been bypassed by the implant electrodes, which stimulate the nerves directly. Consider the essentials of that finely constructed mechanism, the product of eons of evolution: Someone speaks, and the sound waves move the listener's eardrum, which, for faint sounds, may vibrate over a distance equal to the diameter of a hydrogen atom; the drum in turn drives the tiny bones of the middle ear, which amplify the vibration and transmit it to a diaphragm on the inner ear. The diaphragm vibrates in its turn, creating waves in the fluid of the inner ear that travel up the cochlea through a canal formed by membranes. The mechanics of the cochlea are so arranged that it acts like an electronic filter, sorting out the different frequencies in the sound striking the eardrum: the traveling wave deforms the lower, basilar membrane at several places along its coiled extent, each place corresponding to a component frequency of the sound. The auditory nerve runs up through the center of the "snail" and sends offshoots along the extent of the basilar membrane. Resting on that membrane throughout its length are microscopic cells with tiny projecting hairs, some of which are wedged into an overhanging membrane and act as a biological strain gauge. When the traveling wave creates a depression at a certain location on the basilar membrane, that membrane moves with respect to its over-hang, and the projecting hairs are deflected—for weak sounds, less than three one-thousandths of a degree, which corresponds to dis-placing the top of the Eiffel Tower by a thumb's width. The hairs' deflection in turn causes current to flow through the hair cell; the cell then secretes a chemical into the gap that separates it from an adjacent offshoot of the auditory nerve. The chemical travels across the gap and stimulates the nerve cell. From this point on, nature and the implant share the same mechanism: the auditory nerve, with its relay stations and representation on the surface of the brain. But prior to that point, the mechanisms are very different: a microphone, a processor (the pattern of nerve firing in the auditory region of the brain is abnormal with the FDA-approved implant because its processor does some preliminary analysis of the original sound, which does not duplicate processing in the normal ear), and a wire with electrodes, in the one case; in the other, two diaphragms connected by bones, traveling waves in a fluid medium, mechanical separation of component frequencies, which changes current flow in adjacent structures and triggers nerve transmission.

The result of the discrepancies between the implant and the natural mechanism of hearing is a sound that many formerly hearing adults have trouble interpreting and sometimes even localizing. Nevertheless, with experience perhaps a fifth of all formerly hearing adults who have been implanted find that they can connect up the sounds they are hearing with their knowledge of the sounds of English, especially when they can see the speaker's lips, and they do quite well in oral communication. Another three-fifths achieve modest gains in their lip-reading scores; the remainder derive little or no profit at all from the implant.

The success of cochlear implants with children is much more limited. One large study conducted by the Cochlear Corporation examined deaf children before they had surgery for the implant and again a year later, after many hours of training in speaking and listening with the implant. The children were given seven tests of speech perception with words and sentences chosen from a long list and presented clearly in a quiet place; their scores using the implant were reliably higher than before the implant on only two of the seven tests. Worse yet, the children's average scores on those tests where they did improve reliably were only 11 and 13 percent correct, even though many in the sample of about thirty children had become deaf after learning English.* If 90 percent of the children had been born deaf or deafened before learning English, as in the deaf school-age population at large, the average scores would have been even lower.*

Investigators at Indiana University tested the ability of a like number of children with the same implant to understand common phrases like "Close the door." The children were accurate, on the average, on only one sentence in ten, although the task was so easy that profoundly deaf children wearing hearing aids averaged better than eight out of ten. All in all, the Indiana researchers conclude, "children with multi-channel cochlear implants continued to have limited auditory speech perception abilities and required hearing-impaired rehabilitative services." Likewise, implant surgeons at the University of Pittsburgh School of Medicine state: "It is important to stress to the parents that their child will continue to be severely hearing-impaired."

The first and fundamental question that parents have for the doctor is: Can you make my deaf child hear? They generally do not mean: Will implant surgery give him any hearing at all? They mean, rather: Will he be able to hear well enough to learn our language, to communicate with us, with his teachers, and with other hearing people? In short, they want the deafness undone. The otologist who is abreast of the latest research will answer, as we have seen, that the miracle the parents hope for is very unlikely if their child is typical, and that he cannot predict the outcome of the surgery—where the child will place in the range between scarcely any hearing and an ability to understand some speech. There are several reasons for our present ignorance.

• Rigorous experimental reports on children are few and have just begun to trickle in. The longest experience of implant use in children is with single-channel implants inserted in experiments done in the 1980s, but the results were poor indeed;* the manufacturer, 3M, has stopped production, and multichannel implants are coming into general use instead.

• Many reports of research combine indiscriminately results for mixed populations of children, deafened for various reasons, deaf for various periods of time, and measured in various laboratories with various procedures and tests.

• Testing is often conducted by speech therapists and teachers who are "rooting for" the implanted child, and their biases can creep into the scoring.

• It is difficult to test young children in a reliable and valid way, particularly if the experimenter and the child do not have a common language, all the more so if the child has had limited access to a language up to the time of testing—the case with many young deaf children. In order to get any results at all, the experimenter is sometimes forced to suit the test to the child: for example, to present only those few words the deaf child knows; that's like getting to choose among the questions you must answer on an exam—your score will be inflated. Average scores are also inflated when implanted children who do not respond intelligibly to the test are excluded from the results.

• Children are normally tested before receiving the implant and then a year or so later, but during that year they frequently receive oral training and they are continuing to mature, so it is difficult to know how much of their improvement in speech perception, if any, is attributable to the implant and how much would have been achieved without it, through training or maturation alone—or mere readministration of the test.

• Another problem with the research that has been reported is the practice of pooling test findings from a few patients deaf since birth or early childhood, who obtain low scores, and a larger number of patients who became deaf later in life, and who obtain higher scores; the average scores, although they are commonly low, still paint too bright a picture of what the typical deaf child will achieve, since most deaf children are born deaf or become so early in life.

• There are still further problems with the research so far. Different tests of the same perceptual abilities may give different results. There are large unexplained differences in the performances of implanted children who are highly similar in all measured respects. These differences among the children may be due partly to differences in their mental abilities, such as skill in interpreting ambiguous stimulation, or, to go from mind to matter, in the numbers of surviving fibers in their auditory nerve. Both have eluded accurate measurement.

• The few reports available on the effectiveness of the multichannel device, some coming from the implant manufacturer, present results in terms that make it difficult to gauge material gain in speech perception. By "material gain" I mean gains that will really change the child's oral communication with family, neighbors, peers, and teachers. For example, studies report the percent of children who can identify one or more words out of fifty, or the percent of children who showed any improvement at all on any of five quite different perceptual tests. When we learn that half of the children tested in one study improved to some degree on at least one out of seven tests of word recognition, what does this enable us to say about the material gain that Johnny will receive if he is implanted? Almost nothing at all.

In short, cochlear implants for children who have been born deaf or become so early in life are still highly experimental; detailed inspection of the data that are available leads me to conclude that most such children are unlikely to profit materially from implants.

A significant factor in predicting an implanted child's gain in speech perception, as I have told, is the age at which the child became deaf. One study presented twenty-seven children born deaf with words chosen from a large list, once before they received an implant and again a year later. Only four children improved in identifying words on this test, although eleven improved to some degree on a multiple-choice test. The same study tested fifty-three other implanted children who had become deaf at various ages *after* birth. About two-thirds of all the children could not recognize words chosen from a large set; these youngsters had become deaf on the average when they were one and a half years old. The remaining third of the children, who could identify some of the words, had become deaf on the average at age five years, three months. Thus, the children who perform most like deafened, formerly hearing adults and who get the largest gains from the implant are those who are "small adults"— that is, who became deaf starting around age five, after fully mastering English. Children who become deaf in the first few years of life are no more likely to profit from their implant than those born deaf. Likewise, adults who were deaf before school age frequently make very poor gains in speech comprehension after receiving cochlear implants.

Since most deaf children are deaf before reaching school age, and such children are commonly not able to understand speech with the help of an implant, this augurs ill for their mastery of the English language, especially if English teaching is carried out in spoken English. Poor mastery of English brings with it poor mastery of all other subjects when those subjects are taught in English. Even if, in particular cases, the implant was so successful in audiologic terms that a totally deaf child achieved speech discrimination scores typical of children with severe hearing losses using hearing aids, the child's educational prospects would scarcely improve, since children with severe hearing loss have almost as much difficulty understanding even strongly amplified speech as profoundly deaf children; two-thirds of students with "severe hearing losses" rely primarily on the few signs teachers may use in school. An extensive study of the academic achievement of deaf high school leavers finds that profoundly deaf and severely deaf students at the end of their schooling score quite similarly on reading achievement—about the level of a fourth-grade hearing child. And the children in this survey with less than severe hearing losses averaged only about a half grade higher. Likewise, an extensive study of deaf children in oral educational programs found "low correlations between reading scores and measures of hearing acuity, speech perception, and speech production."

It may be that even a modest diminution of hearing during preschool years prevents a child from acquiring English by ear, whether naturally or with intensive training. When sixteen children were tested in reading, spelling, and math before implant surgery with the older, single-channel device and then again six months later, academic progress proved poor; the investigator could only conclude that "the implant did not negatively affect the academic progress of the recipients"—it hadn't made things worse.

Some scholars argue that an implant, providing the deaf child with some spoken-language input in childhood such as hearing children have, could arrive during a "critical period" for language acquisition and might provide a matrix for English-language learning. From their point of view, deaf children should be implanted as early as possible, even before age two if the FDA would allow it. However, the scientific literature does not provide clear guidelines on when such a hypothesized critical period might begin and end; different estimates arise from examining different performances. By some criteria, it ends in the teens or early twenties, after which speech is often little affected by deafening; by other criteria, puberty is the cutoff point, after which second-language learning or delayed learning of one's first language becomes more difficult, as does recovery from damage to language areas of the brain; by still other criteria, the critical period extends to age five or six, by which time the child has fully mastered the grammar of his language; still other scientists set the limit at age two or so, when children are uttering well-formed sentences. According to Kathryn Meadow-Orlans, "more recently, the critical age was reduced to eighteen months and some [scientists] believe that important linguistic information is acquired from the age of six months."

The typical deaf child is discovered to be deaf at about age three. By that time—or even by age two, the earliest permitted age for implantation—the critical period may be over or well advanced, or the nervous system may have made a partially irreversible adaptation to the child's sensory milieu.* It is not even certain that there exists a critical period for language acquisition, if by "critical period" we mean an extended window of opportunity for starting to learn one's native language. The similarities in the stages of language acquisition across unrelated spoken and signed languages suggest that language mastery may unfold developmentally in relatively fixed stages, beginning with babbling in the first year of life. (Deaf children of deaf parents, who acquire ASL as a native language, start out with manual babbling—meaningless repetition of the building blocks of words—suggesting that the activity reflects a stage in the maturation of the brain for language.) To end up with normal language, the child may need to board the nonstop train before it leaves the station.*

Whatever the time limits and suppleness of the critical period, it is highly unlikely that an impoverished auditory signal such as the implant provides will yield the same benefits for later language acquisition that normal hearing does; indeed, the coding carried out by the speech processor of the implant may work against the usefulness of the auditory input for language development, since the human nervous system did not evolve to acquire language from cochlear prostheses. Because children who become deaf early but are implanted some years later do poorly in speech perception, some audiologists urge, when parents present their deaf child, "Let's not wait, let's implant him now." That's the experimental spirit, but it would not be a responsible decision grounded in research findings.

Granted that children deaf since birth or early childhood who are implanted generally don't understand spoken language much better than before—what about their speech? Among deaf children in general, the less a child hears, the less well he speaks. However, among profoundly deaf speakers, there is no clear relation between hearing loss and intelligibility. It is not clear that a little hearing is better than none when a child tries to make himself understood.* Early indications are that implanted children are better able to produce some speech features, such as voicing, than they could without the implant. One investigator has reported that naïve listeners could understand one word in five from totally deaf children before their implant and two words in five a year after they had received their implant and extensive training.* Many children in that sample, however, were late-deafened, so we do not know yet what progress to expect from the typical deaf child, who was born deaf or became so early in life. Nor do we know which children stand to benefit more and which less in this matter. One leading investigator, Mary Joe Osberger of the Indiana University Medical Center, states: "Given the limitations of any cochlear prosthesis at this time, it can be predicted that the performance levels of nonauditory children might match but not exceed those of profoundly hearing-impaired children with residual hearing who use hearing aids."* If the intelligibility of implanted children only comes up to that of profoundly deaf children who wear hearing aids, parents who are trying to undo their child's deafness are bound to be disappointed: three fourths of such children are judged by their teachers to be unintelligible.

It is clear, then, from the research findings on both the speech perception and the speech production of implanted children, that the typical implanted child will rely on some form of manual communication throughout his schooling and his life. The chances are that he will learn American Sign Language, marry a deaf person, and become involved in the deaf community. He may have deaf children. Therefore, the child's mastery of ASL is of great importance.

But the family's commitment of time, emotion, and money to the implant process and the necessity of intensive training in speech and hearing at home, in school, and in the clinic raises the risk that the child will start acquiring ASL later than he might have without the implant. The following case history illustrates the risk. When "Curt" was a year and a half old, his parents' suspicions that he was deaf were confirmed, he was classified "profoundly deaf," and he was fitted with a "body aid"—an amplifier worn on the chest, connected to two ear inserts by a Y-cord. When he was three years old, Curt was placed in a special oral program; two years later, he was transferred to a total communication program, where his communication skills improved. Although he was seeing a speech therapist daily, Curt expressed himself increasingly in ASL, which he was acquiring from contacts with deaf peers. His parents preferred, however, that he read lips, so they tried not to sign to him unless necessary. At their request, Curt underwent cochlear implant surgery; his parents hoped it would help him develop spoken language. His classroom teacher was all for it and promised to help in training his ear after the implant. Nevertheless, when Curt was tested one year after receiving his implant, his speech was unintelligible, and he could not understand words and sentences.

If the child's opportunity to master a language and to use it for fluently exchanging messages and learning about the world is delayed, the normal growth of his intellect may be delayed as well. We know that on average, deaf children of deaf parents, who experience no such delay, have a substantial educational and psychosocial advantage over deaf children with hearing parents.* This is probably because of early language mastery, though other factors may be interwoven, such as closeness between parent and child. One parent whom I know argued that she had no intention of minimizing the role of ASL in the life of her implanted child. But the commitment to the English-speaking community is not an optional feature of cochlear implant programs. Ask an implant team if they would accept one of their patients attending a school for deaf children of the sort envisaged by the Unlocking the Curriculum program, where instruction is conducted in ASL, and English mastery is sought only in the written form. Most implant teams would be reluctant to implant such a child; many would refuse to do so. A recent text on the management of the implanted child states: "A child with a cochlear implant will obtain the best results in a[n] environment where all family members . . . us[e] speech. . . . As the child's auditory skills improve, it may be possible to reduce (or eliminate) signing."

With respect to the child's developing a social identity, a partially successful implant may be worse than none at all. The family's commitment to the implant process, the child's program of speech and hearing training, whatever auditory benefit the implant provides, its visual appearance, and a likely delay in acquiring ASL may all hinder the child's developing an identity as a deaf person. However, it is unlikely that he will be able to develop as a hearing person either. Someone who tries to "pass" as a member of a nonstigmatized group, Erving Goffman predicts, "will feel torn between two attachments. He will feel some alienation from his new 'group' for he is unlikely to be able to identify fully with their attitude to what he knows he can be shown to be." And yet he will probably feel enough loyalty to his original group that things said and done to discredit them will offend him. Thus, the implanted child may "fall between" two potential sets of friends and mates and two "worlds." "Hard-of-hearing adolescents . . . tend to be culturally homeless, belonging to neither the deaf nor the hearing communities," writes Dr. J. William Evans at the University of California Center on Psychosocial and Linguistic Aspects of Deafness.

Hearing parents of a deaf child have some things in common with white couples who adopt a black child. In both cases, the parents have a child who is stigmatized in their culture and whom they cannot provide in the usual way with a sense of his or her own identity as a member of a minority, with pride in that identity and heritage, and with a knowledge of how to thrive while a member of a stigmatized minority. When the parents endeavor to deny that minority identity, to impress on their deaf child that he can be as hearing people are, or on their dark-skinned child that he is "not really different," the child may pay a high price for this denial. A British adoption agency has described the transracial adoption of "Trevor," who as a boy showed signs of "identity confusion" by trying to scratch off his skin in the bath. The first placement broke down when Trevor was nine, but he insisted on another white family. That placement lasted for four years, when it was discovered that he thought he was white and could not relate to other black youths. He also felt rejected by white society. "His confusion," the report continues, "manifested itself in conduct disorder. It was so severe that he was eventually diagnosed as schizophrenic."

Deaf leader Donnell Ashmore describes in his autobiography how the cultural homelessness of oral deaf youngsters develops. A young partially oral deaf person is viewed with reserve by the deaf community. After all, the deaf community, and deaf adults individually, have a history of oppression by professional people who speak and do not sign. Nearly all deaf adults have grown up treated by hearing people as a broken ear with a child attached. If the partially oral young deaf person gives "signs of 'hearism'," Ashmore writes, "evidence of attempts to impose the values of the hearing world on the deaf community, [this will] often result in a hostile or silent reprimand. This reprimand, in turn, is sensed by the young oral deaf person as being rejected." Ashmore relates the case of a young deaf woman, Jennifer, who came to see him for counseling. "I cannot hear but my father tells me that I am not deaf," she said. "I do not know who I am." Since she had great difficulty communicating orally with hearing people and with other deaf people, Jennifer decided to enroll in classes to learn ASL. One evening while she was practicing her ASL at home with videotapes, she told Ashmore, her father broke in. "Jennifer, you are not deaf," he shouted. "You are hearing. You should not be learning that stuff. If you don't stop it, your speech will suffer." "Dr. Ashmore," Jennifer sobbed, "Who am I?"

When deaf students leave the oral programs of home and school, they find that the hearing world no longer sees them as superior to signing deaf adults solely because of their oral skills, Ashmore explains. They find, moreover, that most hearing people, unlike their family and teachers, are untrained to understand their deaf speech. A few stay the course, but most choose to learn ASL, as Sammy Rue did. When they do, they are often confronted by their parents for betraying them. And when they turn to the deaf community for support, they experience discrimination in reverse. Gunned down by both sides, some young oral deaf people refuse to take either side. It's a carryover, Ashmore explains, from the days of faking understanding when lip-reading wasn't conveying the message. Such a person loses connectedness with the social world. "With that follows the downfall of trust, intimacy, happiness, and productivity."

Consistent with Ashmore's account, many cochlear implant teams report with some puzzlement a phenomenon they have labeled "adolescent rejection"—implanted children who refuse to use their implants once in their teens. To head off "teen rejection," one implant team has students enroll in a special preimplant program in an oral school for deaf children. There they wear a Tactaid, a vibratory device for detecting sound, receive psychological counseling, are paired up with an implanted buddy, and receive guidance from school counselors to ensure that they have realistic expectations of the benefit to be had from the cochlear implant. They must understand that they will be severely hearing-impaired and will continue to require special education.

On the average, the later the age at which the child acquires ASL, the less will be his skill. Children born deaf and deprived of language in childhood have more difficulty learning ASL later in life than hearing children do. It is astonishing to think that hearing children could outperform deaf children in learning a manual language, until we recall that in this comparison, the hearing children had the advantage of acquiring a language—albeit spoken—right from birth.

There are some risks associated with cochlear implantation of children that are peculiarly the parents'. If the implant does not live up to the parents' hopes, they may suffer a second cycle of regret and acceptance, like the one incurred on learning their child was deaf. The implant process may also delay the time when the parents improve their own manual communication and therefore their ability to communicate with their child. Parents of children receiving implants have higher levels of stress and poorer psychological adjustment than parents of hearing children. Mothers of children using the newer twenty-two-channel implant reported more stress and more problems in managing their child's behavior than mothers of children implanted with the older and less effective single-channel implant. Some of these mothers were so stressed that their test scores fell within the range typical of psychiatric outpatients. Not surprisingly, the children presenting the greatest behavioral problems had parents who were the most emotionally disturbed.

One source of stress, parents reported, was teaching their child some initial speech skills (if he did not have them previously) so he could qualify as an implant candidate. The next stressful challenge they confronted was raising money for the many medical and paramedical services their child would require. While insurance frequently paid for a good part of this, the rest had to come from personal savings, from raffles, from selling ice cream, from appealing to the generosity of neighbors and relatives, and in many other ways.

Particularly stressful, parents said, were their efforts to have their child's IEP revised to support the implant through auditory and speech training both before and after the operation.

What the FDA Did Wrong

Limited perception and production of speech despite a commitment to oral training and practices, limited command of American Sign Language as well as English, hampered communication at home with parents suffering from stress, inability to communicate and socialize with either hearing or deaf friends, an uncertain identity—is that the quality of life that surgical implantation of early-deafened children promises? Astonishingly, the FDA has approved early implantation and surgeons are proceeding with it in the total absence of research describing the impact of the implant on the deaf child's quality of life—on his integration as an adolescent and an adult into the deaf community, on his social, intellectual, and emotional development and mental health. "One has to inquire into the entire human drama, that surrounds the attacks," writes neurologist Oliver Sacks about medicating migraine, "to explore what they might mean in a particular person. One has to take not just a 'medical history' but to try to construct a complete human narrative." Sacks is articulating a growing conviction in the medical community that treatments should be evaluated "in terms of comprehensive outcomes that are important to the patient." "Biomedical good does not exhaust the good the physician is obliged to do," write medical ethicists Edmund Pellegrino and David Thomasma. It is an error "to make the patient a victim of the medical imperative, to insist that if a procedure offers any physiological or therapeutic benefit then it must be done. . . . It is the obligation of the physician to ascertain, by the most careful method, the consequences that might ensue from a particular treatment. . . . A biomedically or technomedically good treatment is not automatically a good from the patient's point of view. It must be examined in the context of the patient's life situation." Nevertheless, the FDA's summary regarding the safety of the childhood implant only mentions problems arising in the implanted ear and formal patient complaints about battery life and the like. Its summary of effectiveness considers only laboratory tests and counts as a favorable result any improvement, however small, on any of several tests, provided only that the improvement seems unlikely to have occurred by chance according to statistical methods.

In general, thoughtful people favor wariness when considering the use of high technology for life enhancement—as opposed to lifesaving. We know how poor our record is in predicting side effects—as in "a little radiation will get rid of this acne" (radiation treatment for acne was later shown to be a major cause of thyroid cancer). The newer the technology, the more cautious we want to be, for the less sure the results. Many, perhaps most advocates of cochlear implants in children would agree that with the benefit of hindsight, it was an error to implant hundreds of children over the years with the single-channel device that is now increasingly in disuse. However, they see no moral in that acknowledgment for their ongoing implant programs with the twenty-two-channel device. "How are we to find out the benefits of the new devices and to continue improving them, if we don't implant children?" they ask me angrily. This is a tacit admission of what all the evidence I have presented clearly shows: Cochlear implants are highly experimental devices of questionable therapeutic value for most deaf children. On scientific grounds, the FDA should never have given approval for these devices to be taken out of the investigation stage and marketed at will for early-deafened children. Indeed, the FDA has required that the notice accompanying the prosthesis include the warning (easily ignored by medical practitioners) that children who are born deaf or become deaf shortly thereafter may derive less benefit from the device than children who are deafened later in life; however, there is strong evidence that the risk of no benefit is not peculiar to children born deaf or deafened shortly after birth but applies as well to children who become deaf throughout most of the preschool years.

Even a closely regulated program of experimentation with deaf children is difficult to justify ethically. Since the child cannot give informed consent, implanting that child for research purposes is to impose altruism on another person—and that is incompatible with respect for the autonomy of other people as moral agents. An exception to this principle might be justified if the child's life were at risk, if, for example, the only way of respecting his autonomy were to use an experimental drug. However, experimentation on children with prostheses that are arguably life-enhancing for an unidentifiable subgroup is quite another matter. The staunchest advocates of childhood cochlear implants do not dispute deaf parents' decision to abjure this operation for their deaf child; it is clearly elective surgery. Experimentation with deaf children is just what the World Federation of the Deaf warned against when it resolved in 1989 that technical implant developments were "encouraging for persons deafened after some years of hearing" but "experimentation with young deaf children is definitely not encouraged."

The FDA also erred in failing to consult formally with organizations of deaf Americans and with deaf leaders and scholars who have some knowledge of how deaf children acquire language, how they develop socially and emotionally, and how they become an integral part of the American deaf community and its culture. The FDA formally consulted otologists, speech and hearing scientists, manufacturers, parents, and members of its own staff in arriving at its decision; its failure to consult deaf leaders represents, if an oversight, gross ignorance concerning growing up deaf in America, or, if willful, an offense against fundamental American values. Disputing the statement of the National Association of the Deaf branding the FDA action "unsound scientifically, procedurally, and ethically," the American Academy of Otolaryngology, Head and Neck Surgery said in rebuttal that the FDA and its Ear, Nose and Throat Devices Panel make judgments only "on the basis of valid scientific evidence." As if that were not reassurance enough, the letter goes on to point out that the academy itself has long had an official policy endorsing surgical implantation of young deaf children as soon as it is approved by the FDA. Moreover, the academy argued, the FDA panel was made up of experts representing otology, pediatrics, audiology, deaf education, engineering, an industry advocate, and a consumer advocate (we know about her). Further buttressing their argument, the academy notes that experts from those disciplines as well as from statistics and physiology are part of the internal FDA review and had input into the research conducted by the implant manufacturer. Deaf children are in expert hands, seems to be the message, and deaf people should butt out.

I have presented the case that cochlear implants are still highly experimental devices for early-deafened children, with unknown consequences for their quality of life, and that experimentation on such children in these circumstances cannot be justified ethically. There are several other ethical arguments that weigh against the decision of the FDA, the audist establishment, and many parents who promote surgical implantation of children who are born deaf or become deaf early in life.

Since the child is a minor and is not competent to decide whether he shall receive an implant or not, the parent acts as surrogate. For the parents to make a morally valid surrogate decision, however, several conditions must be satisfied. The surrogate must really know the patient and his values. This condition commonly is not met because of prolonged lack of communication between parent and child. If the child has been in touch with other deaf children and deaf adults and has acquired ASL, it may be possible, depending on the child's age, to discuss the implant issues with him or her: If we do nothing, you will grow up like the deaf adults you know; if we perform the operation, here is what we think might happen. Of course, this is risky: The child may not grasp the alternatives, or may be unduly influenced by the parents' wishes or the doctor's. But at least he has been consulted. If the parents have kept their child languageless, however, he cannot participate at all in the process, they cannot know his values, and their burden of a responsible surrogate decision is heavier than ever.

The surrogate must be able to make an informed decision. This condition commonly is not met because the parents are not provided with the information they need with respect to sensory, linguistic, educational, social, and psychological outcomes—the doctor does not possess that information. And they are not provided with information they need about the deaf community because the professionals they consult do not possess the knowledge or are unsympathetic to that community. If physicians knew and disclosed to parents all the relevant information concerning the risks and benefits of cochlear implants for early-deafened children—the poor results for speech perception, the uncertain outcome for communication and English mastery, the unassessed risks of social and psychological development, the widely practiced cultural alternative, the case that cultural deafness is not an infirmity at all—if physicians presented all this, it seems likely that many patients and their parents would withhold consent. Thus it also seems likely that some physicians have opened themselves to the charge of having proceeded without informed consent.

Finally, the morally valid surrogate must not have a conflict of interest with the patient's best interest. Painful as it is to acknowledge, parents may have such a conflict of interest; for example, they put more weight on their child acquiring extremely limited communication in their primary language than on the child acquiring fluent communication in ASL. "I fully respect deaf people and their community," a hearing mother of a deaf child said at a discussion of implants with deaf leaders, "but surely I have a right to want surgery for my child which will make him more like me, a hearing person." Ontario legislator Gary Malkowski replied: "Then presumably you have no objection to deaf parents requesting surgery to make their hearing child deaf." The interests of parent and child are not always identical, and this has given rise to a children's rights movement and a body of law and litigation. The relation of the hearing parent to the young deaf child is a microcosm of the relation of hearing society to the deaf community; it is paternalistic, medicalizing, and ethnocentric.

Children have rights: the parents' authority over the body of their child is not limitless, as child abuse laws testify. It is romantic but untrue to imagine that parents have no other interest in their child than to see him develop into an independent and successful adult. Child labor laws and compulsory education laws arose in the gap between child and parent interests. However, most children would find it very difficult to dissent against the wishes of both their parents and their physician. If the child cannot fully advocate his own position, because he is too young or because he has been kept languageless, the child should have a representative or an advocate. The crucial skill that a child advocate must possess is the ability to interpret information to children. For a deaf child, a deaf adult is in a peculiarly good position to do that. Moreover, with or without the implant, the child is likely to be a deaf adult, to take a deaf spouse, and to enter the deaf community, so the child advocate should be a member of that community.

Far from involving deaf adults in these difficult ethical decisions, however, the medical community and the FDA have avoided them like lepers. True, some parents might protest at first any interference in family matters by an outsider; yet American parents are accustomed to many such agents acting in the interests of their child, including teachers, doctors, social workers, scout leaders, pastors. Why not a deaf child advocate?

The implant devices are highly experimental; the parents who make the decision to have their child implanted are often poorly informed about the alternatives and unable to discuss them with their child; they may have a conflict of interest. There are still further obstacles to an ethically valid decision to implant young deaf children. While some ethicists contend that it is never moral to experiment on a child without the certainty that he will benefit, some pediatricians would allow nontherapeutic intervention provided the risks are low enough. They see nothing wrong, for example, in measuring a healthy child's weight and height for the purpose of gathering statistical data, or even in taking a sample of his blood. Cochlear implantation, however, entails invasive surgery and tissue destruction with new technology, and the outcomes for the child's quality of life are uncertain. It is hard to see how the surgeon can be acting ethically in this case, when the benefits are unpredictable and the comprehensive risks unassessed. Therefore, we would normally prefer to wait until the child is older and can give his informed consent. We are most comfortable delegating that authority to the parents when the intervention cannot wait and when the child, if he grew to adulthood without the intervention, would wish he had had it. Thus, when it comes to lifesaving measures for their child, we expect parents to request them, and if they do not, the courts may order it. When it comes to debatable measures for life enhancement, on the other hand, we prefer to wait; the individual might make a different decision when he is competent to decide.

Neither justification for ethically delegating decision making to the parents applies in childhood cochlear implants. There is no urgent lifesaving issue here, or evidence that the implant must be done while the child is young; implanted early or later, the child will probably rely on manual communication. And we can be confident that the child would *not* reason as his parents do in this matter were he an adult. In order to respect the personhood of someone who is not competent, we decide what is in his best interests by asking someone like him, under similar conditions, what he would choose. What do deaf individuals like the child who are, however, adult and competent choose? They choose overwhelmingly not to have the implant surgery. Nor is there evidence that children implanted young are pleased as adults with the decision their parents made for them.

There is not a moral equivalence between positive and negative duties. Failing to swim toward a drowning person in order to save him is not morally equivalent to killing someone by drowning him. We must be more morally sure when we intervene than when we fail to intervene. Parents and doctors must be more sure they are doing good by implanting than by not implanting. The burden of proof is on the intervention, yet it remains to be shown that it improves rather than degrades the child's quality of life.

Even if the child's surrogates felt they knew the patient's mind well, judged themselves sufficiently informed about the long-term consequences of cochlear implantation to risk it, protested they had only the child's interests at heart, and were convinced their child would thank them one day for their early intervention—even in this case, the ethical physician cannot simply say, as many physicians do, "Let the parent decide." The physician's concern must be for the child, Thomasma and Pellegrino argue, "for the infant, not the family, is the patient." The physician has the obligation "to be sure the surrogate is competent to make the decision and that, in addition, the surrogate is acting in the best interests of the patient."

We seem to have different criteria for respecting the parents' wishes in educational and in medical life enhancement. In the former case, audist professionals have no difficulty in overruling the parents' wishes with respect to the Individualized Educational Plan for their child. The parents can appeal, and if the appeal fails they can go to court, but at both levels of review there is a presumption that the experts have made the right decision. The parents have the burden of proof to overrule the experts. When it comes to cochlear implants, however, the experts say, "Let the parents decide." Perhaps in the foreseeable future, cochlear implantation will become part of the IEP, with which it is closely linked in any case, and the experts will decide (with parents retaining the right of appeal) whether the child should have this prosthesis or not. That would be a logical next step in the state's exercise of bio-power. There is a precedent for this politicization of the body in nations, such as Mexico, that require parents by law to receive genetic counseling before they are allowed to enroll their deaf child in school. And while no school district has yet required parents to have their child implanted with a cochlear prosthesis, school authorities in Concord, New Hampshire, insisted for three years—until overruled in court in 1991—that twelve-year-old Casey Jesson could not return to his classroom unless his parents resumed medicating him with amphetamines for his "attention deficit disorder."

I believe profoundly that the decision to surgically implant a young deaf child is ethically unsound for a reason yet more fundamental than the several I have given. There is now abundant scientific evidence that, as the deaf community has long contended, it constitutes a linguistic and cultural minority. I expect most Americans would agree that our society should not seek the scientific tools or use them, if available, to change a child biologically so he or she will belong to the majority rather than the minority—even if we believe that this biological engineering might reduce the burdens the child will bear as a member of a minority. Even if we could take children destined to be members of the African-American, or Hispanic-American, or Native American, or Deaf American communities and convert them with bio-power into white, Caucasian, hearing males—even if we could, we should not. We should likewise refuse cochlear implants for young deaf children even if the devices were perfect.

I believe that our country is richer for its pluralism. If there could be an end to our diversity, we would have that single voice (an upper-middle-class white male speaking a mid-Atlantic dialect of English) that some Americans seem to yearn for. It might indeed be easier to arrive at a consensus—but can the best consensus arise from a limited range of proposed options? There would be greater unity of purpose, but in behalf of what goals? There would be no voices with which to speak to the other peoples of the world, nor any voices with which their own resonated. There would be one cuisine, presumably steak and potatoes, one school of music and one of art, one kind of literature. The richly diverse nation we once were would be an abstraction recorded in the history books. Indeed, a founding principle of our society was tolerance for other ways of being. Our failure to live up fully to our national ideals of tolerance is not a valid reason to seek to eradicate our human differences or to recast them as deviance.

It is illegitimate to ask, What does our society gain by having a deaf culture and community? if the implication is that a minority must pass a value-added test or otherwise face extinction or attempts at forcing its assimilation. Cultural diversity is central to our understanding of what it means to be a human being; each culture lost, each language allowed to die out, reduces the scope of every person's humanity. Intolerance is also almost laughably shortsighted. If the Arab minority in France, for example, is to be subjected to the value-added test, then the French minority in North Africa must be subjected to it as well. Intolerance always contains within it the seeds of self-destruction.

Members of the American deaf community affirm that what characterizes them as a group is their shared language and culture, and not an infirmity. When Gallaudet University's president, I. King Jordan, was asked if he would like to have his hearing back, he replied: "That's almost like asking a black person if he would rather be white. . . . I don't think of myself as missing something or as incomplete. . . . It's a common fallacy if you don't know deaf people or deaf issues. You think it's a limitation."

So medical intervention is inappropriate, even if a perfect "bionic ear" were available, because invasive surgery on healthy children is morally wrong. We know that as members of a stigmatized minority, these children will live lives full of challenge, but, by the same token, they have a special contribution to make to their own community and the larger society. On the other hand, the more we view the child born deaf as tragically infirm, the more we see his plight as desperate, the more we are prepared to conduct surgery of unproven benefit and unassessed risk. Our representation of deaf people determines the outcome of our ethical judgment.

Scholarship does not provide reliable guides on where to draw the line between valuable diversity and treatable deviance. In the course of American history, health practitioners and scientists have labeled various groups biologically inferior that they no longer consider in that light; these include women, Southern Europeans, blacks, gay men and lesbians, and culturally deaf people. What scholarship does tell us is that there is increasingly the well-founded view in America, as around the globe, that the deaf communities of the world are linguistic and cultural minorities. Logic and morality demand that where there are laws or mores protecting such minorities, they extend to the deaf community. In America, this recognition of the status of the deaf community, fueled by the civil rights movement, is leading to greater acceptance of deaf people. The interests of the deaf child and his parents may best be served by accepting that he is a deaf person, with an elaborate cultural and linguistic heritage that can enrich his parents' life as it will his own. We should heed the advice of the deaf teenager who, when reprimanded by her mother for not wearing the processor of her cochlear prosthesis, hurled back bitterly: "I'm deaf. Let me be deaf."

The Science and Ethics
of Cochlear Implantation in Young Children
(prepared in collaboration with Ben Bahan)*

Nearly eight years have passed since the discussion of cochlear implants in the preceding section was written, shortly after the FDA approved of cochlear implant surgery on children. In that interval, several studies have been published that assess speech perception with implants by the largest group of Deaf* children concerned, those born Deaf. And there has been heated debate in the professional journals about the ethics of this surgical practice, bringing to light some new ways of viewing the ethical issues.[1] Moreover, the surgery has been criticized by numerous organizations of culturally Deaf adults here and abroad,[2] including the World Federation of the Deaf with more than one hundred member nations.[3] Meanwhile, large numbers of Deaf children are receiving cochlear implants. Parents, teachers, doctors, and others want to know if the practice is scientifically and ethically sound.

This chapter answers those questions by reviewing recent findings in audiology and medical ethics. It presents evidence that the main benefits sought are unlikely for most children while the potential risks are serious and not yet assessed. This makes the surgery innovative, not to say experimental, and optional innovative surgery on children is ethically questionable. The chapter shows, further, that the values of Deaf-World cultures conflict with the values of hearing cultures on this issue and that both sets of cultural values have standing. Finally, we show that a social policy allowing large-scale implantation of children in principle conflicts with the right of the Deaf language and cultural minority to exist and to flourish.

*In part adapted from "Ethics of cochlear implantation in young children: A review and a reply from a Deaf-World perspective." *Otolaryngology–Head and Neck Surgery*, 1998, *119*(4), 297–308, 309–312. (H. Lane & B. Bahan).
*Since the first edition of *Mask*, the practice has become more widespread to capitalize *Deaf* when writing about the culture and the children and adults who are its members. The term *Deaf-World* is a gloss on the signs in ASL with which members of that culture refer to it.

Innovative Surgery

Many surgeons claim that cochlear implantation on children is no longer innovative, since clinical trials began in the United States in 1985, more than 4,000 children have received the multichannel implant,[4] and the procedure has been approved by, among other groups, the Food and Drug Administration,[5] a National Institutes of Health Consensus Conference,[6] and the American Academy of Otolaryngology–Head and Neck Surgery.[7] Yet much remains unknown about the language, psychological, and social outcomes of the procedure. Indeed, some of the strongest surgical advocates have nevertheless referred to cochlear implantation as "an emerging technology."[8]

Spoken language acquisition is an important goal of cochlear implantation in children[9]—the more so as an estimated 86% of children with profound hearing losses are born that way and most would be unlikely to acquire spoken language and communicate orally.[10] It is also an important goal of the surgery in the view of many of the parents who give consent, and it is the focus of postsurgical habilitative efforts often lasting several years. Nevertheless, in the twelve years since the clinical trials began with the multichannel implant, the literature has seen a number of reports on individual children's performance with implants but not a single case has been reported of a child acquiring language because of an implant. More importantly, the studies that have been published indicate that congenitally Deaf children do very poorly on tests of unprompted ("open set") word recognition, even after many years of implant use and therapy. If children with implants cannot perceive speech well, even under optimal listening conditions, it seems unlikely they will be able to use speech perception to master the sound system of spoken language (phonology), its grammar, and its semantics. In the words of the developers of the multichannel implant: "It is vital to realize that all measures, such as effects of device use on speech production, educational progress, development of language, and effects on social and communication skills depend on the child being able to accurately perceive speech information through his/her device."[11]

The literature on speech perception benefit in children with implants both in the United States and abroad was screened to identify those studies reporting aural word-recognition scores on an open-set test for groups of four or more children Deaf before age three using a multichannel implant for a specified period of time. Table 3 reports the results.[12]

TABLE 3

Aural open-set word recognition by children Deaf before age three using multichannel cochlear implants.

ROW	REFERENCE	YEAR	NUMBER OF CHILDREN	AGE* AT ONSET	AGE AT FITTING	YEARS OF USE	CHILDREN EXCLUDED	MEAN %	MEDIAN %
1	13	91	28	1.9	7.4	1.7	11	6	0
2	14	92	10	0	~6	2	0	6	0
3	15	93	19	1	6	3	8	8	4e
4	16	94	10	<2	2.3	3	6	19	0
5	17	94	6	0.3	?	5	Some	13	13e
6	18	94	13	1.6	6	3	9	>4	0
7	19	95	5	0.5	10.5	1	0	0	0
8	-	95	9	2.5	4.5	1	0	30	?
9	20	97	18	0	2-5	3	0	44	0
10	-	97	8	0	2-5	4	0	33	?
11	21	97	8	<2.5	2-5	5	0	32	37
12	-	97	11	<2.5	5+	5	4	12	8

*AGE AT ONSET IS THE AVERAGE AGE AT WHICH THE CHILDREN IN THE GROUP WERE BELIEVED TO HAVE BECOME DEAF; AGE AT FITTING, THEIR AGE WHEN THEY BEGAN TO USE THEIR IMPLANTS. MEAN % IS THE AVERAGE GROUP SCORE ON THE TEST; MEDIAN % IS THE SCORE OF THE PERSON WHO RANKED AT THE MIDDLE OF THE GROUP. THE MEDIAN IS LESS INFLUENCED THAN THE MEAN BY INFREQUENT HIGH AND LOW SCORES.

The table gives an indication of how recent and how small is the scientific literature that uses the kind of test considered most predictive of success in oral communication and that involves subjects from the largest group of potential candidates for implants (the 9 out of 10 "profoundly hearing-impaired" Deaf children born Deaf or become so before age three).[22] Studies with fewer than four children have been excluded from the table as their average results would be particularly unreliable, and only the latest years of longitudinal studies are reported, but even if some pertinent studies are absent, this scientific literature clearly pales in size by comparison with those more established literatures concerning less invasive devices such as tactile aids or hearing aids.

Table 3 also presents the word recognition scores achieved by these implanted early-Deaf children on open-set tests.[23] Most of the children scored zero or close to zero. The evidence supports the conclusion of one team of implant researchers: "Children with multichannel cochlear implants generally perform poorly on these ... tests."[24] Another implant team concurs: "Most children receiving cochlear implants before age 5 will ultimately be able to use audition only to repeat some words.... Prelingually deafened children do not have the auditory memory of spoken language to help them interpret the electrical signal of the cochlear implant."[25]

More commonly, implant teams are enthusiastic about the benefits in speech perception and language provided by the surgery. One team of implant advocates has written: "The great majority of children with CI's obtain the ability to hear and understand words without lipreading."[26] The published evidence does not support such enthusiasm. On the contrary, more than 80% of the children reported on in Table 3 scored zero or close to zero. It is possible to be misled on this issue by a cursory reading of those studies that exclude subjects or report the percentage of subjects who recognized some words (that is, at least one) or by the anecdotal report that many children with implants attend mainstream educational programs; after all, four-fifths of all Deaf schoolchildren in the United States today are mainstreamed in some sense.[27] In support of their claim that early Deaf children "obtain the ability to hear and understand words," these implant advocates cite quantitative data from three studies. However, results in those studies do not support the claim. Children in the first of the studies cited, reported in row 4 of Table 3, had a median score of zero on the cited test (PB-K). Those in the second, reported in row 5, had a median score estimated at 13% correct, although there may have been some subjects excluded who could not do the test, which would lower the estimate. Children in the third cited study, reported in row 3, had a median score estimated at 4% correct. The implant advocates state that "the average child in this group had 63% open-set speech understanding"[28] but in fact the study reports that 63% of the children (5 of the group of 8) scored above chance (8%) on the open-set test.

Some of the children reported on in Table 3 do considerably better than zero percent correct word recognition for reasons that have not been established. It might appear from the table that children who are implanted earlier and who have more experience with the prosthesis may have an advantage; however, the sample sizes are so small and the variability among the children so great, that neither this nor any other such inference can be made confidently. For example, the study cited in row 9 [29] reported a decrease in average percent correct from year 3 to year 4, as if speech perception deteriorated with longer implant use. More likely, the difference between the scores obtained in years 3 and 4 is not statistically reliable. Much of the published research interprets differences between the average scores obtained by groups while failing to apply first the necessary statistical tests to assure the reliability of the differences.

All of the following have been advanced as possible reasons for some children outperforming their peers, but supporting evidence is either lacking or conflictual: age at which the child became Deaf; age at implant; years the child was Deaf before implant; language use (English or ASL); length of implant use; processor type[30]; educational placement; residual hearing prior to implantation[31]; methods and frequency of programming processors; nature and frequency of therapy; and parental commitment to oralism and therapy.[32] Some of the advantage that these exceptional children show may not be attributable to the implant and would have been attained with the intensive oral training that they received even if they did not have an implant. Suitable control group studies to estimate the contribution of the implant itself to speech perception have not been conducted.

Consequently, it is not possible to say whether a given candidate for an implant, who was born Deaf or early became so, will behave like the small group in the table who have substantial open-set recognition, or, more probably, like the large group who have little or none. Moreover, we do not know whether even the few who do well on open-set recognition will go on to acquire spoken language and oral communication. A survey of all U.S. educational programs for the hearing-impaired with one hundred or more students, found that half of the children Deaf before age three who received implants were using them on a regular basis and half were not; moreover, two-thirds of those who were users were in oral educational programs where their use was required, and many of the users reported little benefit (only three children had single-channel implants).[33] This high rate of nonutilization is consistent with the poor recorded levels of speech recognition in Table 3. All in all, it seems that most implanted early-Deaf children are deriving little communicative benefit from their implants.

The scientific literature assessing the language benefits of cochlear implants (as opposed to just word perception) is "practically nonexistent."[34] There are, however, two group studies whose results concerning language acquisition are consistent with the low levels of word recognition and of implant use we just described. The first study compared English language progress in early-Deaf implanted children with that in an unimplanted Deaf control group.[35] Both groups were learning English in simultaneous communication (oral + sign) or oral only programs. First, a developmental language scale designed for hearing children was administered to the unimplanted Deaf children of varying ages and their scores were converted into an age-equivalent score using normative data obtained from children with normal hearing. Then, statistics were used to compute the straight line that best described the relation between the ages of the unimplanted Deaf children and the age-equivalent English-language scores that they achieved. The formula for that line was used to predict a language score for each implanted child based on his or her age. Finally, the test was administered to the implanted children and the difference between their predicted and obtained scores noted. The implanted group averaged nearly seven years of age but their English-language age-equivalent score was three years, four months. Thus they were more than three years behind comparable Deaf children learning ASL or hearing children learning English (both progress at the same rate[36]). They outpaced the English language scores they were predicted to have based on the unimplanted children by about five months and they seemed to be making faster progress than their peers.

The advantage of the implanted children over the unimplanted is small. It is not clear whether it is a solid advantage or not: it all depends on how the prediction is calculated. For example, if the implanted children's language age actually grew a little faster than proportionately with the passing years, the predicted scores of the implanted children would be a little higher and their five-month advantage would be reduced or eliminated. Then, too, the language scale used leaves large interpretive leeway to the examiners, who knew which children were implanted and which were not, so their biases might have crept into their scoring. And it may be that the implanted children received a little more attention to their English learning than did their unimplanted peers. Further, we wonder about the numbers of "prelingually Deaf" children in the study who became Deaf some years after birth and after some learning of English by ear. Such children are quite rare and must not be represented disproportionately.

Apparently very few, if any, of the Deaf children in this study had been allowed to use their native language-learning ability from infancy on to acquire a full-blown natural language that was entirely accessible to them, American Sign Language. Forty percent of the unimplanted group used oral communication and the remainder Total Communication (in which, as we have seen, signs borrowed from ASL are used in English word order, without much of the grammar of ASL, frequently accompanied by spoken English). Consequently, the implanted children are apparently being compared not to normal Deaf children but to Deaf children who have been language deprived. Providing Deaf children with the opportunity to acquire ASL normally is a third course available to parents and schools, beyond implant surgery and language deprivation, a course that does not require surgery nor habilitative therapy, and may facilitate English-language acquisition substantially. There is a body of literature showing that mastery of a first language facilitates mastery of a second language later on.[37] Recent reports of correlation between ASL mastery and English mastery in Deaf children support that conclusion. A study with Deaf children ages eight to eleven found that the better they did on a test of ASL production and comprehension, the better they did on a test of English literacy.[38] In a separate study, scores on a test of Imitating Sentences in ASL and on a test of Verb Agreement Production in ASL each correlated with reading scores on the Stanford Achievement Test.[39] It has long been known that Deaf children born to Deaf parents outperform Deaf children born to hearing parents on several measures of English mastery.[40] These studies suggest that they do so because of their earlier and fuller acquisition of manual language. Clearly, the first of the two language studies concerning children with cochlear implants raises many more questions than it provides answers. What is needed for sound assessment of benefits and risk is a large corpus of such studies, with other measures of language acquisition, additional control groups, children who could not have learned English by ear (since they comprise nine out of ten implant candidates), more precautions against examiner bias—in short, a scientific basis for the surgical practice which is proceeding willy nilly without one.

The second language study of children with implants found that they did not differ from comparable children using a tactile aid in expressive and receptive vocabulary nor in linguistic structure and developmental sentence scores based on their spontaneous English.[41] Consistently, when 50 parents of prelingually Deaf children who had used the Nucelus-22 implant for three years were given a list to check off advantages and disadvantages of the implant, none selected "improved vocabulary" and none selected "improved language skills."[42]

Implanted Deaf children who are unable to master spoken language run the risk of remaining communicatively impaired for many years unless they are brought into contact with culturally Deaf people and allowed to acquire a natural signed language such as ASL (in North America). However, many implant programs and books for parents on the management of their implanted child emphasize oral communication, including placement in oral educational programs, and seek to discourage the Deaf child's natural tendency to communicate in a visual/manual language.[43] For example, one team of implant advocates criticizes use of ASL in Deaf education and states: "to best learn English during the critical period of language acquisition, children should be exposed to a rich environment of spoken language."[44]   The implanted Deaf child who cannot master spoken English, but is not allowed to master ASL, pays cognitive and linguistic penalties.[45]

Because there are language risks in cochlear implantation of children, it follows that there are psychosocial and educational risks but these have not been assessed. The implanted child in a mainstream school who is unable to communicate fluently with hearing peers and with Deaf peers (if indeed there are any present) may have problems of identity development and social development more broadly, problems exacerbated if ready communication is not possible in the family setting as well. There is a consensus among experts that implanted children remain "severely hearing-impaired."[46] In fact, most comparisons of implanted children with hearing-aid users place them preponderantly in the category of profoundly hearing-impaired.[47] Severely hearing-impaired children have only a one-half grade advantage academically, on the average, over their profoundly hearing-impaired peers.[48] If implanted Deaf children perform like severely hearing-impaired children without implants, and if severely hearing-impaired children have only a half-grade academic advantage, then implanted Deaf children should be expected to have a half-grade academic advantage over their profoundly hearing-impaired unimplanted peers. Moreover, if many implanted Deaf children encounter problems of language acquisition and psychosocial development, such children may prove to have no academic advantage at all, and even a disadvantage. In the study that quizzed parents of implanted children on the advantages and disadvantages of the implant, only some 12% checked off educational advantages.[49]

A body of carefully conducted research on these linguistic, psychosocial, and educational issues could clarify what the likely consequences are of childhood implantation. That research has not been conducted. Hence it is appropriate to describe childhood implantation as innovative. It is also clearly optional. Certainly Deaf children can and do prosper without it—often achieving high levels of success in life, love, and work. Nor do we view Deaf or hearing parents as neglectful of their Deaf children if they opt not to have the surgery performed on their child. In general, choosing optional innovative surgery for a child is ethically problematic since the patient does not choose to incur the risks to which he or she will be subjected and there is no compelling reason such as life-saving to intercede anyway.[50] One eminent implant surgeon explains that the decision to have their child undergo cochlear implant surgery is difficult for the parents "since it involves major surgery, some degree of pain and risk, significant financial obligations, years of training, and unpredictable benefits."[51] Such innovative optional treatment with children is best conducted as research rather than treatment; as research, it must bear a higher ethical burden, even with parental consent, because the risks and benefits are not sufficiently known. Moreover, the controlled manipulations and systematic long-term data gathering that are part of the research undertaking make the findings generalizable by identifying the populations and conditions under which various balances of risks and benefits are obtained.

Conflicting Values

In Deaf culture, relying primarily on vision for language and the rest of daily life does not bespeak an impairment. On the contrary, there is much that is admirable about it: the intellectual and aesthetic power of ASL; the close bonding with members of the Deaf "family," participation in unique social institutions; enhanced abilities in spatial cognition, and more.[52] Children who are merely Deaf are perfectly healthy, and it is unethical to operate on healthy children. In American hearing culture, however, limited hearing is an impairment; parents and doctors in that culture find that they have an obligation to alleviate that impairment if possible. This is a cross-cultural conflict of values and there does not seem to be a morally valid way of choosing one set over the other. Hence there is an ethical dilemma.

Several surgeons who perform childhood implants have acknowledged the existence of Deaf culture and find that Deaf Americans are rightfully proud of their language and culture. However, once Deaf culture is recognized, the ethical dilemmas around childhood implants and the protests of the Deaf-World follow closely. It is to miss what is most interesting about this controversy, what is most richly human and revealing of the challenges confronted by bioethics, to believe with one team that a few "Deaf advocates have misled the Deaf community" in the matter of cochlear implantation of young Deaf children.[53] Such a view cannot explain the international outcry of organizations of Deaf people* Moreover, it overlooks the obvious explanation for the deep Deaf beliefs about this issue: Deaf culture values being Deaf. Likewise, when these surgeons criticize Deaf people for an apparent intolerance of diversity in failing to welcome implant users to their midst,[54] they seem to overlook the criteria that

---

*A detailed account of the protests and position papers by Deaf organizations may be found in *A Journey into the Deaf-World*. San Diego, CA: DawnSignPress, 1996. (H. Lane, R. Hoffmeister, B. Bahan).

cultures impose for membership, including shared values and language fluency. If the implanted converts learn the new language and culture and genuinely embrace its values, so different from those that guided them throughout childhood, they are likely to be accepted; there is no reason to expect that the Deaf-World will act differently in this matter of converts than any other culture. Indeed, the Deaf-World has traditionally included hard-of-hearing members and deafened adults who learned its language and embraced its values.

The ethical dilemma arising from the conflict of Deaf and hearing values would be resolved if either set of values could be rejected as without standing in the matter. It could be argued (wrongly, we think) that hearing values have no standing when it comes to implanting a Deaf child since the child is Deaf, not hearing, in the first place and since, if implanted children follow the life trajectory of most other severely hearing-impaired children, they will eventually learn manual language and become acculturated to the Deaf-World. Since the child is Deaf and will be a Deaf adult, Deaf-World values are the most relevant. We do not agree with this argument because it minimizes the legitimate interest of (hearing) parents in raising their children according to their own cultural values. On the other hand, it has been argued that Deaf cultural values have no standing when it comes to childhood implants, since Deaf children start out in mainstream hearing society and become part of the Deaf-World only when they are "placed in that community by their parents or voluntarily decide to enter it."[55] We do not agree with this argument, either, because it neglects the role that physical constitution plays in determining cultural membership, and it minimizes the legitimate interest of Deaf adults in the welfare of Deaf children.   One does not say of, for example, Native-American children that they start out in the mainstream society and only become members of the Native-American minority culture when placed there by their parents or their own decision; rather, we would say that the child "is Native-American" and has a Native-American heritage at birth.   Is that because Native-American children normally have Native-American parents—is it the parents' culture that is criterial in ascribing cultural membership to the infant? No, since a Native-American child that is transracially adopted at any age is still considered a Native-

American child. It seems that the cultural membership ascribed to the child is not based on its parents' culture, but rather on the culture the child would enter given its physical makeup. Thus, most Deaf children do not belong to the same culture as their biological parents do.

Does a visual child   (one who relies primarily on vision), however raised, have a Deaf heritage? For members of the Deaf-World, the answer is clearly "yes." They feel a strong bond with that child; they may note that it has "deaf eyes" (eyes that actively scan for information) and, after all, that child's life trajectory, given its constitution, will likely cause him or her to become fully acculturated to the Deaf-World. The Deaf child can be deprived of the opportunity to acculturate to that world, as can the Native-American child or the Black child, but the child's potential for acculturation to that world, which is rooted in his or her physical difference, remains, so we consider children with that difference Deaf, Native-American, or Black right from the start, whether they are in fact able to enter their respective cultures or not. This would explain why adult Deaf, Native-Americans, and Blacks (for example) feel a strong emotional investment in the welfare of, respectively, Deaf, Native-American, or Black children, and identify and empathize with them, even when they are not related to them.

Although some children are Deaf for hereditary reasons, others became Deaf as a sequel to illness prenatally or in childhood. Children in other cultural minorities do not acquire their distinctive physical constitution as a sequel to illness or in childhood, so an examination of the cultural norms for membership in the Deaf-World is particularly interesting. The reasons for which the Deaf constitution arises are irrelevant for those norms but the constitution itself is essential: hearing children of Deaf adults are not considered fully Deaf despite their fluency in ASL and acculturation to the Deaf-World. The situation reminds us of the status of Caucasians who are occasionally raised in a Native-American culture and are considered honorary rather than genuine Native-Americans. However, as with other language minorities, the characteristic constitution is important, we said earlier, in that it predisposes the person to communicate in the language and thus participate in the life of the culture. If that predisposition is undermined by long acculturation to spoken language and culture, as it would be in a deafened hearing adult, it seems that person is not considered Deaf on constitutional grounds alone and must acquire signed language fluency and Deaf-World cultural norms before the Deaf-World will view them as Deaf.[56]

To summarize this ethical dilemma: Following the ordinary language practices by which we ascribe cultural membership to children, all visual children are Deaf, and this is true no matter the means by which they acquired the constitution characteristic of that cultural minority. Therefore, the values of the Deaf culture to which they belong have ethical standing in making plans for their life, as do the values of the hearing culture to which their parents usually belong. Because the two sets of values are ethically opposed on this issue, there is a dilemma.

The Right of the Deaf-World to Exist and Flourish

It is helpful to consider whether cochlear implant surgery performed on young children would be ethical if, contrary to the present facts, implants could deliver close to normal hearing for most implanted children, and the children then proceeded to acquire spoken language. If we conclude that there are serious ethical dilemmas associated even with a perfect implant, then the present practices—far from perfect (we have seen they leave the Deaf child "severely hearing-impaired")—are open to even more serious challenge. With a "perfect implant," the Deaf child would acquire English not ASL (assuming the parents are English speakers) and become acculturated to his or her parents' culture and not that of the Deaf-World. If this surgery were performed on a large scale, many children who would have learned ASL and who would have become acculturated to the Deaf-World would not do so. Some 60,000 schoolchildren receive special services for the hearing-impaired in the United States and, with a perfect implant available, most would be candidates for the surgery. Thus, the population of the Deaf-World in the United States would decline drastically (although most Deaf children of Deaf parents would presumably continue to enter it). The presently thriving culture would diminish as well, and possibly die. If so, the program of cochlear implantation in children, and the parental decisions that implemented it, would have as one effect the diminution or death of a minority culture. This must be a matter of grave ethical concern which is not, in principle, diminished by observing that implants do not now have and are not likely to have for some time to come the ability to provide near-normal hearing. Implant advocates have maintained that Deaf leaders contradict themselves when they object both that implants do not provide language for the Deaf child and that they threaten the survival of Deaf culture.[57] Yet surely a minority is justified in decrying an ineffective social policy that if effective would threaten its existence.

It is widely held as an ethical principle that the preservation of minority cultures is a good. The variety of humankind and cultures enriches all cultures and contributes to the biological, social, and psychological well-being of humankind. Laws and covenants, such as the United Nations Declaration of the Rights of Persons Belonging to National or Ethnic, Religious, and Linguistic Minorities, are founded on a belief in the value of protecting minority cultures.[58] The Declaration calls on states to foster their linguistic minorities and ensure that children and adults have adequate opportunities to learn the minority language. It further affirms the right of such minorities to enjoy their culture and language and participate in decisions on the national level that affect them. Programs that substantially diminish minority cultures are engaged in ethnocide[59] and may constitute crimes against humanity. The United Nations Convention on the Prevention and Punishment of the Crime of Genocide defines as genocide "any of the following acts committed with intent to destroy in whole or in part a national, ethnical, racial or religious group, [including] measures intended to prevent births within the group."[60] Surgical programs that implant Deaf children do not have as their intent the destruction of Deaf-World culture. Ethicists have maintained, however, that a general intent to commit genocide can be established, in the absence of a specific intent, from proof of reasonable forseeability.

Both the UN Declaration and the Convention express humankind's interest in preserving and fostering minority languages and cultures. Once the minority language and culture of the Deaf-World is recognized, those statements of ethical principles for social policies related to language minorities sensitize us to the ethical dilemma posed in principle by programs of childhood cochlear implantation. Articulating a view held by many colleagues,[61] one otologist has written: "We have uppermost in our minds not to harm, let alone destroy the Deaf community; not to do damage to Deaf culture...."[62] How can this goal be reconciled with a program of cochlear implantation in young Deaf children that seeks to endow them with a different language and acculturation? The same otologist has written that implants are "inevitably going to diminish the numbers of young children who would otherwise enter the Deaf community.... The net effect on the Deaf culture may well be a negative one."[63]

Confronted with a related ethical dilemma, some Black leaders and organizations have condemned transracial adoption practices with Black children on the ground (among others) that they promote "cultural genocide."[64] The Congress and the courts of the United States seem to have held both values dear—the best interests of the child and those of the minority culture—in legislating and adjudicating cases under the Indian Child Welfare Act of 1978. Passed at a time when the survival of Native-American cultures was considered threatened by very high rates of transracial adoption, the act was designed to prevent the undermining of Native-American tribes; it states that "it is the policy of this nation to protect the best interests of Indian children and to promote the stability and security of Indian tribes...." The Supreme Court has ruled that lower courts must consider the best interests of the particular Native-American tribe as well as the best interests of the child.[65]

Hearing parents may object that their sole duty is to serve the reasonable best interests of their child, leaving to social institutions the responsibility for defending the interests of minority cultures. Likewise, the surgeons consulted might maintain that their sole responsibility in this matter is the health of their child patient. Relegating the responsibility to society does not provide an entirely satisfactory solution since hearing parents and doctors are members of the larger society to which the responsibility for defending the Deaf-World would be left and if hearing parents elected in large numbers to have their Deaf children surgically implanted, and if surgeons simply abided by parents' wishes, it is hard to see what measures a concerned society might take to ensure the survival of the Deaf-World that would not trammel the primary authority of the parents' decision. Still, the objection has merit: in matters of public health policy, it is not normally the individual patients, their relatives, or their doctors who are expected to consider the ethical implications for society at large; it is instead social organizations, such as associations of doctors and surgeons and, above all, the public health branch of government. It is deeply disquieting that the ethical implications of childhood implant have not been formally considered by those bodies with, of course, the participation of the concerned minority.

Implant advocates have claimed that Deaf people's objection to implantation in young children is invalidated by their conflict of interest in wishing to see their culture survive.[66] In fact, Deaf people seek to promote the interests of individual Deaf children as well as that of their culture in opposing childhood implantation. It is highly implausible to argue that Deaf organizations around the world have adopted their strong anti-implantation stand without regard to the best interests of Deaf children. Deaf adults strongly identify with Deaf children on a personal level, as we have said, and they recognize that the children will become Deaf adults. Moreover, the best interests of the Deaf child and those of the Deaf-World are largely consonant, so neither parents nor Deaf adults, who hold both values dear, need feel divided in their allegiances. In the most likely scenario, visual children will continue to be born to hearing parents and most will become acculturated to the Deaf-World, implanted or not, when finally able to acquire ASL (in the United States). Deaf adults usually take a Deaf spouse and integrate into the social structure of that world. Therefore, those actions that are favorable to Deaf-World interests—such as provision of interpreters, captioning, anti-discrimination legislation, promotion of the Deaf arts and the like—will be favorable to the Deaf child's interests.

Likewise, Deaf leaders have been accused of wishing to pre-empt parental decision-making and even to supplant parents in various roles involved in raising their Deaf children.[67] We find no basis for such attributions in our knowledge of Deaf-World culture or in the many policy statements of national and international Deaf organizations. On the contrary, there is no dispute that parents have the moral and legal responsibility for raising their children and approving measures for their health care. However, a major function of government and of professional organizations is to withhold from parents the option to approve health measures that are unproven in their balance of risks and benefits, or unethical, or both. It is the public health policy decision here that has come under attack, not the parents. Because the Deaf-World is concerned above all with the Deaf child, and such a concern is consonant with the desire to see its culture thrive, it wants to ensure that Deaf children are not penalized for being Deaf. Deaf adults want to see Deaf children enjoy full and easy communication at home and school, and all that that brings with it in socialization and education. Deaf adults want Deaf children to have Deaf role models, so that they can, as can hearing children, envision possible lives for themselves.[68] Clearly these are central parental concerns as well. Therefore, Deaf-World policy has long favored collaboration with hearing parents to promote the best interests of the Deaf child.

We must conclude then that the public health policy which allows cochlear implant surgery on young children is scientifically and ethically flawed. However, the theoretical discussion of the relative standing of Deaf and hearing values, and of the ethical problems presented by a perfect implant, must not obscure the present reality: widespread cochlear implant surgery today is in all likelihood damaging many Deaf children's lives by depriving them of a full language and by placing them at risk socially and psychologically.

Notes for The Science and Ethics of Cochlear Implantation in Young Children

1. Balkany T. The rescuers. *Adv Otorhinolaryngol* 1995; *50*: 4–8. Balkany T, Hodges A. Misleading the Deaf community about cochlear implantation in children. *Ann Otol Rhinol Laryngol* 1994; *114*: 148–9. Cohen N. The ethics of cochlear implants in young children. *Am J Otol* 1994; *15*: 1–2. Cohen N. Medical and surgical perspectives: Issues in treatment and management of severe and profound hearing impairment. *Ann Otol Rhinol Laryngol* 1994; *114*: 149–50. Cohen N. Cochlear implants in young children: Ethical considerations. *Ann Otol Rhinol Laryngol* 1995; *166*: 17–9. Geers A. Closing comments on the decision to implant a Deaf child. *Ann Otol Rhinol Laryngol* 1995; *166*: 20–1. Hyde M. Some ethical dimensions of cochlear implantation of Deaf children. *Ann Otol Rhinol Laryngol* 1995; *166*: 19–20. McCaughey J. Cochlear implants: Some considerations of a more or less ethical character. *Ann Otol Rhinol Laryngol* 1995; *166*: 16–7. Tyler R. Cochlear implants and the Deaf culture. *Am J Audiol* 1993; *2*: 26–32. Balkany T, Hodges A, Goodman K. Ethics of cochlear implantation in young children. *Otolaryngol—Head Neck Surg* 1996; *114*: 748–55.

Lane H, Grodin M. Ethical issues in cochlear implant surgery: An exploration into disease, disability and the best interests of the child. *Kennedy Inst Ethics J* 1997; 7: 231–51. Crouch RA Letting the deaf be deaf. Reconsidering the use of cochlear implants in prelingually deaf children. *Hastings Cent Rep.* 1997 Jul–Aug; *27*(4):14–21.

2. Lane H. The cochlear implant controversy. *World Fed Deaf News* 1994; (2–3): 22-8. NAD. Report of the Task Force on Childhood Cochlear Implants. *Natl Assn Deaf Broadcaster* 1991; *13*: 1.

3. World Federation of the Deaf. Proceedings of the XII World Congress of the World Federation of the Deaf. Vienna, Austria: *Federal Ministry for Labor and Social Affairs* 1995.

4. Nicolai J, Aubert L, Farmer C, von Wallenberg E. A comparative study of the use of FM systems with the Nucleus cochlear implant system. In: Balkany, T editor. Proceedings of the Sixth Pediatric Implant Conference; 1996 Feb 1; Miami, FL.

5. Food and Drug Administration. PMA 890027. June 27, 1990.

6. National Institutes of Health. Cochlear implants in adults and children. *NIH Consensus Conf* 1995; *13*: 1–30.

7. Kveton J, Balkany T. The status of cochlear implantation in children. *J Pediatr* 1991; *118*: 1–7.

8. Balkany T, Hodges A, Goodman K. op. cit. p. 748.

9. Moog JS, Geers AE. Impact of the cochlear implant on the educational setting. *Adv Otorhinolaryngol* 1995; *50*: 174–6.

10. CADS (Center for Assessment and Demographic Studies, Gallaudet University).. Annual Survey of Hearing-Impaired Children and Youth 1991-1992. Age at Onset of Deafness for Students with Profound Hearing Losses. Washington DC: CADS, Gallaudet University, 1992.

11. Cowan RS., Dowell RC, Pyman BC, Dettman SJ, Dawson PW, Rance G, Barker EJ, Sarant JZ, Clark GM. Preliminary speech perception results for children with the 22-electrode Melbourne/cochlear hearing prosthesis. *Adv Otorhinolaryngol* 1993; *48*: 231–5.

12. Studies from the same laboratory that report on subject groups that overlap extensively have been represented by the most comprehensive study. Longitudinal studies are represented by the group(s) with the longest implant use. Studies using modified open-set tests that prompt responses by topic or stress pattern, for example, are not included. The results of such studies are difficult to interpret since there is no measure of the varying degrees of prompting they provide. Open-set tests are considered a better test of the general speech perception benefit to be derived from the implant. (Cf. Tyler RS. editor. Cochlear Implants: Audiological Foundations. San Diego: Singular, 1993.Waltzman S, Cohen NL, Gomolin RH, Green JE, Shapiro WH, Hoffman RA, Roland JT. Open set speech perception in congenitally Deaf children using cochlear implants. *Am J Otol* 1997; *18*: 342–9. Osberger MJ, Kessler D. Issues in protocol design for cochlear implant trials in children: The Clarion pediatric study. *Ann Otol Rhinol Laryngol* 1995; *9*(2) (Suppl): 337–9.) The largest group of studies excluded employed the Common Phrases Test, a modified open-set test with picture-prompted sentence recognition. The mean percent correct in those six studies was 16; the median was zero where it could be determined. (Cf. Osberger MJ., Miyamoto RT, Zimmerman-Phillips S, Kemink JL, Stroer B, Firszt JB, Novak MA. Independent evaluations of the speech perception abilities of children with the Nucleus 22-channel cochlear implant system. *Ear Hear* 1991; *12*(4) (Suppl): 66S–80S. Osberger MJ, Robbins AM,

Miyamoto RT, Berry SW, Myres WA, Kessler KS, Pope ML. Speech perception abilities of children with cochlear implants, tactile aids, or hearing aids. *Am J Otol* 1991; *12* (Suppl): 105–15. Miyamoto RT, Osberger MJ, Robbins AM, Myres WA, Kessler K, Pope ML. Longitudinal evaluation of communication skills of children with single-or multichannel cochlear implants. *Am J Otol* 1992; *13*(3): 215–22. Miyamoto RT, Osberger MJ, Robbins AM, Myres WA, Kessler K. Prelingually deafened children's performance with the nucleus multichannel cochlear implant. *Am J Otol* 1993; *14*: 437–45.) We found no studies of audiovisual open-set word recognition with groups of children born Deaf or early become so that had a lipreading-only condition so that the contribution of the implant could be assessed. However, good lipreading generally requires prior knowledge of the language (Boothroyd A. Profound Deafness. In: Tyler R, editor. Cochlear Implants: Audiological Foundations. San Diego CA: Singular, 1993: 1–33). The study reported in row 6 of Table 3 also had an audio-visual condition in which, using a variety of tests, some of them with prompting, the investigators compared enhancement of lipreading scores in matched groups of children, Deaf before age three, who had used a tactile aid or a multichannel implant or a hearing aid for three years (Geers A, Brenner C. Speech perception results: Audition and lipreading enhancement. *Volta Rev* 1994; *96*: 1–11). The implant users performed at about the level of children with profound losses averaging 95 dB and using hearing aids; they were superior to hearing aid users with 110-dB average losses, and not significantly different from the children using tactile aids.

13. Osberger MJ, Miyamoto RT, Zimmerman-Phillips S, Kemink JL, Stroer B, Firszt JB, Novak MA. Independent evaluations of the speech perception abilities of children with the Nucleus 22-channel cochlear implant system. *Ear Hear* 1991; *12*(4) (Suppl): 66S–80S.

14. Fryauf-Bertschy H, Tyler RS, Kelsay D, Gantz BJ. Performance over time of congenitally and postlingually Deafened children using a multi-channel cochlear implant. *J Speech Hear Res* 1992; *35*: 913–20.

15. Miyamoto RT., Osberger MJ, Robbins AM, Myres WA, Kessler K. Prelingually Deafened children's performance with the nucleus multichannel cochlear implant. *Am J Otol* 1993; *14*: 437–45.

16. Waltzman SB., Cohen NL, Gomolin RH, Shapiro WH, Ozdamar SR, Hoffman RA. Long-term results of early cochlear implantation in congenitally and prelingually Deafened children. *Am J Otol* 1994; *15* (Suppl): 9–13.

17. Gantz BJ., Tyler RS, Woodworth GG, Tye-Murray N, Fryauf-Bertschy H. Results of multi-channel cochlear implants in congenital and acquired prelingual Deafness in children: Five year follow-up. *Am J Otol 1994*; *15* (Suppl): 1–7.

18. Geers A, Brenner C. Speech perception results: Audition and lipreading enhancement. *Volta Rev* 1994; 96: 1–11.

19. van den Borne B, van denBroek P, Snik A, Vermeulen A, Brokx J. Pediatric cochlear implantation in The Netherlands. Selection criteria and initial results. *Adv Otorhinolaryngol* 1995; *50*: 108–13.

20. Waltzman S, Cohen NL, Gomolin RH, Green JE, Shapiro WH, Hoffman RA, Roland JT. Open set speech perception in congenitally Deaf children using cochlear implants. *Am J Otol* 1997; *18*: 342–9.

21. Fryauf-Bertschy H, Tyler RS, Kelsay DMR, Gantz BJ, Woodworth GG. Cochlear implant use by prelingually Deafened children: The influences of age at implant and length of device use. *J Speech Lang Hear Res* 1997; *40*: 183–99.

22. Waltzman S, Cohen NL, Gomolin RH, Green JE, Shapiro WH, Hoffman RA, Roland JT. Open set speech perception in congenitally Deaf children using cochlear implants. *Am J Otol* 1997; *18*: 342–9.

23. In some respects the mean scores are expected to be overestimates of speech perception capability: (1) A correct response generally requires only a subjectively scored "correct" repetition of the test word, not an objectively scored measure that the word was understood. (2) Listening conditions are usually more favorable in the laboratory than elsewhere. (3) Some of the children were quite practiced on the lists, which were restricted in length or content in some studies. (4) Some subjects were excluded from testing because they could not understand the verbal instructions. (If it could be determined that this was the case from the report, these were conservatively assigned a score of zero, following the procedure of Waltzman *et al.*(Waltzman S, Cohen NL, Gomolin RH, Green JE, Shapiro WH, Hoffman RA, Roland JT. Open set speech perception in congenitally Deaf children using cochlear implants. *Am J Otol* 1997; *18*: 342–9) and the discussion in Tyler (Tyler RS. Speech perception by children. In: Tyler RS, editor. Cochlear Implants: Audiological Foundations. San Diego: Singular, 1993: 191–256) and their data were included in computing the mean and median. The number of such subjects is listed in the column "children excluded." (5) Some studies include children deafened as late as age three, who would thus have considerable fluency in English before implantation. These comprise an estimated 1 in 14 children with profound hearing losses (CADS (Center for Assessment and Demographic Studies, Gallaudet University). Annual Survey of Hearing-Impaired Children and Youth 1991-1992. Age at Onset of Deafness for Students with Profound Hearing Losses. Washington DC: CADS, Gallaudet University, 1992) but have a much higher incidence in the test populations. (6) The distributions of scores are frequently right-skewed—that is, the mean is disproportionately influenced by a few outlying scores when they occur. In these circumstances, the median score, also shown where it could be derived, is a better measure of central tendency of the scores. The median is obtained by rank-ordering the scores of individual children and identifying the score located at the 50th percentile (i.e., at the mid-point of the distribution). In some cases (marked "e") the median had to be estimated from the information supplied; in other cases, it could be determined only by reading individual scores from graphs.

24. Kirk KI, Pisoni DB, Osberger MJ. Lexical effects on spoken word recognition by pediatric cochlear implant users. *Ear Hear* 1995; *16*: 470–81.

25. Fryauf-Bertschy H, Tyler RS, Kelsay DMR, Gantz BJ, Woodworth GG. Cochlear implant use by prelingually deafened children: The influences of age at implant and length of device use. *J Speech Lang Hear Res* 1997; *40*: 183–99.

26. Balkany T, Hodges A, Goodman K. op. cit. p. 752.

27. Holt J. Classroom attributes and achievement test scores for Deaf and hard of hearing students. *Am Ann Deaf* 1994; *139*: 430–7

28. Balkany T, Hodges A, Goodman K. op. cit. p. 752.

29. Waltzman S, Cohen NL, Gomolin RH, Green JE, Shapiro WH, Hoffman RA, Roland JT. Open set speech perception in congenitally Deaf children using cochlear implants. *Am J Otol* 1997; *18*: 342–9.

30. Miyamoto RT, Osberger MJ, Todd SL, Robbins AM, Stroer BS, Zimmerman-Phillips S, Carney AE. Variables affecting implant performance in children. *Laryngoscope* 1994; *104*: 1120–4.

31. Cowan RS, Dowell RC, Pyman BC, Dettman SJ, Dawson PW, Rance G, Barker EJ, Sarant JZ, Clark GM. Preliminary speech perception results for children with the 22-electrode Melbourne/cochlear hearing prosthesis. *Adv Otorhinolaryngol* 1993; *48*: 231–5.

32. Waltzman S, Cohen NL, Gomolin RH, Green JE, Shapiro WH, Hoffman RA, Roland JT. Open set speech perception in congenitally Deaf children using cochlear implants. *Am J Otol* 1997; *18*: 342–9.

33. Rose DE., Vernon M, Pool A. Cochlear implants in prelingually Deaf children. *Am Ann Deaf* 1996; *141*: 258—61

34. Geers A, Moog J. Spoken language results: Vocabulary, syntax, and communication. *Volta Rev* 1994; *96*: 131–48.

35. Miyamoto R, Svirsky M, Robbins A. Enhancement of expressive language in prelingually Deaf children with cochlear implants. *Acta Otolaryngol* 1997; *117*: 154–7. We discuss here the results of the most recent in a series of published studies on the same population from the same laboratory.

36. Petitto LA. On the ontogenetic requirements for early language acquisition. In: de Boysson-Bardies E, de Schonen S, Jusczyk P, Morton J, editors. Developmental neurocognition: Speech and Face Processing in the First Year of Life. New York: Kuwer Academic, 1993: 365–83.

37. Cummins J. Linguistic interdependence and the educational development of bilingual children. *Rev Ed. Rese.* 1979; *49*: 222–51.

38. Strong M, Prinz P. A study of the relationship between American Sign Language and English literacy. *J Deaf Stud Deaf Ed* 1997; *2*: 37–46.

39. Padden C. American Sign Language and reading ability in Deaf children. In: Chamberlain C, Morford J, Mayberry R, editors. Language Acquisition by Eye. Mahwah NJ: Lawrence Erlbaum, in press.

40. Moores D, Sweet C. Factors predictive of school achievement. In: Moores DF, Meadow-Orlans K, editors. Educational and Developmental Aspects of Deafness. Washington DC: Gallaudet University Press, 1990: 154–201. Strong M . Language Learning and Deafness. New York: Cambridge University Press, 1988.

41. Geers A, Moog J. Spoken language results: Vocabulary, syntax, and communication. *Volta Rev* 1994; *96*: 131–48.

42. Kelsay D, Tyler R. Advantages and disadvantages expected and realized by pediatric cochlear implant recipients as reported by their parents. *Am J Otol* 1996; *17*: 866–73.

43. Tye-Murray N. Cochlear Implants and Children: A Handbook for Parents, Teachers and Speech Professionals. Washington DC: AG Bell Assn, 1992

44. Balkany T, Hodges A, Goodman K. op. cit. p. 754.

45. Petitto LA. On the ontogenetic requirements for early language acquisition. In: de Boysson-Bardies E, de Schonen S, Jusczyk P, Morton J, editors.

Developmental Neurocognition: Speech and Face Processing in the First Year of Life. New York: Kuwer Academic, 1993: 365–83. Mayberry R, Eichen E. The long-lasting advantage of learning sign language in childhood: another look at the critical period for language acquisition. *J Mem Lang* 1991; *30*: 486–512.

46. Osberger MJ, Kessler D. Issues in protocol design for cochlear implant trials in children: The Clarion pediatric study. *Ann Otol Rhinol Laryngol* 1995; *9*(2) (Suppl): 337–9.

47. Osberger MJ, Miyamoto RT, Zimmerman-Phillips S, Kemink JL, Stroer B, Firszt JB, Novak MA. Independent evaluations of the speech perception abilities of children with the Nucleus 22-channel cochlear implant system. *Ear Hear* 1991; *12*(4) (Suppl): 66S–80S. Boothroyd A. Profound Deafness. In: Tyler R, editor. Cochlear Implants: Audiological Foundations. San Diego CA: Singular, 1993: 1–33. Geers A, Brenner C. Speech perception results: Audition and lipreading enhancement. *Volta Rev* 1994; *96*: 1–11. Horn RM, Nozza RJ, Dolitsky JN. Audiological and medical considerations for children with cochlear implants. *Am Ann Deaf* 1991; *136*: 82–6. Miyamoto RT, Kirk KI, Todd SL, Robbins AM, Osberger MJ. Speech perception skills of children with multichannel cochlear implants or hearing aids. *Ann Otol Rhinol Laryngol* 1995; *104* (Suppl)l: 334–7.

48. Schildroth AN, Karchmer MA, editors. Deaf Children in America. San Diego CA: College-Hill, 1986.

49. Kelsay D, Tyler R. Advantages and disadvantages expected and realized by pediatric cochlear implant recipients as reported by their parents. *Am J Otol* 1996; *17*: 866–73.

50. Grodin MA, Glantz LH. Children as Research Subjects. New York: Oxford, 1994.

51. Cohen N. op. cit. 1995, p. 18.

52. Lane H, Hoffmeister R, Bahan B. A Journey into the Deaf-World. San Diego CA: DawnSignPress, 1996.

53. Balkany T, Hodges A, Goodman K. op. cit. p. 750.

54. Balkany T, Hodges A, Goodman K. op. cit. p. 753.

55. Cohen N. The ethics of cochlear implants in young children. *Am J Otol* 1994; *15*: 1–2.

56. Bahan B. Comment on Turner. *Sign Lang Stud* 1994; *84*: 241–9.

57. Balkany T, Hodges A, Goodman K. op. cit. p. 751.

58. United Nations. Rights of persons belonging to national, or ethnic, religious and linguistic minorities. Resolution 47/135. *UN Handbook* 1992.

59. Diamond S. [Who killed Biafra]. *Les Temps modernes* 1970; *283*: 1194–206.

60. United Nations. Convention on the Prevention and Punishment of the Crime of Genocide. Resolution 96/I. 1948.

61. NIDCD. National Strategic Research Plan for Hearing and Hearing Impairment and Voice and Voice Disorders. NIH pub. 93-3443. Bethesda MD: National Institutes of Health, 1992. Tyler R. Cochlear implants and the Deaf culture. *Am J Audiol* 1993; *2*: 26–32.

62. Cohen N. op. cit. 1995, p. 19.

63. Cohen N. op. cit. 1995, p. 19.

64. Simon RJ, Altstein H. Adoption, Race and Identity: From Infancy through Adolescence. New York: Praeger, 1992.

65. Simon RJ, Altstein H. op. cit.
66. Balkany T, Hodges A, Goodman K. op. cit. p.750, 753.
67. Balkany T, Hodges A, Goodman K. op. cit. p. 749.
68. Bloch N. Early Childhood Implants: American Deaf Community Concerns. Address to the Conference on Childhood Implants: Ethical Issues in Debate. Portland State University. 1993.

Notes

Part One. *Representations of Deaf People: The Infirmity and Cultural Models*

Page xiii "our reports." Y. Andersson (1990). Who should make decisions on communication among deaf people? *Deaf American, 40,* 1–4.

3   "to speak." G. Weiss (1990). New hope for deaf children: implant gives them hearing and speech. *American Health, 9,* 17.

"and ethically." National Association of the Deaf, Cochlear Implant Task Force, Cochlear implants in children: A position paper of the National Association of the Deaf. February 2, 1991. Reprint: *The National Association of the Deaf Broadcaster, 13,* March 1991, p. 1.

6   "who try to." C. Padden and T. Humphries (1988). *Deaf in America: Voices from a Culture.* Cambridge, MA: Harvard University Press.

"THINK-HEARING is . . . just as insulting as ORAL but can be used to label any Deaf person, even those who are not ORAL . . . HEARING is not just a category of people who hear; it is a category of those who are the opposite of what Deaf people are; e.g., students at schools for Deaf children sometimes call their football opponents HEARING even when the team is from another school for Deaf children" T. Humphries (1990). An introduction to the culture of deaf people in the United States: content notes and reference materials for teachers. *Sign Language Studies, 72,* 209–40, p. 222.

7   "and tribal." E. Goffman (1963). *Stigma: Notes on the Management of Spoiled Identity.* Englewood Cliffs, NJ: Prentice-Hall.

"gesturing is not." C. Padden and T. Humphries (1988). *Deaf in America: Voices from a Culture.* Cambridge, MA: Harvard University Press.

"*Lonely Hunter.*" C. McCullers (1967). *The Heart Is a Lonely Hunter.* Boston: Houghton Mifflin. Also see I. Turgenev, *Mumu.* Reprinted in T. Batson and E. Bergman (1985). *Angels and Outcasts: An Anthology of Deaf Characters in Literature,* 3rd ed. Washington, DC: Gallaudet University Press, p. 86.

8   "*In This Sign.*" J. Greenberg (1970). *In This Sign.* New York: Holt, Rinehart & Winston.

"his misery." Charles Dickens' *Dr. Marigold* and Guy de Maupassant's *The Deaf-Mute* are reprinted in *Angels and Outcasts: An Anthology of Deaf Characters in Literature,* 3rd ed. Washington, DC: Gallaudet University Press.

Page 8   *"Pig Outdoors."* H. Kisor (1990). *What's That Pig Outdoors?* New York: Hill and Wang.

9   "hearing people's." J. G. Kyle and G. Pullen (1988). Cultures in contact: Deaf and hearing people. *Disability, Handicap and Society, 3,* 49–61, p. 56.

"further demands." E. Goffman (1963). *Stigma: Notes on the Management of Spoiled Identity.* Englewood Cliffs, NJ: Prentice-Hall, p. 121.

11   "to despair." A. Memmi (1984). *Dependence.* Boston: Beacon Press, p. 108.

"without meaning." C. Padden and T. Humphries (1988). *Deaf in America: Voices from a Culture.* Cambridge, MA: Harvard University Press.

"Susan Sontag." S. Sontag (1989). *Illness as Metaphor and AIDS and Its Metaphors.* New York: Anchor.

"that they do." Undergraduates studying education were asked, "How do you feel when you meet someone who is disabled?" The strongest reaction encountered was unease and uncertainty as to how to behave, and therefore embarrassment. The next most common response was: It is not different from meeting anyone else when you get used to the situation. In third place by frequency came emotions such as pity, guilt, and "thank goodness it's not me." Students were disinclined to share a house with someone disabled, but living next door they found acceptable. From L. Barton, ed. (1988). *The Politics of Special Educational Needs.* Philadelphia: Falmer Press, p. 138.

"and freshness." L. H. Sigourney (1866). *Letters of Life.* New York: Appleton, pp. 222–33. Also see A. de Musset, *Pierre et Camille,* reprinted in T. Batson and E. Bergman (1985). *Angels and Outcasts: An Anthology of Deaf Characters in Literature,* 3rd ed. Washington, DC: Gallaudet University Press.

"properly buried." A. Naniwe (1991). *L'enfant sourd et la société burundaise.* Ph.D. dissertation, University of Brussels.

"spirit aggression." Cf. G. P. Murdock (1980). *Theories of Illness.* Pittsburgh: University of Pittsburgh Press.

12   "three wives?" R. Shweder (1984). Anthropology's romantic rebellion against the enlightenment. In R. Shweder and R. A. LeVine, eds., *Culture Theory* (pp. 27–66). New York: Cambridge University Press, p. 55.

"and empathy." Z. Vendler (1984). Understanding people. In R. Shweder and R. A. LeVine, eds., *Culture Theory* (pp. 200–13). New York: Cambridge University Press, p. 209. Also see C. Geertz (1984). "From the native's point of view." On the nature of anthropological understanding. In R. Shweder and R. A. LeVine, eds., *Culture Theory* (pp. 123–36). New York: Cambridge University Press, p. 135.

14   "two languages." U. Bellugi and S. Fischer (1972). A comparison of sign language and spoken language. *Cognition, 1,* 173–200.

15   "Salk Institute." See E. Klima and U. Bellugi (1979). *The Signs of Language.* Cambridge, MA: Harvard University Press.

Page 16 "much more." S. Rutherford (1988). The culture of American deaf people. *Sign Language Studies, 59*, 128–47.

17 "cultural group." J. Schein (1987). The demography of deafness. In P. C. Higgins and J. E. Nash, *Understanding Deafness Socially*. Springfield, IL: Charles C Thomas, pp. 3–27. Also see J. Schein (1989). *At Home Among Strangers*. Washington, DC: Gallaudet University Press, p. 106.

"important role." J. Schein (1989). *At Home Among Strangers*. Washington, DC: Gallaudet University Press. Deaf people feel that their clubs are "a piece of their own land in exile—an oasis in the world of sound" (B. Bragg and E. Bergman [1981]. *Tales from a Clubroom*. Washington, DC: Gallaudet University Press, p. vii.) One deaf club member explained to a hearing person: "For Deaf people, the Deaf club is like a second home. Hearing people don't have anything like that. They go home from work, put on headphones, and listen to their stereos or [they] watch television. But the Deaf get together and socialize at their club. It's like a second home" (S. Hall [1991]. Door into deaf culture: Folklore in an American Deaf social club. *Sign Language Studies, 73*, 421–29, p. 421). This author elaborates: "More than just a social gathering place, Deaf clubs are where the Deaf look for adult guidance in their youth, where they can obtain information and advice about employment, where they may meet the one they will marry, or where a Deaf stranger in town may find aid and friendship" (p. 422).

"left out." G. Becker (1980). *Growing Old in Silence*. Berkeley: University of California Press, p. 65.

18 "such contact." My authority for the information about values and mores is the videotape series *An Introduction to American Deaf Culture* by MJ Bienvenu and B. Colonomos (1989). Burtonsville, MD: Sign Media, Inc. The videotape series *American Culture: The Deaf Perspective* (S. Rutherford, Deaf Media, Inc., 1986) was also very helpful. I am indebted to Ms. Alma Bournazian for reviewing many aspects of American deaf culture with me.

19 "and who not." B. Heyman, B. Bell, M. R. Kingham, and E. C. Handyside (1990). Social class and the prevalence of handicapping conditions. *Disability, Handicap and Society, 5*, 167–84, p. 169.

"who is not." D. A. Gerber (1990). Listening to disabled people: the problem of voice and authority in Robert B. Edgerton's "The Cloak of Competence." *Disability, Handicap and Society, 5*, 3–23, p. 8. Also see S. A. Gelb (1987). Social deviance and the "discovery" of the moron. *Disability, Handicap and Society, 2*, 247–58; B. Heyman, B. Bell, M. R. Kingham, and E. C. Handyside (1990). Social class and the prevalence of handicapping conditions. *Disability, Handicap and Society, 5*, 167–84, p. 169. The mental retardation profession also claimed that the United States was being flooded with immigrants who required custodial care: W. S. Barnett (1986). The transition from public residential schools for retarded people to custodial facilities: an economic explanation. *Disability, Handicap and Society, 1*, 53–71, p. 61.

Page 19   "their race." *Larry P.* v. *Riles*, 495F, Supp. 926 (N.D. Cal. 1979), affirmed 793F 2nd 969 (9th Cir. 1984).

20   "the impairment." P. Abberley (1987). The concept of oppression and the development of a social theory of disability. *Disability, Handicap and Society*, 2, 5–20.

"what to do.'" G. Becker (1980). *Growing Old in Silence.* Berkeley: University of California Press, p. 55.

"*Globe.*" R. Saltus (1989). Returning to the world of sound. *Boston Globe*, July 10, 1989, pp. 27, 29.

"precious gift." M. Oliver (1989). Conductive education: if it wasn't so sad it would be funny. *Disability, Handicap and Society*, 4, 197–200, p. 199.

"deaf minority." National Institute on Deafness and Other Communication Disorders, *The Working Group on Research and Training at the National Institute on Deafness and Other Communication Disorders from a Deaf Community Perspective: Report to Dr. James B. Snow, Director.* September 7, 1990.

21   "cultural frame." R. D'Andrade (1984). Cultural meaning systems. In R. Shweder and R. A. LeVine, eds., *Culture Theory* (pp. 88–122). New York: Cambridge University Press.

22   "the ADA." J. Gansberg (1990). What does the ADA mean to deaf Americans? *Deaf Community News, 13(8)*, p. 1. " 'Disabled' is a label that has not historically belonged to deaf people. It suggests political self-representations and goals unfamiliar to the group." C. Padden and T. Humphries (1988). *Deaf in America: Voices from a Culture.* Cambridge, MA: Harvard University Press, p. 44. "Deaf peoples' enduring concerns have been these: finding each other and staying together, preserving their language, and maintaining lines of transmittal of their culture. These are not the goals of disabled people. Deaf people do know, however, the benefits of this label and make choices about alignment with these people politically." T. Humphries (1990). An introduction to the culture of deaf people in the United States: content notes and reference materials for teachers. *Sign Language Studies, 72,* 209–40, p. 220.

" 'common sense' position." Rorty calls the thinker who has doubts about his vocabulary, since he is impressed with those of others and has seen all such vocabularies change in time, an ironist. The opposite of the ironist view is called common sense. "The ironist takes the unit of persuasion to be a vocabulary rather than a proposition." R. Rorty (1989). *Contingency, Irony and Solidarity.* New York: Cambridge University Press, p. 78.

23   "her abilities." R. Rorty (1989). *Contingency, Irony and Solidarity.* New York: Cambridge University Press, p. 84.

"deaf children." S. Mather (1990). Is America really a free country for us all? *Deaf American, 40,* 87–89, p. 88.

24   "perception and thought." U. Bellugi, L. O'Grady, D. Lillo-Martin, M. O'Grady-Hines, K. van Hoek, and D. Corina (1990). Enhancement

of spatial cognition in deaf children. In V. Volterra and C. Erting, eds., *From Gesture to Language in Hearing and Deaf Children* (pp. 279–98). Berlin: Springer Verlag.

"point of view." Dr. Simon Parisier, speaking at the meeting convened by the Cochlear Corporation in Boston, October 29, 1990.

25 "social order." R. A. Scott has made a similar observation concerning blind men: "The current definition of blindness is based upon a meaningless demarcation among those with severely impaired vision." R. A. Scott (1981). *The Making of Blind Men.* New Brunswick: Transactions, p. 42. On p. 73 he describes how the stigma of "blind" is attached by the ophthalmologist.

"serve them." H. Lane (1984). *When the Mind Hears: A History of the Deaf.* New York: Random House.

26 "hearing classroom." A 1985 survey found only one deaf child in four in integrated school settings had a teacher who used signs. "Using signs" is not the same thing as using ASL. T. Allen and M. Karchmer (1990). Communication in classrooms for deaf students: student, teacher, and program characteristics. In H. Bornstein, ed., *Manual Communication: Implications for Education.* Washington, DC: Gallaudet University Press, pp. 45–66.

"his fate." J.-P. Sartre, Introduction. In A. Memmi (1966). *Portrait du colonisé.* Paris: Pauvert, pp. 35–36.

" 'modern' initiative." G. List. Oralistic tradition and written history: Deaf in German-speaking countries. Address to the Deaf Way Congress, July 11, 1989, Washington, DC.

27 "and powerless." R. Rorty (1989). *Contingency, Irony and Solidarity.* New York: Cambridge University Press, p. 89.

28 "been through." Quoted in J. Grémion (1990). *La Planète des sourds.* Paris: Messinger, p. 79.

Part Two. Representations of Deaf People: Colonialism, "Audism," and the "Psychology of the Deaf"

32 "primary school." International Bank for Reconstruction and Development (1981). *World Tables*, 3rd ed. Volume II: *Social Data.* Washington, DC: World Bank, p. 15.

33 "throughout the land." J. P. Chrétien (1980). Vocabulaire et concepts tirés de la féodalité occidentale et administration indirecte en Afrique orientale. In D. Nordman and J. P. Raison, eds., *Sciences de l'Homme.* Paris: Presse de l'ENS. J. P. Chrétien (1983). Féodalité ou féodalisation du Burundi sous le Mandat Belge. In *Etudes Africaines offertes à Henri Brunschwig.* Paris: EHESS.

"cunning and lazy." J. Gahama (1983). *Le Burundi sous administration Belge (1919–1939).* Paris: Karthala, pp. 62, 68.

35 "psychiatrically devastating." B. Harry and P. E. Dietz (1985). Offend-

ers in a silent world: hearing-impairment and deafness in relation to criminality, incompetence, and insanity. *Bulletin of the American Academy of Psychiatry and Law*, *13(1)*, 85–96.

Page 35 "these judgments." S. Chess and P. Fernandez (1980). Do deaf children have a typical personality? *Journal of the American Academy of Child Psychiatry*, *19*, 654–64, p. 655.

"is delayed." F. P. Lebuffe and L. A. Lebuffe (1979). Psychiatric aspects of deafness. *Primary Care*, *6(2)*, 295–310, p. 301.

"social ineptness." E. Levine (1981). *Ecology of Early Deafness*. New York: Columbia University Press, p. 196.

"psychology of the deaf." In calling the list in Table 2 "a distillation" of the psychometric literature on deafness in the 1970s and 1980s, I mean that I examined a very large sample of that literature without bias in selection with respect to positive or negative ascriptions to deaf people. I began with major reviews of the literature and then proceeded to the studies they cited and to other studies cited in turn. If another investigator should be foolish enough to undertake an independent survey of this scope, I believe that fundamentally the same picture of deaf people would emerge from the distilled list. I am not concerned here with the (much smaller) psychological literature that engages not in psychometric evaluation and trait attribution but in experimental studies of language and cognition in deaf children and adults.

37 "of their own." R. Brown (1986). *Social Psychology*, 2d ed. New York: Free Press.

38 "native policy." R. C. F. Maugham (1929). *Africa as I Have Known It*. London: Murray (reprint: Negro Universities Press, 1969).

"deaf children." C. E. Williams (1970). Some psychiatric observations on a group of maladjusted deaf children. *Journal of Child Psychology and Psychiatry*, *11*, 1–18.

"mental hospitals." S. Dubow and L. J. Goldberg (1981). Legal strategies to improve mental health care for deaf people. In L. K. Stein, E. D. Mindel, and T. Jabaley, eds., *Deafness and Mental Health*. New York: Grune & Stratton, p. 195.

"with them." "Government primary schools were established with the idea of training an African elite to serve as clerks, teachers, or to govern the masses. This elite would have to be literate, able to perform bureaucratic tasks, and loyal to the colonial state and its policies." P. Manning (1988). *Francophone Sub-Saharan Africa*. New York: Cambridge University Press, p. 100.

40 "modern world." D. Thébault (1959). Langue arabe et parlers maghrébins. *Cahiers nord-africains*, *74*, août-septembre.

"this decree." K. McCracken (1987). 85 at TSD suspended in sign language dispute. *Knoxville Journal*, October 5, 1987, pp. 1, 10.

41 "Tables 1 and 2, respectively." L. Ndoricimpa and C. Guillet (1984). *L'Arbre-mémoire. Traditions orales du Burundi*. Paris: Karthala. C. Padden and T. Humphries (1988). *Deaf in America: Voices from a Culture*. Cambridge, MA: Harvard University Press.

"*Deaf Persons.*" G. Braddock (1975). *Notable Deaf Persons.* Washington, DC: Gallaudet College Alumni Association.

"*Speaks Out.*" L. Jacobs (1980). *A Deaf Adult Speaks Out,* 2d ed. Washington, DC: Gallaudet University Press.

"deaf playwrights." For example, G. Eastman (1974). *Sign Me Alice.* Washington, DC: Gallaudet College, 1974; B. Bragg and E. Bergman (1981). *Tales from a Clubroom.* Washington, DC: Gallaudet University Press.

"performing groups." B. Bragg (1989). *Lessons in Laughter: The Autobiography of a Deaf Actor.* Washington, DC: Gallaudet University Press. Also see B. Bragg and E. Bergman (1981). *Tales from a Clubroom.* Washington, DC: Gallaudet University Press; G. Eastman (1974). *Sign Me Alice.* Washington, DC: Gallaudet University Press; D. Miles (1976). *A Play of Our Own*; *Gestures: Poetry by Dorothy Miles.* Northridge, CA: Joyce Motion Picture Co.

"*Lesser God.*" M. Medoff (1980). *Children of a Lesser God.* Clifton, NJ: J. White.

42   "states across the nation." S. Wilcox (1989). Teaching American Sign Language as a foreign language. *ERIC Digest,* EDO-FL-8901. At the present writing, sixteen states have such laws.

"registers, poetry." See, for example, the journal *Sign Language Studies*; M. L. Sternberg (1990). *American Sign Language: A Comprehensive Dictionary.* New York: Harper & Row; C. Lucas (1989). *The Sociolinguistics of the Deaf Community.* New York: Academic Press; R. Wilbur (1987). *American Sign Language,* 2d ed. Boston: Little, Brown.

"videotapes abound." For example: G. C. Eastman (1989). *From Mime to Sign.* Silver Spring, MD: TJ Publishers; C. Baker and D. Cokely (1980). *American Sign Language: A Teacher's Resource Text on Grammar and Culture.* Silver Spring, MD: TJ Publishers.

"1987–1991." What do these people have in common? *Deaf Life,* September 1991, pp. 19–31.

"hearing people." Convention of American Instructors of the Deaf (1991). Programs and services summary. *American Annals of the Deaf, 136,* 126–54.

"classes across the nation." J. Gannon (1981). *Deaf Heritage.* Silver Spring: National Association of the Deaf; J. Gannon (1989). *The Week the World Heard from Gallaudet.* Washington, DC: Gallaudet University Press.

43   "the Deaf." H. Lane (1984). *When the Mind Hears: A History of the Deaf.* New York: Random House.

"deaf culture." J. V. Van Cleve, ed. (1987). *Gallaudet Encyclopedia of Deaf People and Deafness.* New York: McGraw-Hill; J. Van Cleve and B. Crouch (1989). *A Place of Their Own: Creating the Deaf Community in America.* Washington, DC: Gallaudet University Press.

"*From a Culture.*" C. Padden and T. Humphries (1988). *Deaf in America: Voices from a Culture.* Cambridge, MA: Harvard University Press; S. Wilcox (1989a). *American Deaf Culture: An Anthology.* Silver Spring, MD: Linstok.

Page 43   *"Deaf Culture."* S. Wilcox (1989a). *American Deaf Culture: An Anthology.*
Silver Spring, MD: Linstok.

"United States." J. Schein (1989). *At Home Among Strangers.* Washington,
DC: Gallaudet University Press.

"Deaf Community." C. Lucas (1989). *The Sociolinguistics of the Deaf Community.* New York: Academic Press.

"audism." The term "audism" was coined by Tom Humphries in
T. Humphries (1977). *Communicating Across Cultures (Deaf/Hearing) and
Language Learning.* Ph.D. dissertation, Union Graduate School, Cincin-
nati, Ohio.

"deaf community." I have paraphrased Edward Said's definition of
Orientalism. See E. Said (1989). Representing the colonized: anthropology's interlocutors. *Critical Inquiry, 15,* 205–25. E. Said (1978). *Orientalism.* New York: Pantheon.

44   "political dominance." E. Said (1989). Representing the colonized:
Anthropology's interlocutors. *Critical Inquiry, 15,* 205–25.

"deaf education." Commission on the Education of the Deaf (1988).
Toward Equality: Education of the Deaf. Washington, DC: Government
Printing Office.

"restrictive environment." J. Champie (1986). Toward a less restrictive
"least restrictive environment." *Gallaudet Today, 16,* 19–21; National
Association of the Deaf (1987). NAD recommends to the Commission
on Education of the Deaf. *NAD Broadcaster, 5,* 1–8; O. Wrigley and
M. Suwanarat (1987). Issues of significance to deaf people: findings
and recommendations for an action agenda through the UN Decade
of Disabled Persons. In *Proceedings of the Global Meeting of Experts to
Review Implementation of the World Programme of Action.* Stockholm:
United Nations.

"deaf people." National Association of the Deaf (1987). NAD recommends to the Commission on Education of the Deaf. *NAD Broadcaster,
5,* 1–8.

"job vacancies." T. E. Allen and J. Woodward (1987). Teacher charac-
teristics and the degree to which teachers incorporate features of
English in their sign communication with hearing students. *American
Annals of the Deaf, 132,* 61–67. These investigators sampled 50,000
deaf students and found that 85 percent of the 609 teachers were
hearing females; only 3 percent were deaf. None used ASL. Also see
H. Lane (1984). *When the Mind Hears: A History of the Deaf.* New York:
Random House; H. Lane (1987). Listen to the needs of deaf children.
New York Times, July 17, 1987, p. A35. *TBC Newsletter,* 1990, p. 3.

"the profession." D. S. Martin (1984). Can deafness be a teaching
advantage? *Journal of the Rehabilitation of the Deaf, 17,* 17–22.

45   "to eradicate." C. B. Wallis (1903). *The Advance of Our West African
Empire.* London: Fisher Unwin, pp. 2, 119.

"savage adversaries." R. Acuña (1988). *Occupied America: A History of
Chicanos,* 3rd ed. New York: Harper & Row, p. 41.

"symbol system." M. Myklebust (1964). *Psychology of Deafness.* New
York: Grune & Stratton, p. 158.

46 "similar pairs." D. Colin (1978). *Psychologie de l'enfant sourd*. Paris: Masson, p. 10.

"is valid." J. K. Reeves (1976). The whole personality approach to oralism in the education of the deaf. In Royal National Institute for the Deaf, *Methods of Communication Currently Used in the Education of Deaf Children*. Letchworth, Hertfordshire: Garden City Press, p. 12.

"extremely weak." A. van Uden (1986). *Sign Languages Used by Deaf People and Psycholinguistics*. Lisse: Swets & Zeitlinger, p. 89.

"sophisticated ideas." I. Rapin (1979). The effects of early blindness and deafness on cognition. In R. Katzman, ed., *Congenital and Acquired Cognitive Disorders* (pp. 189–245). New York: Raven Press, pp. 209, 223.

"so on." K. Klima and U. Bellugi (1979). *The Signs of Language*. Cambridge, MA: Harvard University Press; R. Wilbur (1987). *American Sign Language*, 2nd ed. Boston: Little, Brown.

"other languages." *Consultation sur les différentes approches de l'éducation des sourds*, ED-84/ws/102. Paris: UNESCO, 1985.

47 "speak it intelligibly." E. Levine (1981). *Ecology of Early Deafness*. New York: Columbia University Press, p. 84. Also see C. Smith (1975). Residual hearing and speech production in deaf children. *Journal of Speech and Hearing Research, 18*, 795–811; R. Stark (1979). Speech of the hearing-impaired child. In L. J. Bradford and W. G. Hardy, eds., *Hearing and Hearing Impairment*. New York: Grune & Stratton; R. Conrad (1979). *The Deaf Schoolchild*. London: Harper & Row; R. Conrad (1977). Lipreading by deaf and hearing children. *British Journal of Educational Psychology, 47*, 60–65; L. Evans (1981). Psycholinguistic perspectives on visual communication. In B. Woll, J. Kyle and M. Deuchar, eds., *Perspectives on British Sign Language and Deafness*. London: Croom Helm, pp. 151, 157.

"as native palaver." UNESCO (1979). *Sociopolitical Aspects of the Palaver in Some African Countries*. Paris: UNESCO.

"likely explanation." T. E. Allen (1986). Patterns of academic achievement among hearing-impaired students: 1974 and 1983. In A. N. Schildroth and M. A. Karchmer, eds., *Deaf Children in America* (pp. 161–206). San Diego, CA: College-Hill; R. J. Trybus and M. A. Karchmer (1977). School achievement scores of hearing-impaired children: national data on achievement status and growth patterns. *American Annals of the Deaf, 122*, 62–69.

48 "naturally inclined." J. D. Schein and M. T. Delk (1974). *The Deaf Population of the United States*. Silver Spring, MD: National Association of the Deaf.

"the purchase." C. Erting (1985). Cultural conflict in a school for deaf children. *Anthropology and Education Quarterly, 16*, 225–43.

"speech at all." P. Ries (1986). Characteristics of hearing-impaired youth in the general population and of students in special education programs for the hearing-impaired. In A. N. Schildroth and M. A. Karchmer, eds., *Deaf Children in America*. San Diego, CA: College-Hill; S. C. Brown (1986). Etiological trends, characteristics, and distributions. In A. N. Schildroth and M. A. Karchmer, eds., *Deaf Children in America* (pp. 33–54). San Diego, CA: College-Hill.

Page 48   "was dismissed." G. Vollmar (1991). Standing up for my son cost my job. *TBC News, 35,* 2–3.

50   "do it." E. S. Levine (1971). Mental assessment of the deaf child. *Volta Review, 73,* 80–105; R. Trybus (1973). Personality assessment of entering hearing-impaired college students using the 16PF form E. *Journal of Rehabilitation of the Deaf, 6,* 34–40; M. Vernon and P. Ottinger (1981). Psychological evaluation of the deaf and hard of hearing. In L. K. Stein, E. D. Mindel, and T. Jabaley, eds., *Deafness and Mental Health* (pp. 49–64). New York: Grune & Stratton; D. Watson (1979). Guidelines for the psychological and vocational assessment of deaf rehabilitation clients. *Journal of Rehabilitation of the Deaf, 13,* 27–57.

51   "the test." M. Vernon (1968). Fifty years of research on the intelligence of the deaf and hard of hearing. *Journal of Rehabilitation of the Deaf, 1,* 1–11; B. W. Heller and R. I. Harris (1987). Special considerations in the psychological assessment of hearing impaired persons. In B. W. Heller, L. M. Flohr, and L. S. Zegans, eds., *Psychosocial Interventions with Sensorially Disabled Persons* (pp. 53–77). Orlando, FL: Grune & Stratton.

"IQ scores." E. Graham and E. Shapiro (1953). Use of the performance scale of the WISC with the deaf child. *Journal of Consulting Psychology, 17,* 396–98. Goetzinger and Proud support this conclusion: C. P. Goetzinger and G. O. Proud (1975). The impact of hearing impairment upon the psychological development of children. *Journal of Auditory Research, 15,* 1–60.

"thirty points." R. F. Dillon (1980). Cognitive style and elaboration of logical abilities in hearing-impaired children. *Journal of Experimental Child Psychology, 30,* 389–400.

"different tests." C. Dwyer and S. Wincenciak (1977). A pilot investigation of three factors of the 16PF Form E, comparing the standard written form with an Ameslan videotape revision. *Journal of Rehabilitation of the Deaf, 10,* 17–23.

"either test." J. D. Rainer and K. Z. Altshuler (1967). *Psychiatry and the Deaf. U.S. Department of Health, Education and Welfare, Social and Rehabilitation Service.* Washington, DC: U.S. Government Printing Office.

52   "rarely fulfilled." E. Levine (1977). The preparation of psychological service providers for the deaf. *Journal of Rehabilitation of the Deaf,* Monograph 4; F. C. Orr, A. DeMatteo, B. Heller, M. Lee, and M. Nguyen (1987). Psychological assessment. In H. Elliott, L. Glass, and J. W. Evans, eds., *Mental Health Assessment of Deaf Clients: A Practical Manual* (pp. 93–106). San Diego, CA: College-Hill; M. Vernon and P. Ottinger (1981). Psychological evaluation of the deaf and hard of hearing. In L. K. Stein, E. D. Mindel, and T. Jabaley, eds., *Deafness and Mental Health* (pp. 49–64). New York: Grune & Stratton; D. Wat-

son (1979). Guidelines for the psychological and vocational assessment of deaf rehabilitation clients. *Journal of Rehabilitation of the Deaf, 13,* 27–57.

"their education." B. Heller (1987). Mental health assessment of deaf persons: a brief history. In H. Elliott, L. Glass, and J. W. Evans, eds., *Mental Health Assessment of Deaf Clients: A Practical Manual* (pp. 9–20). San Diego, CA: College-Hill.

"state of mind." B. W. Heller and R. I. Harris (1987). Special considerations in the psychological assessment of hearing impaired persons. In B. W. Heller, L. M. Flohr, and L. S. Zegans, eds., *Psychosocial Interventions with Sensorially Disabled Persons* (pp. 53–77). Orlando, FL: Grune & Stratton.

"learning disabled." E. Levine (1981). *Ecology of Early Deafness.* New York: Columbia University Press; F. C. Orr, A. DeMatteo, B. Heller, M. Lee, and M. Nguyen (1987). Psychological assessment. In H. Elliott, L. Glass, and J. W. Evans, eds., *Mental Health Assessment of Deaf Clients: A Practical Manual* (pp. 93–106). San Diego, CA: College-Hill. Rudner (1980) analyzed deaf and hearing responses on the Stanford Achievement Test, which measures English vocabulary and reading comprehension, mathematics concepts, and computation. He found many questions on the test markedly biased against deaf students, and these all fell into six categories—not of knowledge but of language use: questions on the test proved difficult for deaf students if they were long or if they contained subordinate clauses, comparatives, negatives, auxiliary verbs, or pronouns. L. Rudner (1978). Using standard tests with the hearing-impaired. *Volta Review, 80,* 31–40. Clearly, reading ability in English decides the outcome in all academic areas of the test; S. Quigley and R. Kretschmer (1982). *The Education of Deaf Children.* Baltimore: University Park Press. The validity of the test is thus highly questionable. See D. F. Moores (1986). Public education: implications for the deaf community. In R. Rosen, ed., *Life and Work in the 21st Century: The Deaf Person of Tomorrow. Proceedings of the 1986 NAD Forum.* Silver Spring, MD: National Association of the Deaf, pp. 33–42. Likewise, it comes as no surprise to learn that deaf students score lower on the verbal Scholastic Aptitude Test than all handicapped groups, lower even than students classified as learning disabled. See R. E. Bennett, D. A. Rock, and B. A. Kaplan (1985). *The Psychometric Characteristics of the SAT for Nine Handicapped Groups.* Princeton, NJ: Educational Testing Service. The SAT is the test that most high school seniors in America take who seek admission to college. Eighty-five percent of the deaf students taking the test have lower scores than the average hearing applicant. See M. Ragosta (1987). *Students with Disabilities. Four Years of Data from Special Test Administrations of the Scholastic Aptitude Test 1980–1983* (Report 87-2). New York: College Board. Of course this is not an accurate measure of the aptitude of deaf high school students, as their high scores on nonverbal IQ tests remind us. See R. Conrad and B. C. Weiskrantz (1981). On the cognitive ability of deaf children with deaf parents. *American Annals of the Deaf, 126,* 995–1003. F. H. Sisco and R. J. Anderson (1980). Deaf children's performance on the WISC-R relative to hearing status of parents and child-rearing experiences. *American Annals of the Deaf, 125,* 923–30. The Scholastic Aptitude Test does not predict the scholastic achievement of deaf students, who outperform its sorry predictions. See H. Braun, M. Ragosta, and B. Kaplan (1986). *The Predictive Validity of the Scholastic Aptitude Test for Disabled Students.* Princeton, NJ: Educational Testing Service. Nonetheless, the test is widely used with deaf students. The situation is analogous to giving an immigrant whose primary language is not English a verbal test battery or interview in English—test scores might well show mental retardation or psychosis. American authorities on Ellis Island used this method to label as idiots and reject large numbers of immigrants arriving from Southern Europe earlier in this century. H. H. Goddard (1917). Mental tests and the immigrant. *The Journal of Delinquency, 2,* 243–77.

Page 52   "tests meaningfully." G. Montgomery (1978). Towards a viable surdotherapy: mental hygiene in schools. In G. Montgomery, ed., *Of Sound and Mind* (pp. 75–87). Edinburgh: Scottish Workshop. Smith, 1986, estimates eighth grade conservatively for the MMPI: D. Smith (1986). Mental health research enters realm of linguistics. *Research at Gallaudet,* 3–5.

"of English." S. Quigley and R. Kretschmer (1982). *The Education of Deaf Children.* Baltimore, MD: University Park Press; S. Wolk and T. E. Allen (1984). A five-year follow-up of reading comprehension achievement of hearing-impaired students in special education programs. *Journal of Special Education, 18,* 161–76.

"reported earlier." "Questionnaires are not good instruments for the assessment of a deaf person's personality. . . . We would not recommend [them]." F. C. Orr, A. DeMatteo, B. Heller, M. Lee, and M. Nguyen (1987). Psychological assessment. In H. Elliott, L. Glass, and J. W. Evans, eds., *Mental Health Assessment of Deaf Clients: A Practical Manual* (pp. 93–106). San Diego, CA: College-Hill, p. 101.

53   "or joiners." G. Montgomery (1978). Towards a viable surdotherapy: mental hygiene in schools. In G. Montgomery, ed., *Of Sound and Mind* (pp. 75–87). Edinburgh: Scottish Workshop, p. 79.

"from them." J. H. Kahn, ed. (1969). *Psychiatry and the Deaf Child.* London: Lewis.

"are not." E. Jones (1974). Social class and psychotherapy: a critical review of research. *Psychiatry, 37,* 307–20.

"through speaking." R. R. Grinker (1969). *Psychiatric Diagnosis, Therapy, and Research on the Psychotic Deaf* (USHEW Report SRS-RSA-192-1971). Washington, DC: U.S. Government Printing Office; J. D. Rainer, K. Z. Altshuler, and F. J. Kallmann, eds. (1963). *Family and Mental Health Problems in a Deaf Population.* Rockland, NY: N.Y. State Psychiatric Institute.

"in mania?" G. Montgomery (1978). Towards a viable surdotherapy:

mental hygiene in schools. In G. Montgomery, ed., *Of Sound and Mind* (pp. 75–87). Edinburgh: Scottish Workshop; J. W. Evans and H. Elliott (1987). The mental status examination. In H. Elliott, L. Glass, and J. W. Evans, eds., *Mental Health Assessment of Deaf Clients: A Practical Manual* (pp. 83–92). San Diego: College-Hill.

"good evidence." S. Dubow and L. J. Goldberg (1981). Legal strategies to improve mental health care for deaf people. In L. K. Stein, E. D. Mindel, and T. Jabaley, eds., *Deafness and Mental Health* (pp. 195–209). New York: Grune & Stratton; J. W. Evans (1987). Mental health treatment of hearing-impaired adolescents and adults. In B. W. Heller, L. M. Flohr, and L. S. Zegans, eds., *Psychosocial Interventions with Sensorially Disabled Persons* (pp. 167–86). Orlando, FL: Grune & Stratton; B. Goldberg, H. Lobb, and H. Kroll (1975). Psychiatric problems of the deaf child. *Canadian Psychiatric Association Journal*, *20*, 75–83; B. W. Heller and R. I. Harris (1987). Special considerations in the psychological assessment of hearing impaired persons. In B. W. Heller, L. M. Flohr, and L. S. Zegans, eds., *Psychosocial Interventions with Sensorially Disabled Persons* (pp. 53–77). Orlando, FL: Grune & Stratton; W. C. Stokoe and R. M. Battison (1981). Sign language, mental health, and satisfactory interaction. In L. M. Stein, E. D. Mindel, and T. Jabaley, eds., *Deafness and Mental Health* (pp. 179–94). New York: Grune & Stratton; R. J. Trybus (1977). The future of mental health services for the deaf. *Mental Health in Deafness* (experimental journal, St. Elizabeth's Hospital, National Institutes of Health), *1*, 1–5; M. Vernon (1976). Psychological evaluation of hearing-impaired children. In L. Lloyd, ed., *Communication Assessment and Intervention Strategies* (pp. 195–223). Baltimore: University Park Press; D. Watson (1979). Guidelines for the psychological and vocational assessment of deaf rehabilitation clients. *Journal of Rehabilitation of the Deaf*, *13*, 27–57.

"or staff." A second chance but 57 years are gone. *New York Times*, June 14, 1987, p. 28.

"State Hospital." Sister sues California for misplacing brother. *New York Times*, November 5, 1983, p. 10.

"the list." R. R. Grinker (1969). *Psychiatric Diagnosis, Therapy, and Research on the Psychotic Deaf* (USHEW Report SRS-RSA-192-1971). Washington, DC: U.S. Government Printing Office.

54   "were hearing." N. Tinbergen (1974). Ethology and stress diseases. *Science*, *185*, 24–27.

"and insight." J. D. Rainer and K. Z. Altshuler (1967). *Psychiatry and the Deaf*. Washington, DC: USDHEW, p. 86.

"have no language." D. Colin (1978). *Psychologie de l'enfant sourd*. Paris: Masson, p. 82.

"of misunderstanding." Editorial (1977). Deafness and mental health. *British Medical Journal*, *1* (*6055*), 191.

55   "but themselves." Discussed in E. Levine (1981). *Ecology of Early Deafness*. New York: Columbia University Press; B. W. Heller and R. I. Harris (1987). Special considerations in the psychological assessment

of hearing impaired persons. In B. W. Heller, L. M. Flohr, and L. S. Zegans, eds., *Psychosocial Interventions with Sensorially Disabled Persons* (pp. 53–77). Orlando, FL: Grune & Stratton.

Page 55 "deaf Americans." Discussed in M. Rodda and C. Grove (1987). *Language, Cognition and Deafness*. Hillsdale, NJ: Lawrence Erlbaum Associates.

"in adulthood." Editorial (1977). Deafness and mental health. *British Medical Journal, 1 (6055)*, 191; R. R. Grinker (1969). *Psychiatric Diagnosis, Therapy, and Research on the Psychotic Deaf* (USHEW Report SRS-RSA-192-1971). Washington, DC: U.S. Government Printing Office.

"healthy adults." S. Chess and P. Fernandez (1980). Do deaf children have a typical personality? *Journal of the American Academy of Child Psychiatry, 19*, 654–64; A. F. Cooper (1976). Deafness and psychiatric illness. *British Journal of Psychiatry, 129*, 216–26; A. F. Cooper, R. F. Garside, and D. W. Kay (1976). A comparison of deaf and nondeaf patients with paranoid and affective psychoses. *British Journal of Psychiatry, 129*, 532–38; J. W. Evans (1987). Mental health treatment of hearing-impaired adolescents and adults. In B. W. Heller, L. M. Flohr, and L. S. Zegans, eds., *Psychosocial Interventions with Sensorially Disabled Persons* (pp. 167–86). Orlando, FL: Grune & Stratton; J. W. Evans and H. Elliott (1987). The mental status examination. In H. Elliott, L. Glass, and J. W. Evans, eds., *Mental Health Assessment of Deaf Clients: A Practical Manual* (pp. 83–92). San Diego: College-Hill; B. Harry and P. E. Dietz (1985). Offenders in a silent world: hearing-impairment and deafness in relation to criminality, incompetence, and insanity. *Bulletin of the American Academy of Psychiatry and Law, 13*, 85–96; J. D. Rainer and K. Z. Altshuler (1967). *Psychiatry and the Deaf*. U.S. Department of Health, Education and Welfare, Social and Rehabilitation Service. Washington, DC: U.S. Government Printing Office; H. Schlesinger (1985). Deafness, mental health, and language. In F. Powell, T. Finitzo-Hieber, S. Friel-Patti, and D. Henderson, eds., *Education of the Hearing-Impaired Child* (pp. 103–19). San Diego, CA: College-Hill; M. Vernon (1976). Psychological evaluation of hearing-impaired children. In L. Lloyd, ed., *Communication Assessment and Intervention Strategies* (pp. 195–223). Baltimore, MD: University Park Press. Elliott, Glass, and Evans state: "Our clinical experience shows that the prevalence of schizophrenia in deaf patients is comparable with that in the hearing population." H. Elliott, L. Glass, and J. W. Evans, eds. (1987). *Mental Health Assessment of Deaf Clients*. San Diego, CA: College-Hill, p. 95.

"developing schizophrenia." F. P. Lebuffe and L. A. Lebuffe (1979). Psychiatric aspects of deafness. *Primary Care, 6*, 295–310, p. 299.

"or teacher." K. P. Meadow (1981). Studies of behavior problems of deaf children. In L. K. Stein, E. D. Mindel, and T. Jabaley, eds., *Deafness and Mental Health* (pp. 3–22). New York: Grune & Stratton; M. F. Hoyt, E. Y. Siegelman, and H. S. Schlesinger (1981). Special issues regarding psychotherapy with the deaf. *American Journal of Psychiatry, 138*, 807–11.

" 'middle class' patients." W. Haase (1964). The role of socioeconomic class in examiner bias. In F. Riessman, ed., *Mental Health of the Poor* (pp. 241–48). New York: Free Press.

56   "residential school." A. D. Evans and W. W. Falk (1986). *Learning to Be Deaf*. New York: Mouton de Gruyter, p. 13. Also see: G. Bachara, P. Raphael, and W. Phelan (1980). Empathy development in deaf preadolescents. *American Annals of the Deaf, 125,* 38–41.

"emotional disturbance." H. Schlesinger (1985). Deafness, mental health, and language. In F. Powell, T. Finitzo-Hieber, S. Friel-Patti, and D. Henderson, eds., *Education of the Hearing-Impaired Child* (pp. 103–119). San Diego, CA: College-Hill, p. 106.

"other authors." For example, J. W. Evans and H. Elliott (1987). The mental status examination. In H. Elliott, L. Glass, and J. W. Evans, eds., *Mental Health Assessment of Deaf Clients: A Practical Manual* (pp. 83–92). San Diego: College-Hill; K. P. Meadow-Orlans (1987). Psychosocial intervention with deaf children. In B. W. Heller, L. M. Flohr, and L. S. Zegans, eds., *Psychosocial Interventions with Sensorially Disabled Persons* (pp. 115–30). Orlando, FL: Grune & Stratton.

"years earlier." H. Schlesinger and K. Meadow (1972). *Sound and Sign: Childhood Deafness and Mental Health.* Berkeley: University of California Press.

"and colleagues." Reviewed in R. Brown (1986). *Social Psychology,* 2d ed. New York: Free Press.

57   "beyond deafness." A. B. Wolff and J. E. Harkins (1986). Multihandi-capped students. In A. N. Schildroth and M. A. Karchmer, eds., *Deaf Children in America* (pp. 55–82). San Diego, CA: College-Hill; C. Jensema and J. Mullins (1974). Onset, cause, and additional handicaps in hearing-impaired children. *American Annals of the Deaf, 119,* 701–705.

"handicapping condition." R. Conrad (1977). Facts and fantasies about the verbal abilities of deaf school leavers. *The British Deaf News, 11,* 145–47.

"regular schoolroom." C. E. Williams (1970). Some psychiatric observations on a group of maladjusted deaf children. *Journal of Child Psychology and Psychiatry, 11,* 1–18.

"female students." C. Jensema and J. Mullins (1974). Onset, cause, and additional handicaps in hearing-impaired children. *American Annals of the Deaf, 119,* 701–705.

"emotionally disturbed." "It is probable that being both black and deaf constitutes a double jeopardy with respect to standardized testing and subsequent labeling." A. B. Wolff and J. E. Harkins (1986). Multihandi-capped students. In A. N. Schildroth and M. A. Karchmer, eds., *Deaf Children in America* (pp. 55–82). San Diego, CA: College-Hill, p. 68. From the reported high incidence of emotional disturbance among profoundly deaf children compared to those with mild hearing impairment, I infer this inverse relation with English mastery, which has not been directly tested.

"in Berkeley." M. Vernon (1969). *Multiply-Handicapped Deaf Children:*

Medical, Educational, and Psychological Considerations. (C.E.C. Research Monographs). Washington, DC: Council for Exceptional Children.

Page 57   "classroom situation." T. J. Goulder and R. J. Trybus (1977). *The Classroom Behavior of Emotionally Disturbed Hearing Impaired Children* (Office of Demographic Studies Report, Series R, Number 3). Washington, DC: Gallaudet College, p. 21.

"comparable size." C. Jensema and R. J. Trybus (1975). *Reported Emotional/Behavioral Problems Among Hearing-Impaired Children in Special Education Programs. United States 1972–1973* (Office of Demographic Studies Report, Series R, Number 1). Washington, DC: Gallaudet College.

"and labeling." A. B. Wolff and J. E. Harkins (1986). Multihandicapped students. In A. N. Schildroth and M. A. Karchmer, eds., *Deaf Children in America* (pp. 55–82). San Diego, CA: College-Hill, p. 73.

58   "or more." C. Jensema and R. J. Trybus (1975). *Reported Emotional/Behavioral Problems Among Hearing-Impaired Children in Special Education Programs. United States 1972–1973* (Office of Demographic Studies Report, Series R, Number 1). Washington, DC: Gallaudet College, p. 1.

"health testing." Welfare Planning Board of Los Angeles County (1960). *Mental Health Survey of Los Angeles County*. Sacramento: Welfare Planning Board.

"IQ scores." J. Mercer (1973). *Labeling the Mentally Retarded*. Berkeley: University of California Press.

"classroom problems." K. P. Meadow-Orlans (1987). Psychosocial intervention with deaf children. In B. W. Heller, L. M. Flohr, and L. S. Zegans, eds., *Psychosocial Interventions with Sensorially Disabled Persons* (pp. 115–30). Orlando, FL: Grune & Stratton, p. 124; B. M. Gerber and H. K. Goldberg (1980). Psychiatric consultation in a school program for multiply handicapped deaf children. *American Annals of the Deaf*, *125*, 579–85.

"Dr. Schlesinger." H. Schlesinger (1987). Effects of powerlessness on dialog and development: Disability, poverty and the human condition. In B. W. Heller, L. M. Flohr, and L. S. Zegans, eds., *Psychosocial Interventions with Sensorially Disabled Persons* (pp. 1–28). Orlando, FL: Grune & Stratton, p. 11.

59   "the child." M. Greenberg (1980). Hearing families with deaf children: stress and functioning as related to communication method. *American Annals of the Deaf*, *125*, 1063–71.

"95 percent of the time." I obtained this rule of thumb in the following way. It is generally accepted that test reliability should reflect agreement in test scores exceeding a correlation of 0.8. For the case of two dichotomous variables, namely, rater 1 and rater 2 and disturbed or not disturbed, the ratio of agreements to disagreements must exceed 15 for the estimated value of r to be 0.8, based on Pearson's cosine method. For a sample with 100 ratings there must therefore be at least 93.75 agreements and 6.25 disagreements. See A.

Edwards (1967). *Statistical Methods*. New York: Holt, Rinehart & Winston, p. 131.

"40 percent of the time." R. D. Freeman, S. F. Malkin, and J. O. Hastings (1975). Psychosocial problems of deaf children and their families: a comparative study. *American Annals of the Deaf*, *121*, 391–405. The authors found that mother and father agree r = 0.63, mother and teacher r = 0.45, and father and teacher r = 0.16. The percent agreement figures were inferred from these correlations.

"test results." M. Rodda and C. Grove (1987). *Language, Cognition and Deafness*. Hillsdale, NJ: Lawrence Erlbaum.

"be discarded." K. Altshuler, W. E. Deming, J. Vollenweider, J. D. Rainer, and R. Tendler (1976). Impulsivity and profound early deafness: a cross-cultural inquiry. *American Annals of the Deaf*, *121*, 331–45, p. 333.

"by Altshuler." K. P. Meadow and B. Dyssegaard (1983). Teachers' ratings of deaf children: an American Danish comparison. *American Annals of the Deaf*, *128*, 900–98, p. 907.

"in impulsivity." K. Z. Altshuler (1964). Personality traits and depressive syndromes in the deaf. In J. Wortis, ed., *Recent Advances in Biological Psychiatry* (pp. 63–73). New York: Plenum.

"use ratings." K. Altshuler, W. E. Deming, J. Vollenweider, J. D. Rainer, and R. Tendler (1976). Impulsivity and profound early deafness: a cross-cultural inquiry. *American Annals of the Deaf*, *121*, 331–45.

61 "and learning disabled." S. Tomlinson (1982). *A Sociology of Special Education*. Boston: Routledge and Kegan Paul, pp. 69ff., 149.

"multiply-handicapped." W. N. Craig and H. B. Craig (1981). Directory of services for the deaf. *American Annals of the Deaf*, *126*, 191.

"face value." M. Vernon (1967). Characteristics associated with postrubella deaf children: psychological, educational and physical. *Volta Review*, *69*, 176–85; M. Vernon (1967). Rh factor and deafness: the problem, its psychological, physical, and educational manifestations. *Exceptional Children*, *34*, 5–12; M. Vernon (1967). Meningitis and deafness: The problem, its physical, audiological, psychological and educational manifestations in deaf children. *Laryngoscope*, *77*, 1856–74; M. Vernon (1982). Multi-handicapped deaf children: types and causes. In D. Tweedie and E. H. Shroyer, eds., *The Multi-Handicapped Hearing Impaired* (pp. 11–28). Washington, DC: Gallaudet University Press; M. Vernon (1967). Prematurity and deafness: the magnitude and nature of the problem among deaf children. *Exceptional Children*, *33(1)*, 289–98.

"learning disabled." G. O. Bunch (1973). Canadian services for multiply handicapped deaf children. *Canadian Teacher of the Deaf*, *2*, 27–31.

"hearing-impaired group." G. O. Bunch and T. L. Melnyk (1989). A review of the evidence for a learning-disabled, hearing-impaired subgroup. *American Annals of the Deaf*, *134*, 297–300, p. 298.

"hearing parents." F. H. Sisco and R. J. Anderson (1980). Deaf children's performance on the WISC-R relative to hearing status of parents and child-rearing experiences. *American Annals of the Deaf, 125,* 923–30; R. Conrad and B. C. Weiskrantz (1981). On the cognitive ability of deaf children with deaf parents. *American Annals of the Deaf, 126,* 995–1003; M. A. Karchmer, R. J. Trybus, and M. M. Paquin (1978). Early manual communication, parental hearing status, and the academic achievement of deaf students. In *Proceedings of the American Educational Research Association,* Toronto; M. Vernon (1969). *Multiply-Handicapped Deaf Children: Medical, Educational, and Psychological Considerations* (C.E.C. Research Monographs). Washington, DC: Council for Exceptional Children; R. G. Brill (1974). The superior IQs of deaf children of deaf parents. In P. J. Fine, ed., *Deafness in Infancy and Early Childhood* (pp. 151–61). New York: Medcom.

Page 61   "in age." U. Bellugi, L. O'Grady, D. Lillo-Martin, M. O'Grady-Hines, K. van Hoek, and D. Corina (1990). Enhancement of spatial cognition in deaf children. In V. Volterra and C. Erting, eds., *From Gesture to Language in Hearing and Deaf Children* (pp. 279–98). Berlin: Springer Verlag.

"hearing children." J. Belmont and M. Karchmer (1978). Deaf people's memory: there are problems testing special populations. In M. Gruneberg, P. Morris, and R. Sykes, eds., *Practical Aspects of Memory* (pp. 581–88). London: Academic Press.

62   "hearing adults." H. Neville and D. Lawson (1987). Attention to central and peripheral visual space in a movement detection task. An event-related potential and behavioral study. II. Congenitally deaf adults. *Brain Research, 405,* 268–83.

"or adults." C. S. Holm (1987). Testing for values with the deaf: the language/cultural effect. *Journal of Rehabilitation of the Deaf, 20,* 7–19.

63   "have been published." F. R. Zieziula (1982). *Assessment of Hearing-Impaired People.* Washington, DC: Gallaudet University Press; D. Smith (1986). Mental health research enters realm of linguistics. *Research at Gallaudet,* 3–5.

"a test." A. N. Schildroth and M. A. Karchmer, eds., *Deaf Children in America* (pp. 1–32). San Diego, CA: College-Hill.

"the case." P. Ries (1986). Characteristics of hearing-impaired youth in the general population and of students in special education programs for the hearing-impaired. In A. N. Schildroth and M. A. Karchmer, eds. (1986). *Deaf Children in America.* San Diego, CA: College-Hill; H. Schlesinger (1985). Deafness, mental health, and language. In F. Powell, T. Finitzo-Hieber, S. Friel-Patti, and D. Henderson, eds., *Education of the Hearing-Impaired Child* (pp. 103–119). San Diego, CA: College-Hill.

64   "deaf children." D. Moores (1982). *Educating the Deaf,* 2d ed. New York: Houghton-Mifflin: H. Schlesinger (1987). Effects of power-lessness on dialog and development: Disability, poverty and the human condition. In B. W. Heller, L. M. Flohr, and L. S. Zegans, eds., *Psychosocial Interventions with Sensorially Disabled Persons* (pp. 1–28). Orlando, FL: Grune & Stratton.

"of hearing." M. Vernon (1969). *Multiply-Handicapped Deaf Children: Medical, Educational, and Psychological Considerations* (C.E.C. Research Monographs). Washington, DC: Council for Exceptional Children; M. Vernon (1982). Multi-handicapped deaf children: types and causes. In D. Tweedie and E. H. Shroyer, eds., *The Multi-Handicapped Hearing Impaired* (pp. 11–28). Washington, DC: Gallaudet University Press.

"audist establishment." A number of scholars in the professions serving deaf people have sounded the alarm that the field is improperly lending the weight of science to common stereotypes. "Valid procedures for personality assessment of deaf children and adults are lacking. . . . All research studies are suspect." B. Bolton, ed. (1976). *Psychology of the Deaf for Rehabilitation Counselors*. Baltimore, MD: University Park Press, p. 8. "The judgment as to whether the deaf child has specific deviant personality characteristics is still inconclusive." S. Chess and P. Fernandez (1980). Do deaf children have a typical personality? *Journal of the American Academy of Child Psychiatry, 19,* 654–64, p. 656. A leading educator dismissed the literature of the "psychology of the deaf " in his textbook, *Educating the Deaf*: "For the most part, inappropriate tests have been administered under unsatisfactory conditions and results have been compared with unrealistic norms." D. Moores (1982). *Educating the Deaf*, 2d ed. New York: Houghton-Mifflin, p. 146. And most recently, this indictment appeared in the *Journal of Rehabilitation of the Deaf*: "Professionals who work closely with deaf people have responded to the inconsistencies between these biases and their own experience with deaf people by writing off the whole field of testing." C. S. Holm (1987). Testing for values with the deaf: the language/cultural effect. *Journal of Rehabilitation of the Deaf, 20,* 7–19, p. 15.

65 "make them so." A. Memmi (1966). *Portrait du colonisé*. Paris: Pauvert.

Part Three. Representations of Deaf People: Power, Politics, and the Dependency Duet

69 "appear necessary." The development of special education was made possible by the technology of educational psychology. See J. Quicke (1984). The role of the educational psychologist in the post-Warnock era. In L. Bartson and S. Tomlinson, eds., *Special Education and Social Interests*. London: Croom Helm, p. 123.

"to treat." Overly active and inattentive children did not receive amphetamines for more than a decade after this class of drugs had been shown to calm such children; this medical intervention, promoted by the drug manufacturer, required a syndrome to become widely practiced; hyperkinetic impulse disorder was conveniently "discovered." P. Conrad and J. Schneider (1980). *Deviance and Medicalization: From Badness to Sickness*. Columbus: Merrill.

71 "pre-college education." G. Senior (1980). Temporal orientation in

hearing-impaired people. *Disability, Handicap and Society*, 1988, *3*, 277–90, p. 277.

Page 72   "other reasons." R. A. Scott (1981). *The Making of Blind Men*. New Brunswick: Transaction, p. 103.

"special education." S. Tomlinson (1982). *A Sociology of Special Education*. Boston: Routledge and Kegan Paul, pp. 67ff.

"for failure." L. Barton (1986). The politics of special education needs. *Disability, Handicap and Society*, *1*, 273–90.

"so forth." J. M. De Gérando (1827). *De l'education des sourds-muets de naissance*. Paris: Mequignon.

"or both." A. Memmi (1966). *Portrait du colonisé*. Paris: Pauvert.

73   "in the metropole." A. Memmi (1966). *Portrait du colonisé*. Paris: Pauvert, p. 98.

"audist establishment." F. Berthier (1852). *Sur l'Opinion de feu le Dr. Itard*. Paris: Michel Lévy frères.

"are unreal." R. A. Sicard (1800). Preface. *Cours d'instruction d'un sourd-muet de naissance*. Paris: LeClere.

"it may be." J. M. G. Itard (1821). Sourd. In N. P. Adelon, ed., *Dictionnaire des sciences médicales* (pp. 210–15). Paris: Panckoucke, p. 212.

74   "to communication." R. A. C. Sicard (1800). *Cours d'instruction d'un sourd-muet de naissance*. Paris: Le Clère. Second edition: Paris: Le Clère, 1803. English translation (abridged): F. Philip (1984). *The Deaf Experience: Classics in Language and Education*. Cambridge, MA: Harvard University Press.

"their voyages." J. M. De Gérando (1800). *Considérations sur les diverses méthodes à suivre dans l'observation des peuples sauvages*. Paris: Société des Observateurs de l'Homme. Reprint: J. Copans and J. Jamin, eds. (1978). *Aux origines de l'anthropologie française*. Paris: Le Sycomore. English translation: F. C. T. Moore (1969). *The Observation of Savage People*. Berkeley: University of California Press.

"Deaf-Mutes." H. Lane (1976). *The Wild Boy of Aveyron*. Cambridge, MA: Harvard University Press.

"the forests." C. B. Wallis (1903). *The Advance of Our West African Empire*. London: Fisher Unwin, p. 119.

"as babies." Cited in V. G. Kiernan (1969). *The Lords of Human Kind*. Boston: Little, Brown, p. 217.

"of contempt." P. Bruckner (1986). *The Tears of the White Man*. New York: Free Press, p. 123.

"onto them." D. O. Mannoni (1964). *Prospero and Caliban: The Psychology of Colonization*. New York: Praeger.

75   "missed it." A. Freeman (1988). Parents: dilemmas for professionals. *Disability, Handicap and Society*, *3*, 79–85, p. 85.

"dependency duet." A. Memmi (1984). *Dependence*. Boston: Beacon Press.

76   "to die." Quoted in H. Lane (1976). *The Wild Boy of Aveyron*. Cambridge, MA: Harvard University Press, p. 271.

77   "a father." Quoted in H. Lane (1984). *When the Mind Hears: A History of the Deaf*. New York: Random House, p. 147.

"are women." J. Treesberg (1990). Teacher backgrounds. *The Bicultural Center News*, *29*, 3. A report of a study by James Woodward, Thomas Allen, and Arthur Schildroth, Gallaudet Research Institute. See J. Woodward, T. Allen, and A. Schildroth (1985). Teachers and deaf students: an ethnography of classroom communication. In S. DeLancey and R. Tomlin, eds., *Proceedings of the First Annual Pacific Linguistics Conference* (pp. 479–93). Eugene: University of Oregon Press. J. Woodward and T. Allen (1988). Classroom use of artificial sign systems by teachers. *Sign Language Studies*, *61*, 405–18.

"external criteria." J. McKnight (1981). Professionalized services and disabling help. In A. Brechin, P. Liddiard, and J. Swain, eds., *Handicap in a Social World* (pp. 24–33). Sevenoaks, England: Holder & Stoughton.

78 "What conquest!" J. M. De Gérando (1800). *Considérations sur les diverses méthodes à suivre dans l'observation des peuples sauvages*. Paris: Société des Observateurs de l'Homme. Reprint: J. Copans and J. Jamin, eds. (1978). *Aux origines de l'anthropologie française*. Paris: Le Sycomore, p. 163. English translation: F. C. T. Moore (1969). *The Observation of Savage People*. Berkeley: University of California Press.

"further mystification." S. Tomlinson (1982). *A Sociology of Special Education*. Boston: Routledge and Kegan Paul.

"14.8 percent." Cited in F. Fanon (1967). *Black Skins, White Masks*. New York: Grove.

"as slaves." M. McCarthy (1983). *Dark Continent: Africa as Seen by Americans*. Westport, CT: Greenwood.

"white males." J. Q. Wilson and R. Herrnstein (1985). *Crime and Human Nature*. New York: Simon & Schuster. "Among whites, being a mesomorph is an indicator of a predisposition to crime. Young black males are more mesomorphic (5.14 on Sheldon's scale) than are young white males (4.29) . . ." (p. 469). The authors also qualify these remarks; see chapters 3 and 18.

79 "as dynamite." I am indebted to Dr. Leon Kamin, Chair, Psychology Department, Northeastern University, for providing me with this information. W. H. Sheldon, E. M. Hartl, and E. McDermott (1949). *Varieties of Delinquent Youth*. New York: Harper.

"their race." A. R. Jensen (1969). How much can we boost IQ and scholastic achievement? *Harvard Educational Review*, *39*, 1–123; A. R. Jensen (1981). *Straight Talk about Mental Tests*. New York: Free Press; A. R. Jensen (1985). The nature of the black-white difference on various psychometric tests: Spearman's hypothesis. *The Behavioral and Brain Sciences*, *8*, 193–263.

"IQ test." M. L. Manion and H. Bersani (1987). Mental retardation as a Western sociological construct: a cross-cultural analysis. *Disability, Handicap and Society*, *2*, 231–45, p. 235; W. Shockley (1971). Models, mathematics and the moral obligation to diagnose the origin of Negro IQ deficits. *Review of Educational Research*, *41*, 369–77.

"observes Memmi." A. Memmi (1984). *Dependence*. Boston: Beacon Press, p. 107.

Page 79   "the deafness." M. Vernon (1982). Multi-handicapped deaf children: types and causes. In D. Tweedie and E. H. Shroyer, eds., *The Multi-Handicapped Hearing Impaired* (pp. 11–28). Washington, DC: Gallaudet University Press, p. 24.

"one survey." A. B. Wolff and J. E. Harkins (1986). Multihandicapped students. In A. N. Schildroth and M. A. Karchmer, eds., *Deaf Children in America* (pp. 55–82). San Diego, CA: College-Hill, p. 65.

"deafness itself." A. Webster (1985). "The Deaf Experience," edited by Harlan Lane. *History of Education, 14,* 237–50.

80   "effect change." S. Moscovici, G. Mugny, and E. van Avermaet (1985). *Perspectives on Minority Influence.* New York: Cambridge University Press, p. 124.

81   "and subjection." M. Foucault (1977). *Discipline and Punish.* New York: Pantheon. Excerpted in P. Rabinow, ed. (1984). *The Foucault Reader.* New York: Pantheon, p. 203.

"our deafness." J. Grémion (1990). *La Planète des sourds.* Paris: Messinger, p. 38.

82   "entire culture." B. Jewsiewicki and D. Newbury (1985). *African Historiographies.* Beverly Hills, CA: Sage, p. 77.

"this century." A. Mazrui (1986). *The Africans: A Triple Heritage.* Boston: Little, Brown, p. 112.

83   "deaf pupil." M. Foucault (1979). *Discipline and Punish.* New York: Vintage.

"they speak." M. Foucault (1972). *The Archeology of Knowledge.* New York: Harper Colophon, p. 49.

84   "*Proceedings.*" L. Stewart (1990). The great Rochester snub of 1990. *NAD Broadcaster, 12(11),* 1.

"and improved." M. Foucault (1979). *Discipline and Punish.* New York: Vintage, p. 136.

85   "the norm." M. Foucault (1978). *History of Sexuality.* New York: Random House, pp. 143–44.

"IQ tests." S. A. Gelb (1987). Social deviance and the "discovery" of the moron. *Disability, Handicap and Society, 2,* 247–58, p. 252.

"human comedy." A. Binet and T. Simon (1914). *Mentally Defective Children.* London: Edward Arnold, p. 10.

"five decades." J. Kivirauma and O. Kivinen (1988). The school system and special education: causes and effects in the twentieth century. *Disability, Handicap and Society, 3,* 153–65, p. 154.

"grown fifteenfold." G. Fulcher (1986). Australian policies on special education: towards a sociological account. *Disability, Handicap and Society, 1,* 19–52, p. 37.

"in 1978." Department of Education and Science (1978). *Special Educational Needs* (Warnock Report). London: Her Majesty's Stationery Office.

"education establishment." L. Barton (1986). The politics of special educational needs. *Disability, Handicap and Society, 1,* 273–90.

"Foucault writes." M. Foucault (1983). The subject and power. In

H. Dreyfus and P. Rabinow, eds., *Beyond Structuralism and Hermeneutics*, 2d ed. Chicago: University of Chicago Press, p. 216.

86   "aesthetic idioms." E. Said (1989). Representing the colonized: anthropology's interlocutors. *Critical Inquiry*, *15*, 205–25, p. 212.

"is not." B. Hudson (1988). Do people with a mental handicap have rights? *Disability, Handicap and Society*, *3*, 227–37, p. 228.

"community expectations." D. Moores (1991). *Dissemination of a Model to Create Least Restrictive Environments for Deaf Students*. Unpublished report to the National Institute on Disability and Rehabilitation Research, Center for Studies in Education and Human Development, Gallaudet Research Institute, Gallaudet University.

"she conducted." K. P. Meadow (1981). Burnout in professionals working with deaf children. *American Annals of the Deaf*, *126*, 13–22.

87   "formulated them." M. Foucault (1980). *The History of Sexuality*. Volume 1: *An Introduction*. New York: Random House, p. 95.

"they do does." M. Foucault (1983). In H. Dreyfus and P. Rabinow, eds., *Beyond Structuralism and Hermeneutics*, 2d ed. Chicago: University of Chicago Press, p. 187.

"he enjoys." A. Memmi (1966). *Portrait du colonisé*. Paris: Pauvert, p. 58.

88   "in 1894." R. Acuña (1988). *Occupied America: A History of Chicanos*, 3rd ed. New York: Harper & Row, p. 37.

"Deaf leaders." J. McWhinney (1991). Deaf consciousness. *Signpost*, *2*, 13–15.

"surname, Anglo." R. Acuña (1988). *Occupied America: A History of Chicanos*, 3rd ed. New York: Harper & Row, p. 56.

89   "called hearing-impaired." D. Castle (1990). Employment bridges cultures. *Deaf American*, *40*, 19–21; M. Ross and D. R. Calvert (1967). Semantics of deafness. *Volta Review*, *69*, 644–49; G. B. Wilson, M. Ross, and D. R. Calvert (1974). An experimental study of the semantics of deafness. *Volta Review*, *76*, 408–14.

"our world." J. Grémion (1990). *La Planète des sourds*. Paris: Messinger, p. 38.

90   "gaining knowledge." J. Rabasa (1990). Dialogue as conquest: mapping spaces for counter-discourse. In A. R. JanMohamed and D. Lloyd, *The Nature and Context of Minority Discourse* (pp. 187–215). New York: Oxford, p. 214.

"his provider." A. Memmi (1984). *Dependence*. Boston: Beacon Press, p. 37.

92   "the classroom." A. Freeman (1988). Who's moving the goal posts and what game are we playing anyway: social competence examined. In L. Barton, ed., *The Politics of Special Educational Needs* (pp. 123–44). Philadelphia: Falmer Press, p. 139.

"court intervention." As I explain later in this book, the Individualized Educational Plan that is drawn up for deaf children includes a school placement. When parents disagree with the placement, as frequently happens, the school district generally has the final say, for several reasons. First, some parents are intimidated by and defer to the judgment of the "experts." Second, the effort and costs associated with appeals at several levels often discourage parents from pursuing the issue. Third, the general presumption in the appeals process and in the courts is that local authorities are best qualified to decide. See S. Tomlinson (1982). *A Sociology of Special Education*. Boston: Routledge and Kegan Paul, p. 120.

Page 92   "with TALK." Based on an account of my friend's story in C. Padden and T. Humphries (1988). *Deaf in America: Voices from a Culture*. Cambridge, MA: Harvard University Press, p. 15.

93   "pitiful disease." V. G. Kiernan (1969). *The Lords of Human Kind*. Boston: Little, Brown, p. 242, n. 156.

"nigger!" F. Fanon (1967). *Black Skins, White Masks*. New York: Grove, p. 191.

"not salient." I owe this observation to the distinguished French sociologist of deafness, Bernard Mottez.

"bored me." J. Champie (1991). The potter's hand. *Deaf American, 41*, 37–41, p. 38.

94   "at home." E. Booth (1881). Thomas Hopkins Gallaudet. *Iowa Institution Hawkeye*. Reprinted in *American Era, 30*, 1943, 23–25. Excerpted in *American Annals of the Deaf, 26*, 1971, 200–201. Also see E. Booth (1953). *Edmund Booth, Forty-Niner, the Life Story of a Deaf Pioneer*. Stockton, CA: San Joaquin Pioneer and Historical Society.

95   "each other." Quotation from S. Foster (1989). Social alienation and peer identification: a study of the social construction of deafness. Reprinted by permission of the Society for Applied Anthropology from *Human Organization, 48*, 226–35.

96   "with the deaf." S. Foster (1989). Social alienation and peer identification: a study of the social construction of deafness. Reprinted by permission of the Society for Applied Anthropology from *Human Organization, 48*, 226–35, p. 233.

"looks down." Cited in T. Smith (1973). Idealism and people's war: Sartre on Algeria. *Political Theory, 1*, 426–49, p. 437.

"African inferiority." M. McCarthy (1983). *Dark Continent: Africa as Seen by Americans*. Westport, CT: Greenwood, p. 146.

97   "hearing people." J. McWhinney (1991). Deaf consciousness. *Signpost, 2*, 13–15.

"they have." In *The Making of Blind Men* (New Brunswick: Transaction, 1981), sociologist R. A. Scott makes a similar observation concerning blind men and women.

"from attention." E. Goffman (1963). *Stigma: Notes on the Management of Spoiled Identity*. Englewood Cliffs, NJ: Prentice-Hall, p. 102.

98   "be recruited." D. A. Gerber (1990). Listening to disabled people: the problem of voice and authority in Robert B. Edgerton's "The Cloak of Competence." *Disability, Handicap and Society, 5*, 3–23, p. 14.

"deaf person." A. Ballin (1930). *A Deaf-Mute Howls*. Los Angeles: Grafton, p. 66; R. V. Bruce (1973). *Bell: Alexander Graham Bell and the Conquest of Solitude*. Boston: Little, Brown, p. 321.

"among them." R. V. Bruce (1973). *Bell: Alexander Graham Bell and the Conquest of Solitude.* Boston: Little, Brown, p. 380.

"is born." T. Smith (1973). Idealism and people's war: Sartre on Algeria. *Political Theory, 1,* 426–49, p. 437.

"more intolerable." D. O. Mannoni (1964). *Prospero and Caliban: The Psychology of Colonization.* New York: Praeger, p. 84.

99 "the oppressors." J.-P. Sartre (1968). Introduction. In F. Fanon, *The Wretched of the Earth.* New York: Grove, p. 25.

Part Four. Language Bigotry and Deaf Communities

103 "are spoken." T. Skutnabb-Kangas and J. Cummins, eds. (1988). *Minority Education.* Philadelphia: Multilingual Matters, p. 11.

104 "to us." Quoted in F. Grosjean (1982). *Life with Two Languages.* Cambridge, MA: Harvard University Press, p. 28.

"to wear." Quoted in F. Grosjean (1982). *Life with Two Languages.* Cambridge, MA: Harvard University Press, p. 209.

"it out." N. Dorian (1981). *Language Death.* Philadelphia: University of Pennsylvania Press, p. 18.

"made us say." H. Lane (1984). *When the Mind Hears: A History of the Deaf.* New York: Random House, p. 404.

"down upon." F. Grosjean (1982). *Life with Two Languages.* Cambridge, MA: Harvard University Press, p. 213.

105 "be evasive." H. Lane (1984). *When the Mind Hears: A History of the Deaf.* New York: Random House, p. 284.

"the capital." M. Certeau, D. Julia, and J. Revel, eds. (1975). *Une politique de la langue. La Révolution Française et les patois: l'Enquête de Grégoire.* Paris: Gallimard.

"speak English." N. Dorian (1981). *Language Death.* Philadelphia: University of Pennsylvania Press.

106 "educational process." Department of Education and Science (1985). *Education for All* (Swann Report). London: Her Majesty's Stationery Office.

"of legislation." R. P. Porter (1990). *Forked Tongue: The Politics of Bilingual Education.* New York: Basic Books, p. 207.

"minority identity." R. G. Tucker (1990). Developing a language-competent American society: The role of language planning. In A. G. Reynolds, ed., *Bilingualism, Multiculturalism, and Second Language Learning.* Hillsdale, NJ: LEA, pp. 65–80; T. Skutnabb-Kangas (1988). Multilingualism and the education of minority children. In T. Skutnabb-Kangas and J. Cummins, *Minority Education.* Philadelphia: Multilingual Matters, pp. 9–44; A. Willig (1985). A meta-analysis of selected studies on the effectiveness of bilingual education. *Review of Educational Research, 55,* 269–317; K. Hakuta (1986). *Mirror of Language: The Debate on Bilingualism.* New York: Basic Books.

107 "to school." National Council for Mother Tongue Teaching (1985).

The Swann Report: Education for All? *Journal of Multilingual and Multicultural Development*, 6, 497–508, p. 501.

Page 107 "whole creation!" A. Ballin (1930). *A Deaf-Mute Howls*. Los Angeles, CA: Grafton. Quoted in H. Lane (1984). *When the Mind Hears: A History of the Deaf*. New York: Random House, p. 372.

"sign language." P. Desloges (1779). *Observations d'un sourd et muet . . .* Paris: Morin. Translated in H. Lane and F. Philip (1984). *The Deaf Experience*. Cambridge, MA: Harvard University Press.

"with education." H. Lane (1984). *When the Mind Hears: A History of the Deaf*. New York: Random House.

"from animals." H. Lane (1984). *When the Mind Hears: A History of the Deaf*. New York: Random House, p. 100.

108 "we think." E. G. Valentine (1870). The proper order of signs. *Proceedings of the Convention of American Instructors of the Deaf*, 44–80, p. 58.

"abstract ideas." A. L. Blanchet (1850). *La Surdi-Mutité*. Paris: Labé.

109 "less complete." H. Kloss (1967). Bilingualism and nationalism. *Journal of Social Issues*, 23, 39–47, p. 46.

111 "to remember." C. M. Epée (abbé de l') (1784). *La véritable manière d'instruire les sourds-muets, confirmée par une longue expérience*. Paris: Nyon. English translation: F. Green (1801). *The Method of Educating the Deaf and Dumb Confirmed by Long Experience*. London: Cooke. Reprint: (Parts I and II): *American Annals of the Deaf*, 12, 1860, 1–132.

"of a verb." C. M. Epée (abbé de l') (1784). *La véritable manière d'instruire les sourds-muets, confirmée par une longue expérience*. Paris: Nyon. English translation: F. Green (1801). *The Method of Educating the Deaf and Dumb Confirmed by Long Experience*. London: Cooke. Reprint (Parts I and II): *American Annals of the Deaf*, 12, 1860, 1–132, p. 22 of the 1860 translation.

"more primitive." R. A. Sicard (1790). *Second mémoire sur l'art d'instruire les sourds et muets de naissance*. Paris: Knapen.

112 "their discussions." The book is translated in H. Lane and F. Philip (1984). *The Deaf Experience: Classics in Language and Education*. Cambridge, MA: Harvard University Press.

"wholly discarded." H. P. Peet (1834). *Fifteenth Report of the New York Institution for the Instruction of the Deaf and Dumb*. New York: New York Institution, pp. 29–30.

"is recognized." F. A. P. Barnard (1835). Existing state of the art of instructing the deaf and dumb. *Literary and Theological Review*, 2, 367–98, p. 389. Dr. Donald Moores writing in the *Deaf American*, 40, 1990, pp. 91–95, acknowledges that the New York school moved away from methodical signing in 1834 but disputes that the Hartford and other schools did. He states that Lewis Weld, principal at the Hartford school, claimed, in its 1835 17th Annual Report, that the school used methodical signs. (The correct reference is the 20th report in 1836.) In fact, Weld states that "almost all direct instruction of the schoolroom is thus communicated [in] the natural language of signs employed by the Deaf and Dumb"; he makes an exception for the teaching of

English, for which he indicates that methodical signs were used. Moores also cites artist John Carlin, principal John Jacobs, and writer John Burnet as advocating signed English. That is correct, but they did so from a peripheral position in deaf education. Jacobs, head of the Kentucky school, was seen as an eccentric advocate of this view. Carlin was respected as a deaf leader, but he was not an educator. His advocacy of methodical signs (he also advocated articulation training and was opposed to using ASL in the classroom) reveals nothing about actual practices. Burnet was employed as a teacher during the 1830–31 school year, and then regularly after 1867; he joined Jacobs in his defense of methodical signs in articles published in the 1850s.

Dr. Moores cites Burnet, writing in 1854: "the prevailing opinion among the more experienced American teachers is that these [methodical] signs are useful, at least to some extent and in the earlier lessons." (J. Burnet. The necessity of methodical signs considered: further experiments. *American Annals of the Deaf*, 7, 1–15, p. 2.) However, the preceding phrase is : "Mr. Stone thinks that they should be 'dispensed with or but sparingly used . . . ' and Mr. Rae pronounces Sicard's system of methodical signs 'a complete piece of charlatanry from beginning to end.' Judging, however, from the proceedings of the second and third conventions . . ." In the proceedings of the Second Convention of American Instructors of the Deaf, Stone (director of the Hartford school) summarized the debate as follows: "The only question is, whether we shall use methodical signs to any great extent, and we all answer, No" (p. 101). The debate in the third convention was actually concerned with whether signs can be dispensed with entirely at later stages of teaching written English, but the value of methodical signs for that purpose came up. The consensus was that they are not useful for classroom instruction in general but may be useful in the earlier stages of teaching English grammar. Rae stated that the Paris and most other French institutions had entirely discarded methodical signs but that the United States had not yet done so in all its schools (p. 167).

When Harvey Peet, superintendent of the New York Institution and first president of the Convention of American Instructors of the Deaf, addressed that convention in 1859, he was the dean of American educators of the deaf and had long been the intellectual leader of his profession. This is his summary of the status of this issue as it appeared in that address: "While Mr. Jacobs, in his zeal for methodic signs, has exemplified the advance in one direction, most of our other schools show progress in an opposite direction; relying mainly on the colloquial language of signs as the best means of mental development and instrument of instruction for deaf-mutes" (p. 340).

"the United States." H. P. Peet (1859). Memoir on the history of the art of instructing the deaf and dumb—second period. In: Convention of American Instructors of the Deaf, *Proceedings*, 277–341, p. 339; J. Williams (1893). A brief history of the American Asylum at Hartford. In E. A. Fay, ed., *Histories of American Schools for the Deaf (1817–1893)*. Washington, DC: Volta Bureau, pp. 22–23.

Page 113 "in 1928." H. Kloss (1967). Bilingualism and nationalism. *Journal of Social Issues*, *23*, 39–47.

114 "congress began." S. Hull (1880). Letter to Miss Rogers on the international congress held at Milan. In Clarke School for the Deaf, *Reports*, 35–43. Reprinted: *Education*, *1*, 1881, 286–93.

"disadvantages of methods." R. Elliott (1911). Reminiscences of a retired educator. *Volta Review*, *13*, 240–44, 303–306, 358–61, 416–19, 478–82, 534–36, p. 241.

"divine thought." Congrès international pour l'amelioration du sort des sourds-muets (1881). *Compte-rendu . . .* Rome: Botta. Quoted in H. Lane (1984). *When the Mind Hears: A History of the Deaf*. New York: Random House, p. 392.

"his soul." Quoted in H. Lane (1984). *When the Mind Hears: A History of the Deaf*. New York: Random House, p. 393.

"prudence and truth." Quoted in H. Lane (1984). *When the Mind Hears: A History of the Deaf*. New York: Random House, p. 394.

115 "divine matters." Quoted in H. Lane (1984). *When the Mind Hears: A History of the Deaf*. New York: Random House, p. 394.

"ultimate results." George Veditz (1933). The genesis of the National Association of the Deaf. *Deaf-Mutes Journal*, *62(22)*.

"native languages." A. Leibowitz (1976). Language and the law: The exercise of political power through official designation of language. In W. O'Barr and J. O'Barr, eds., *Language and Politics* (pp. 449–66). The Hague: Mouton.

"Indian languages." F. Barringer (1991). Faded but vibrant, Indian languages struggle to keep their voices alive. *New York Times*, January 8, 1991, p. A14.

116 "handicapped children." H. Lane, Jean Massieu and deaf teachers of the deaf (1981). In *Proceedings of the National Symposium on Sign Language Research and Teaching. Boston, 1981*. Silver Spring, MD: National Association of the Deaf; J. Woodward, T. Allen, and A. Schildroth (1985). Teachers and deaf students: an ethnography of classroom communication. In S. DeLancey and R. Tomlin, eds., *Proceedings of the First Annual Pacific Linguistics Conference* (pp. 479–93). Eugene, OR: University of Oregon Press; J. Woodward and T. Allen (1987). Classroom use of ASL by teachers. *Sign Language Studies*, *54*, 1–10.

117 "of criminals." Convention of American Instructors of the Deaf (1909). *Proceedings of the Convention of American Instructors of the Deaf*, pp. 38–56.

"answered satisfactorily." H. Lane (1984). *When the Mind Hears: A History of the Deaf*. New York: Random House, p. xvi.

"deaf-mute children." L. Limosin (1886). Les vautours du Prométhée des sourds-muets. *Défense des sourds-muets*, *2*, 127–29.

"of society." V. G. Chambellan (1884). *De L'Importance incontestable du langage mimique dans l'enseignement des sourds-muets de naissance*. Paris: author, p. 18.

118 "the deaf!" Congress of Deaf—International—First (1889). See V. Chambellan, ed. (1890). *Compte-rendu. Congrès international des sourds-muets.* Paris: Association Amicale des Sourds-Muets de France.
"readily corrupted." L. Goguillot (1889). *Comment on fait parler les sourds-muets. Précédé d'une préface par M. le Dr. Ladreit de Lacharrière.* Paris: Masson.

119 "of language." Congress on Deaf—International—Fourth (1900). L. Ladreit de Lacharrière, ed., *Exposition universelle de 1900. Congrès international pour l'étude des questions d'éducation et d'assistance des sourds-muets tenu les 6, 7, et 8 août, 1900, au Palais des Congrès de l'Exposition. Compte-rendu des travaux de la section des entendants.* Paris: Imprimerie d'Ouvriers Sourds-Muets; Congress on Deaf—International—Fourth (1900). H. Gaillard and H. Jeanvoine, eds., *Congrès international pour l'étude des questions d'éducation et d'assistance des sourds-muets (section des sourds-muets). Compte-rendu des débats et relations diverses.* Paris: Imprimerie d'Ouvriers Sourds-Muets; Congress on Deaf—International— Fourth (1900). *Exposition universelle de 1900. Congrès international pour l'étude des questions d'éducation et d'assistance des sourds-muets. Tenu à Paris du 6 au 8 août 1900. Relation des travaux de l'Educazione dei Sordomuti [G. C. Ferreri, ed.], traduit par J. Auffray . . . Suivi des procès verbaux sommaires par le Dr. Martha.* Asnières: Institut Départemental de Sourds-Muets et de Sourdes-Muettes, 1901. *Relation* reprint: A. Martha and H. Gaillard. Paris: Imprimerie nationale, 1901; Congress on Deaf— International—Fourth (1900). Resolutions adopted by the hearing section of the Paris Congress of 1900. *American Annals of the Deaf, 46,* 1901, 329–31; Congress on Deaf—International—Fourth (1900). Resolutions adopted by the deaf section of the Paris Congress of 1900. *Association Review, 3,* 1901, 43–50; Congress on Deaf—International—Fourth (1900). Resolutions adopted by the deaf section of the Paris Congress of 1900. *American Annals of the Deaf, 46,* 1901, 108–11.
"leader observed." H. Gaillard and H. Jeanvoine, eds. (1900). *Congrès international pour l'étude des questions d'éducation et d'assistance des sourds-muets (section des sourds-muets). Compte-rendu des débats et relations diverses.* Paris: Imprimerie d'Ouvriers Sourds-Muets, pp. 332–36.

120 "of discussion." F. W. Booth (1900). Editorial. *Association Review, 2,* 451–52.
"Act of 1968." That is, Title VII of PL 90-247, January 2, 1968; 81 stat. 783, esp. section 704.

121 "grammatical inflections." J. Greene (1975). *Thinking and Language.* New York: Methuen.

122 "spatial concepts." R. Jackendorf (1990). *Semantic Structures.* Cambridge, MA: M.I.T. Press; J. Carrier and J. Randall (1991). *From Conceptual Structure to Syntax.* Dordrecht, Holland: Foris Publications.
"above-below." See the discussion in W. Levelt (1984). Some perceptual limitations in talking about space. In A. J. van Doorn, ed., *Limits in Perception.* Utrecht: VNU Science Press, pp. 323–58.

Part Five. The Education of Deaf Children: Drowning in the Mainstream and the Sidestream

Page 129 "at home." S. C. Brown (1986). Etiological trends, characteristics, and distributions. In A. N. Schildroth and M. A. Karchmer, eds., *Deaf Children in America* (pp. 33–54). San Diego CA: College-Hill; Jensema reports 90 percent before age three in 1974: C. Jensema and J. Mullins (1974). Onset, cause, and additional handicaps in hearing-impaired children. *American Annals of the Deaf, 119,* 701–705.

"decade of training." R. Conrad (1979). *The Deaf Schoolchild.* London: Harper & Row. 1979. Hearing high school students made up the control group.

"utterly unintelligible." R. Conrad (1979). *The Deaf Schoolchild.* London: Harper & Row. Twenty percent of the speech of deaf persons is understood by inexperienced listeners; Allen and Karchmer (1990) found teachers rated three out of four of their own profoundly deaf students nonintelligible. The smaller number of students with severe hearing loss received this rating 44 percent of the time. T. Allen and M. Karchmer (1990). Communication in classrooms for deaf students: student, teacher, and program characteristics. In H. Bornstein, ed., *Manual Communication: Implications for Education.* Washington, DC: Gallaudet University Press, pp. 45–66, p. 53; Jensema, Karchmer, and Trybus (1978) examined teacher ratings of speech intelligibility in a random sample of 479 profoundly deaf children in a variety of educational settings; 25 percent had intelligible speech and intelligibility did not increase with age. C. Jensema, M. Karchmer, and R. Trybus (1978). *The Rated Speech Intelligibility of Hearing-Impaired Children.* Washington, DC: Gallaudet Office of Demographic Studies; C. Smith (1975). Residual hearing and speech production in deaf children. *Journal of Speech and Hearing Research, 18,* 795–811. Forty children born deaf or early deafened proved 18 percent intelligible on word recognition in sentences. According to Stark, even with hearing aids and speech training, the average speech intelligibility of severely and profoundly deaf children is not more than 20 percent for the naive listener: R. Stark (1979). Speech of the hearing-impaired child. In L. J. Bradford and W. G. Hardy, eds., *Hearing and Hearing Impairment* (pp. 229–48). New York: Grune & Stratton. Markides found deaf children 31 percent intelligible to their teachers, 19 percent to strangers: A. Markides (1970). The speech of deaf and partially hearing children with special reference to factors affecting intelligibility. *British Journal of Disorders of Communication, 5,* 126–40. T. Gold (1980). Speech production in hearing-impaired children. *Journal of Communication Disorders, 13,* 397–418. According to Lionel Evans, the speech sounds of English reduce to four homophonous (i.e., visually indistinguishable) groups of consonants and four of vowels. Perhaps half of English words are homophonous and cannot be identified purely visually in isolation. Conrad's 1979 findings (see list p. 157) were consistent with

American studies showing that children with normal hearing perform as well or better than deaf children. L. Evans (1981). Psycholinguistic perspectives on visual communication. In B. Woll, J. Kyle, and M. Deuchar, eds., *Perspectives on British Sign Language and Deafness* (pp. 150–62). London: Croom Helm.

130 "grades behind." T. E. Allen (1986). Patterns of academic achievement among hearing-impaired students: 1974 and 1983. In A. N. Schildroth and M. A. Karchmer, eds., *Deaf Children in America* (pp. 161–206). San Diego, CA: College-Hill; T. Allen (1986). *Understanding the Scores: Hearing-Impaired Students and the Stanford Achievement Test*, 7th ed. Washington DC: Gallaudet College Press; S. Wolk and T. E. Allen (1984). A five-year follow-up of reading-comprehension achievement of hearing-impaired students in special education programs. *Journal of Special Education, 18*, 161–76; R. Trybus (1978). What the Stanford Achievement Test has to say about the reading abilities of deaf children. In H. Reynolds and C. Williams, eds., *Proceedings of the Gallaudet Conference on Reading in Relation to Deafness*. Washington, DC: Gallaudet College Press, pp. 213–21; R. J. Trybus and M. A. Karchmer (1977). School achievement scores of hearing-impaired children: national data on achievement status and growth patterns. *American Annals of the Deaf, 122*, 62–69; C. Jensema (1975). The relationship between academic achievement and the demographic characteristics of hearing-impaired children and youth, Series R, no. 2. Washington, DC: Gallaudet Office of Demographic Studies. Ewoldt (1987) points out that standardized tests do not measure the deaf child's ability to understand text in contextually real situations where the child has background knowledge and contextual cues. C. Ewoldt (1987). Reading tests and the deaf reader. Can we measure how well deaf students read? *Perspectives for Teachers of the Hearing-Impaired, 5*, 21–24.

131 "twenty-five." R. Conrad (1977). Facts and fantasies about verbal abilities of deaf school leavers. *British Deaf News*, 11, 145–47.

"functional level." J. G. Kyle and G. Pullen (1988). Cultures in contact: Deaf and hearing people. *Disability, Handicap and Society, 3*, 49–61, p. 54.

"or sixteen." J. Kyle. Deaf people and minority groups in the U.K. Paper presented at the second European Congress in Sign Language Research, Netherlands, July 1985. The examinations specified were "O" level and "CSE."

"a nine-year-old." Personal communication, Prof. Y. Nakano. Also see Y. Nakano (1975). Communication for hearing-handicapped people in Japan. In H. Oyer, ed. *Communication for the Hearing Handicapped: An International Perspective*. Baltimore: University Park Press, pp. 497–522.

"illiterate adults." United States Senate, *Oversight of Gallaudet College and the National Technical Institute for the Deaf*. Senate Hearing 99-131, June 11, 1985. Washington, DC: U.S. Government Printing Office, 1985.

Page 131 "a paycheck." R. C. Smith *et al.*, eds. *America's Shame, America's Hope: Twelve Million Youth at Risk.* Chapel Hill, NC: MDC, 1988.

"reasoning skills." United States Senate, *Oversight of Gallaudet College and the National Technical Institute for the Deaf.* Senate Hearing 99-131, June 11, 1985. Washington, DC: U.S. Government Printing Office, 1985; J. G. Kyle and G. Pullen (1988). Cultures in contact, deaf and hearing people. *Disability, Handicap, and Society, 3,* 49–61. According to E. Mindel and M. Vernon (1971). *They Grow in Silence.* Silver Spring, MD: National Association of the Deaf, 1970 survey data showed an estimated 87 percent of the deaf population engaged in manual labor (p. 103). J. Schein and M. Delk (1974). *The Deaf Population of the United States.* Silver Spring, MD: National Association of the Deaf, report in Table V.8 the percent of their sample in various occupations, from which I estimate approximately 75 percent were in manual trades. See J. B. Christiansen and S. N. Barnartt (1987). The silent minority: the socioeconomic status of deaf people. In P. C. Higgins and J. Nash, eds., *Understanding Deafness Socially.* Springfield, IL: Charles C Thomas, 1987, pp. 171–96. These authors state that by 1977 30 percent of deaf men were in white-collar positions. However, the deaf male unemployment rate rose to 10 percent by that year. Both figures probably reflect a shift from the industrial to the human services sectors in the work force. According to U.S. Department of Education (1988). *Youth Indicators 1988: Trends in the Well-Being of American Youth.* Washington, DC: U.S. Government Printing Office, 35 percent of whites aged 25 to 29 had matriculated in college. In the 1970s, the proportion of hearing students who went on to college was approximately 15 percent; the proportion of deaf students who did so was about 5 percent. See J. Schein (1989). *At Home Among Strangers.* Washington, DC: Gallaudet University Press, p. 166; J. Christiansen and J. Egelston-Dodd (1982). Socioeconomic status of the deaf population. In Conference, Sociology of Deafness. *Social Aspects of Deafness.* Vol. 4. Washington, DC: Gallaudet College.

132 "semi-skilled employment." J. G. Kyle and G. Pullen (1988). Cultures in contact: Deaf and hearing people. *Disability, Handicap and Society, 3,* 49–61, p. 54.

"Unacceptably so." Commission on the Education of the Deaf (1988). *Toward Equality: Education of the Deaf.* Washington, DC: U.S. Government Printing Office, p. viii.

"years earlier." United States Department of Health, Education and Welfare (1965). *Education of the Deaf: A Report to the Secretary of Health, Education and Welfare by His Advisory Committee on the Education of the Deaf.* March 15, 1965. Washington, DC: U.S. Government Printing Office.

"hands slapped." S. Foster (1989). Reflections of a group of deaf adults on their experiences in mainstream and residential school programs in the United States. *Disability, Handicap and Society, 4,* 37–56, p. 49.

133 "oralist regime." D. Moores (1978). *Educating the Deaf.* New York: Houghton Mifflin, p. 257.

"deaf people." A. M. Holmes (1991). Is there a place for deaf teachers of the deaf? A view from Scotland. *Deaf American, 41,* 67–70, p. 68.

"entered the deaf community." J. D. Schein (1989). *At Home Among Strangers.* Washington, DC: Gallaudet University Press.

"the century." J. Van Cleve (1991). The academic integration of deaf children: A historical perspective. In R. Fischer and H. Lane. *Looking Back: A Reader on the History of Deaf Communities and Their Sign Languages.* Hamburg: Signum.

134 "drawing—whatever." Deaf educator Roy Holcomb introduced the term in 1968. The term was adopted for the educational approach at the Maryland School for the Deaf under David Denton; see D. Denton (1972). A rationale for total communication. In T. J. O'Rourke, ed., *Psycholinguistics and Total Communication: The State of the Art.* Silver Spring, MD: American Annals of the Deaf, pp. 53–61.

"total communication." I. K. Jordan, G. Gustason, and R. Rosen (1979). An update on communication trends and programs for the deaf. *American Annals of the Deaf, 124,* 350–357.

"on the hands." W. Newell, M. Stinson, D. Castle, D. Mallery-Ruganis, B. R. Holcomb (1991). Simultaneous communication: a description by deaf professionals working in an educational setting. *Sign Language Studies, 69,* 391–413; I. K. Jordan and M. A. Karchmer (1986). Patterns of sign use among hearing-impaired students. In A. N. Schildroth and M. A. Karchmer, eds., *Deaf Children in America* (pp. 125–38). San Diego, CA: College-Hill; J. Woodward and T. Allen (1987). Classroom use of ASL by teachers. *Sign Language Studies, 54,* 1–10. A review of the literature on simultaneous communication will be found on pp. 41–47 of N. Israelite, C. Ewoldt, and R. Hoffmeister (1989). A review of the literature on effective use of native sign language on the acquisition of a majority language by hearing-impaired students. Unpublished report, Boston University Center for the Study of Communication and Deafness.

"deaf children." R. Johnson and S. Liddell (1990). The value of ASL in the education of deaf children. *Deaf American, 40,* 59–69.

"in America." There may have been a half-grade improvement from second grade to midway between second and third grades in reading ability at high school leaving from 1974 to 1983 measures. See T. E. Allen (1986). Patterns of academic achievement among hearing-impaired students: 1974 and 1983. In A. N. Schildroth and M. A. Karchmer, eds., *Deaf Children in America* (pp. 161–206). San Diego, CA: College-Hill.

135 "bimodal performances." C. Baker (1979). How does "sim-com" fit into a bilingual approach to education. In F. Caccamise and D. Hicks, eds., *American Sign Language in a Bilingual Context: Proceedings of the Second National Symposium on Sign Language Research and Teaching* (pp. 13–26). Silver Spring, MD: NAD; G. Marmor and L. Petito (1979). Simultaneous communication in the classroom: how well is English grammar represented? *Sign Language Studies, 23,* 99–136.

"in 1977." Public Law 94-142, The Education for All Handicapped

Children Act, was passed in 1975; it requires a free appropriate education for all handicapped children in the least restrictive environment; the law went into effect in 1977. On the failure of earlier mainstreaming efforts in France, Germany, and England, see H. Lane (1984). *When the Mind Hears: A History of the Deaf.* New York: Random House. J. Van Cleve (1992). The academic integration of deaf children. In R. Fischer and H. Lane. *Looking Back: A Reader on the History of Deaf Communities and Their Sign Languages.* Hamburg: Signum.

Page 135 "multiply-handicapped children." P. Ries (1986). Characteristics of hearing-impaired youth in the general population and of students in special education programs for the hearing-impaired. In A. N. Schildroth and M. A. Karchmer, eds., *Deaf Children in America* (pp. 1–32). San Diego, CA: College-Hill, p. 22; T. E. Allen and T. I. Osborn (1984). Academic integration of hearing-impaired students: demographic, handicapping, and achievement factors. *American Annals of the Deaf, 129,* 100–13; Convention of American Instructors of the Deaf (1990). Schools and classes for the deaf in the United States. *American Annals of the Deaf, 135,* p. 135.

136 "in basements." H. Goodstein (1988). What is mainstreaming? Paper prepared for the Gallaudet Research Institute Roundtable on Mainstreaming. Washington, DC: Gallaudet University.

"other deaf children." Cited in L. Siegel (1991). The least restrictive environment? *Deaf American, 41,* 135–39.

"an ASL interpreter." C. Estes (April 1991). Bestest from Estes. *The National Association of the Deaf Broadcaster, 13,* p. 3.

"deaf person." J. Thomas, testimony, National Council on Disabilities. Special Schools. June 8, 1989.

"social isolation." S. Foster (1989). Reflections of a group of deaf adults on their experiences in mainstream and residential school programs in the United States. *Disability, Handicap and Society, 4,* 37–56, p. 44.

137 "deaf students." T. Booth (1988). Challenging conceptions of integration. In L. Barton, ed., *The Politics of Special Educational Needs* (pp. 99–122). Philadelphia: Falmer Press. Also see M. G. Gaustad and T. Kluwin (1991). Patterns of communication among deaf and hearing adolescents in public school programs. In T. Kluwin, D. F. Moores, and M. G. Gaustad, *Defining the Effective Public School Program for Deaf Students.* Unpublished ms., Gallaudet University, pp. 124–46.

"I am deaf." Cited in T. Booth (1988). Challenging conceptions of integration. In L. Barton, ed., *The Politics of Special Educational Needs* (pp. 97–122). Philadelphia: Falmer Press, p. 113.

"residential setting," E. B. Emerson and G. M. H. Pretty (1987). Enhancing the social relevance of evaluation practice. *Disability, Handicap and Society, 2,* 151–62, p. 152. Moores (1991) cites some demographic factors influential in the shift from residential schools to mainstream programs. He points out that the rubella epidemic of 1964–65 caused an influx of deaf pupils in a single age group, many of them with additional physical or mental handicaps which the residential schools were ill prepared to cope with. Moreover, this "rubella bulge" occurred at the same time as a decline in the national birthrate, causing many local school classrooms, which had been built in large numbers to accommodate the post–World War II baby boom, to go empty. D. Moores (1991). An historical perspective on school placement of deaf students. In T. Kluwin, D. F. Moores, and M. G. Gaustad, *Defining the Effective Public School Program for Deaf Students*. Unpublished ms., Gallaudet University, pp. 7–34.

"as a deaf person." Mertens (1989) distributed a questionnaire to some fifty Gallaudet University students, roughly half of whom had attended residential high schools for deaf pupils, and the others, mainstream programs. The former group described their social experiences more positively; they cited their ability to socialize with other deaf students, to participate in extracurricular activities, and to communicate more fluently with their teacher. D. Mertens (1989). Social experiences of hearing-impaired high school youth. *American Annals of the Deaf, 134,* 15–19. With regard to participation in sports, Stewart and Stinson (1991) point out: "Deaf sport is perhaps the best organized social institution in the deaf community. A deaf volleyball player could play for the Greater Vancouver Association of the Deaf, participate in a tournament sponsored by the British Columbia Deaf Sports Federation, compete in the Canada Summer Games, and ultimately represent Canada in the World Games for the Deaf" (p. 164). D. A. Stewart and M. S. Stinson (1991). The role of sport and extracurricular activities in shaping the socialization patterns of deaf and hard of hearing students. In T. Kluwin, D. F. Moores, and M. G. Gaustad, *Defining the Effective Public School Program for Deaf Students*. Unpublished ms., Gallaudet University, pp. 147–70.

138 "out of reach." See T. Kluwin (1991). "What does 'local public school program' mean? Also T. Kluwin (1991). Some reflections on defining the effective program. In T. Kluwin, D. F. Moores, and M. G. Gaustad, *Defining the Effective Public School Program for Deaf Students*. Unpublished ms., Gallaudet University, pp. 35–55; 272–82.

"residential schools." Teachers described four out of five of their hearing impaired students who were extensively integrated as having intelligible or very intelligible speech. T. Allen and M. Karchmer (1990). Communication in classrooms for deaf students: student, teacher, and program characteristics. In H. Bornstein, ed., *Manual Communication: Implications for Education* (pp. 45–66). Washington, DC: Gallaudet University Press, p. 55.

"academic disadvantage." In 1981, Allen and Karchmer examined the reading and mathematics scores on the Stanford Achievement Test of a random sample of 330 deaf students in elementary and high school who were deafened because their mothers contracted German measles during pregnancy. Those students who were partially integrated into mainstream settings had higher achievement scores to begin with (as well as lesser hearing losses), so this difference between them and deaf students in specialized programs had to be factored out statistically. When that was done, there was no reliable advantage to mainstreaming. T. Allen and M. Karchmer (1981). Influences on academic achievement of hearing-impaired students born during the 1963–65 rubella epidemic. *Directions*, 2, 40–54. Holt and Allen (1989), as part of a larger study, examined the reading and mathematics achievement of about sixty deaf students in special schools and in mainstream settings for whom prior achievement scores were available. When students were, in effect, matched statistically on this and several other variables, there was no difference in reading scores obtained in the two settings. However, deaf students who were fully integrated with hearing students for mathematics instruction achieve lower mathematics scores than their peers in special schools. J. Holt and T. Allen (1989). The effects of schools and their curricula on the reading and mathematics achievement of hearing-impaired students. *International Journal of Educational Research*, 13, 547–62.

Four studies have been cited by some authors as supporting mainstreaming of deaf children. That conclusion, however, does not withstand close inspection. With an avowedly strong mainstreaming bias, Van der Horst (1971) published a report in the British journal *The Teacher of the Deaf* (69, 398–414) on matched groups of twelve "auditory defectives," enrolled in a special school (DS) or in a local school for hearing children (HS). The groups were matched on average hearing loss, age, sex, and nonverbal IQ; they were not matched with respect to the socioeconomic level of their homes, nor with respect to the training their teachers had received, although both factors are known to influence academic achievement. The two groups did not differ on one verbal IQ test, but they did differ, in favor of the HS pupils, on a second; we are told the difference was statistically significant but we are not told its size. Moreover, three of the five subtests on this second IQ test showed no difference between the groups. A comparison of the two groups on writing tests showed no difference, but the DS pupils showed less improvement from age eight to age eleven on one writing measure. Using personal records and psychological tests they fail to identify, the authors assigned emotional stability ratings to pupils. These data favor the special school children, who were labeled normal 86 percent of the time compared with only 54 percent for the deaf children in the hearing school. Because of its failure to control important variables, and the finding of no difference on the first verbal IQ test and three of the five subtests of the second IQ test, I believe it is inappropriate to cite this study as showing an advantage to mainstreaming. A 1975 study published by the Toronto Board of Education (C. Reich, R. Hambleton, and B. Klein, *The Integration of Hearing-Impaired Children in Regular Classrooms*) found higher raw scores on reading, language, and speech intelligibility from HS students than from DS, but "when hearing loss as well as other differences in background were taken into account, there was little remaining difference between groups to unequivocally attest to the superiority of one method over another. . . . However, the results do not support the view that integration is *harmful*." [italics theirs]. As was evident in the first study mentioned, a problem that bedevils comparisons of the achievement of HS and DS deaf students is the lack of comparability of the students who attend the two kinds of schools. In 1984, Allen and Osborne (Academic integration of hearing impaired students. *American Annals of the Deaf, 129,* 100–13) made a sophisticated attempt to render comparable by statistical methods noncomparable samples of deaf students taught in HS and DS environments. If one knew the contribution of, say, socioeconomic background to reading achievement in deaf students, and if the HS group on the average came from more upper-class homes, one could lower their average reading scores appropriately in order to render them comparable to the DS students. A problem with this approach arises, however, when the groups differ in several important respects, for it is not obvious that the advantage arising from a wealthier background and that arising from, say, residual hearing are simply additive. This statistical issue would be less critical if a substantial difference remained after the corrections, but in fact "the actual proportion of achievement variance accounted for by integration status alone was very small for all three variables" (a reading test and two math tests). The authors go on to point out, moreover, that such differences as remain "cannot be interpreted as representing a causal relationship between integration status and achievement." They also recognize that there were many uncontrolled variables, such as prior academic ability, not imputable to the demographic variables controlled for. Moreover, there may have been differences between the groups compared in math and language aptitude and in the preparation of their teachers— to mention just two more unexamined factors. Since the slight difference in scores could be attributed to the correction procedures or to uncontrolled variables, and cannot be causally attributed to integration status, it is inappropriate to cite this study as supporting mainstreaming. Kluwin and Moores (1985) studied the effects of mainstreaming on mathematics achievement in a nonrandom sample of eighty deaf students in three high schools. T. Kluwin and D. Moores. The effects of integration on the mathematics achievement of hearing-impaired adolescents. *Exceptional Children, 52,* 153–61. The authors used a different method of post hoc corrections for some but not all of the group differences, leaving a small residual (one third of a standard deviation) advantage for the integrated students. They conclude "that the greatest amount of variance may be accounted for by the fact that regular mathematics teachers are subject matter specialists and have more teaching experience." None of the teachers in the special school, who averaged six years experience, were math specialists; all of the teachers in the hearing school had master's degrees in mathematics, except one who had a Ph.D.; they averaged eighteen years of experience. The same authors again found only trivial effects of placement on the academic achievements of deaf students in a later study: T. Kluwin and D. Moores (1989). Mathematics achievement of hearing-impaired adolescents in different placements. *Exceptional Children*, 55, 327–35. Kluwin has concluded: "Mainstreaming per se is not a solution to improving the academic achievement of deaf students" (p. 274). T. N. Kluwin (1991). Some reflections on defining the effective program. In T. Kluwin, D. F. Moores, and M. G. Gaustad, *Defining the Effective Public School Program for Deaf Students*. Unpublished ms., Gallaudet University, pp. 272–82.

To the best of my knowledge there are no studies that support the premise that a deaf child will fare substantially better in a mainstream school than in a special school for deaf children. One study that compared hearing-impaired students in the mainstream with hearing students in the same classes found that hearing-impaired seniors had "greater academic difficulties, took fewer academic courses, evidenced less school motivation, did even less homework, and appeared less goal-oriented . . . than their normally hearing peers" (p. 16) (J. F. Gregory, T. Shanahan, and H. J. Walberg [1984]. Mainstreamed hearing-impaired high school seniors: a reanalysis of a national survey. *American Annals of the Deaf*, 129, 11–16).

Page 138 "language skills." Earlier studies are reviewed in E. D. Mindel and M. Vernon, *They Grow in Silence*. Silver Spring, MD: National Association of the Deaf, 1971. Also see A. E. Geers and B. Schick (1988). Acquisition of spoken and signed English by hearing-impaired children of hearing-impaired or hearing parents. *Journal of Speech and Hearing Disorders*, 53, 136–43. Deaf children of deaf parents score more than 20 percent higher on sentence production tests than deaf children of hearing parents. They also demonstrate better English skills in manual, oral and combined modes. Also see K. E. Brasel (1975). The influence of early language and communication environments on the development of language in deaf children. Ph.D. dissertation, University of Illinois; H. Corson (1973). Comparing deaf children of oral deaf parents and deaf parents using manual communication with deaf children of hearing parents on academic, social, and communicative functioning. Ph.D. dissertation, University of Cincinnati; N. Israelite, C. Ewoldt, and R. Hoffmeister (1989). A review of the literature on effective use of native sign language on the acquisition of a majority language by hearing-impaired students. Unpublished report, Boston University Center for the Study of Communication and Deafness; A. Weisel and J. Reichstein (1987). Parental hearing status, reading comprehension skills, and socio-emotional adjustment. In R. Ojala, ed., *Proceedings of the Tenth World Congress of the World Federation of the Deaf*. Helsinki: Finnish Association of the Deaf; A. Zweibel (1987). More on the effects of early manual communication on the cognitive development of deaf children. *American Annals of the Deaf*, 132, 16–20.

"effective communication." E. D. Mindel and M. Vernon, *They Grow in Silence*. Silver Spring, MD: National Association of the Deaf, 1971. A list of recent references will be found in R. E. Johnson, S. K. Liddell, and C. J. Erting (1989). Unlocking the curriculum: principles for achieving access in deaf education. *Gallaudet Research Institute Working Papers*, p. 10. Also see R. Harris (1978). Impulse control in deaf children. In L. Liben, ed., *Deaf Children: Developmental Perspectives*. New York: Academic Press.

"with peers." V. Kourbetis (1987). Deaf children of deaf parents and deaf children of hearing parents in Greece: a comparative study. Ph.D. dissertation, Boston University. Also see B. Hansen and R. Kjaer-Sorensen (1976). *The Sign Language of Deaf Children in Denmark*. Copenhagen, Denmark: The School for the Deaf. A. Weisel and J. Reichstein (1987). Parental hearing status, reading comprehension skills, and social-emotional adjustment. In R. Ojala, ed., *Proceedings of the Tenth World Congress of the World Federation of the Deaf*. Helsinki: Finnish Association of the Deaf. It stands to reason that deaf children of deaf parents possess all these advantages because they have acquired a natural language in the natural way, during the first years of their lives; but we cannot rule out other factors that are intertwined with language learning, such as the intimacy of relations possible with their parents, or their parents' expectations concerning their children's academic and social achievement.

139 "permit this." B. White (1990). Deaf education: A game people play. *DCARA News*, January 1990, p. 2.

"brute force." Conference of Executives of American Schools for the Deaf (1977). Statement on "least restrictive" placements for deaf students. *American Annals of the Deaf*, *122*, 62–69. Also see National Association of the Deaf (1987). NAD recommends to the Commission on Education of the Deaf. *NAD Broadcaster*, *9*, suppl., 1–8; National Association of the Deaf (1986). Public Law 94-142 and the least restrictive environment: a position paper of the National Association of the Deaf. *NAD Broadcaster*, *8*, 1.

140 "local school." Commission on the Education of the Deaf (1988). *Toward Equality, Education of the Deaf*. Washington, DC: U.S. Government Printing Office, p. 30.

"handicapped children." J. G. Duncan (1984). Recent legislation affecting hearing-impaired persons. *American Annals of the Deaf*, *129*, 83–94.

"achieved satisfactorily." 34C.F.R. 300.550, 300.552, 300.550(b)(2). Cited in L. Siegel (1991). The least restrictive environment? *Deaf American*, *41*, 135–39.

"for wisdom." *Visco by Visco* v. *School District of Pittsburgh* (684F. Supp. 1310, 1314 Wj.D. Pa. 1988). Cited in L. Siegel (1991). The least restrictive environment? *Deaf American*, *41*, 135–39, p. 137.

"their child." A. T. Bennett (1988). Gateway to powerlessness: incorporating Hispanic deaf children and families into formal schooling. *Disability, Handicap and Society*, *3*, 119–51, p. 127.

141 "Department of Education." S. Dutton (1991). Deaf education: Who

decides. *The Bicultural Center News, 33*, 1–2; L. Levitan (1991). Mark
Dutton: An educational tragedy. *Deaf Life*, December 1991, 10–17.

Page 142 "the U.N. Convention." National Union of the Deaf (1982). *Charter of
the Rights of the Deaf*. Bedfort, Middlesex, England.

143 "specific purposes." MJ Bienvenu (1990). Letter to the editor. *Deaf
American, 40*, 133.

144 "spoken French." Mr. Harry Johnson, the treasurer of the mission,
and his wife received me with great warmth and helpfulness and
have been a friend to all our efforts in Burundi. It is a pleasure to
acknowledge my great debt to them and the devoted staff of their
school.

146 "rector agreed." The plane ticket to America was provided by the
Christoffelblindenmission, a charitable organization that sponsors
schools for blind and deaf children throughout Africa, including the
mission school in Bujumbura. Professor Prime Nyamoya, formerly
dean of the Faculty of Economics at the University of Burundi, extended me every hospitality and assistance, without which I could not
have succeeded in my undertaking.

153 "in 1992." The funds were provided by the United Nations High
Commission for Refugees. The UNHCR public information officer in
Washington, DC, Patricia Fagen, has been an invaluable ally. Claudine
first entered the Model Secondary School as an exchange student
under the aegis of the American Field Service. It is a pleasure to
acknowledge the support of these organizations and the assistance
of many members of the faculty and staff of Gallaudet University,
especially Dr. Robert Davila, now assistant secretary, U.S. Department
of Education, who was Gallaudet University vice-president for pre-
college programs at the time of Claudine's application and arranged
for her admission to the high school. Several very generous families
opened their homes to Claudine as host parents during her stay:
Cathryn Carroll, Caroline Newsome, Mr. and Mrs. Giansanti, and Mr.
and Mrs. Kona.

155 "be *deaf*." T. S. Spradley and J. P. Spradley (1978). *Deaf Like Me*. New
York: Random House, p. 158.
"million members." J. Schein (1989). *At Home Among Strangers*. Washington, DC: Gallaudet University Press, pp. 8–9.
"other children?" H. Lane (1984). *When the Mind Hears: A History of
the Deaf*. New York: Random House, p. 264.

156 "him orally." K. Meadow-Orlans (1987). An analysis of the effectiveness of early intervention programs for hearing impaired children.
In M. J. Guralnick and F. C. Bennett, eds., *The Effectiveness of Early
Intervention for At Risk and Handicapped Children* (pp. 325–57). New
York: Academic Press, p. 334.
"concrete objects." M. T. Greenberg (1980). Social interaction between
deaf preschoolers and their mothers: The effects of communication
method and communicative competence. *Developmental Psychology, 16*,
465–74.

157 "of persecution." A. Ballin, *A Deaf-Mute Howls* (1930). Los Angeles: Grafton, p. 242.

158 "the word." A. Binet and T. Simon (1910). An investigation concerning the value of the oral method. *American Annals of the Deaf*, 55, 4–33.
"the pupil." H. Lane (1984). *When the Mind Hears: A History of the Deaf.* New York: Random House, p. 330.
"is intensified." D. Moores (1982). *Educating the Deaf.* New York: Houghton-Mifflin, p. 257.

159 "less responsive." K. Meadow-Orlans (1987). An analysis of the effectiveness of early intervention programs for hearing-impaired children. In M. J. Guralnick and F. C. Bennett, eds., *The Effectiveness of Early Intervention for At Risk and Handicapped Children* (pp. 325–57). New York: Academic Press.
"social barriers." F. Grosjean (1982). *Life with Two Languages.* Cambridge, MA: Harvard University Press. A. A. Teraoka (1990). *Gastarbeiterliteratur*: The other speaks back. A. R. JanMohamed and D. Lloyd, *The Nature and Context of Minority Discourse.* New York: Oxford, pp. 294–318.

160 "they have received." J. Schein (1989). *At Home Among Strangers.* Washington, DC: Gallaudet University Press, p. 106. Schein calls the coincidence of these numbers the "90-percent rule."

161 "born hearing." R. Thomas, personal communication, 1991.

162 "English language." L. Clerc (1952). *The Diary of Laurent Clerc's Voyage from France to America in 1816.* Hartford, CT: American School for the Deaf.

Part Six: Bilingual Education and Deaf Power

165 "other professions." Cf. H. Lane (1984). *When the Mind Hears: A History of the Deaf.* New York: Random House, pp. 277–78.

166 "that development." Several studies have shown that the deaf child is able to use an innate capacity for language to create grammatical structure from degraded sign input: J. Gee and J. L. Mounty (1990). Nativization, variability, and style shifting in the sign language development of deaf or hearing children. In S. Fischer and P. Siple, eds., *Theoretical Issues in Sign Language Research.* Chicago: University of Chicago Press; S. Goldin-Meadow (1983). Language development under atypical learning conditions. In K. Nelson, ed., *Children's Language.* Hillsdale, NJ: Lawrence Erlbaum; S. Goldin-Meadow and C. Mylander (1984). The development of morphology without a conventional language model. *Chicago Linguistic Society*, 20, 119–35; S. Livingston (1983). Levels of development in the language of deaf children. *Sign Language Studies*, 40, 193–286.
"deaf child." *Consultation sur les différentes approches de l'éducation des sourds.* ED-84/ws/102. Paris: UNESCO, 1985.

167 "Education Act." P.L. 89-10, Title VII, 1965, as amended 1968.

Page 167   "rights statutes." P.L. 88-352, Title VI, 1964; P.L. 93-380, 1974.
           "American children." 20 USCS 3222.
           "the act." 500.4; 34 CFR Ch. V 7-1-87 edition.
     168   "exclusively English." 414 US at 566.
           "instructional program." 20 USC sec 1703f 1976.
           "equal opportunity." 118 Cong Rec 8928 1972.
           "matter instruction." 480 F Supp at 22, E.D.N.Y., 1978; cf. 648 F.2d
           989, 5th Cir., 1981.
     169   "City alone." *The New York Times*, November 10, 1985, Section 12.
           "in 1987." *Official Gazette of the European Community*, July 18, 1988, Doc.
           A2-302/87.
     170   "is the law." Commission on the Education of the Deaf (1988). *Toward
           Equality: Education of the Deaf*. Washington, DC: U.S. Government
           Printing Office, p. 42.
           "school and self." A. Willig (1985). "A meta-analysis of selected studies
           on the effectiveness of bilingual education." *Review of Educational Re-
           search*, 55, 269–317.
           "that curriculum." J. Cummins (1986). Empowering minority stu-
           dents: a framework for intervention. *Harvard Educational Review*, 56,
           18–36, p. 25.
           "solving problems." K. Hakuta (1986). *Mirror of Language: The Debate
           on Bilingualism*. New York: Basic Books. Also see W. Lambert (1977).
           Culture and language as factors in education. In F. Eckman, ed.,
           *Current Themes in Linguistics: Bilingualism, Experimental Linguistics, and
           Language Typologies*. Washington, DC: Hemisphere Publishing;
           M. Swain and J. Cummins (1979). Bilingualism, cognitive functioning,
           and education. *Language Teaching and Linguistics: Abstracts*, 12, 4–18.
     171   "minority-language users." J. D. Haft (1983). Assuring equal educa-
           tional opportunity for language-minority students: bilingual educa-
           tion and the Equal Educational Opportunity Act of 1974. *Columbia
           Journal of Law and Social Problems*, 18, 209–93.
     174   "successful program." Adapted from T. Skutnabb-Kangas (1988).
           Multilingualism and the education of minority children. In T. Skut-
           nabb-Kangas and J. Cummins, *Minority Education*. Philadelphia: Multi-
           lingual Matters, pp. 9–44.
     177   "of acquisition." H. Lane and J.-Y. Dommergues (1976). On two inde-
           pendent sources of error in learning the syntax of a second language.
           Language Learning, 111–23. Also see V. Charrow and J. D. Fletcher
           (1974). English as the second language of deaf children. *Developmental
           Psychology*, 10, 436–70; V. Charrow and R. Wilbur (1975). The deaf
           child as a linguistic minority. *Theory into Practice*, 14, 353–59.
     178   "their language." S. Crain and D. Shankweiler (1991). Modularity and
           learning to read. In I. Mattingly and M. Studdert-Kennedy, eds.,
           Modularity and the Motor Theory of Speech Perception (pp. 375–92). Hills-
           dale, NJ: Lawrence Erlbaum.
           "reading achievement." V. Hanson (1989). Phonology and reading:
           Evidence from profoundly deaf readers. In D. Shankweiler and I. Y.

Liberman, eds., *Phonology and Reading Disability: Solving the Reading Puzzle*. Ann Arbor: University of Michigan Press; V. L. Hanson (1986). Access to spoken language and the acquisition of orthographic structure: evidence from deaf readers. *Quarterly Journal of Experimental Psychology, 38(2)*, 193–212; D. Lillo-Martin, V. Hanson, and S. T. Smith (1989). Deaf readers' comprehension of complex syntactic structure. In D. S. Martin, ed., *Working Papers of the Second International Symposium on Cognition, Education and Deafness* (pp. 258–82). Washington, DC: Gallaudet University Press. The low correlation is reported in A. E. Geers and J. S. Moog (1987). Factors predictive of the development of reading and writing skills in the congenitally deaf: report of the oral sample. Final report to NINCDS. St. Louis, MO: Central Institute for the Deaf. Likewise, Moores and Sweet (1990) find "little relationship between the reading of severely to profoundly deaf adolescents with deaf parents and their hearing and speech skills" (p. 182). They reached the same conclusion with respect to deaf children of hearing parents: "Measures of hearing and fluency in oral . . . communication are not predictive of literacy" (p. 197). D. Moores and C. Sweet (1990). Factors predictive of school achievement. In D. F. Moores and K. Meadow-Orlans, eds., *Educational and Developmental Aspects of Deafness* (pp. 154–201). Washington, DC: Gallaudet University Press. The following study reports that deaf students are sensitive to the underlying regularities of English spelling, and that many subjects with poor speech were, nevertheless, good spellers: V. L. Hanson, D. Shankweiler, and F. W. Fischer (1983). Determinants of spelling ability in deaf and hearing adults: access to linguistic structure. *Cognition, 14*, 323–44.

179 "of letters." V. Hanson (1982). Use of orthographic structure by deaf adults: recognition of fingerspelled words. *Applied Psycholinguistics, 3*, 343–56.

"write it." C. Padden (1990). The acquisition of fingerspelling in deaf children. In P. Siple and S. Fischer, eds., *Theoretical Issues in Sign Language Research* (pp. 2–22). Chicago: University of Chicago Press; V. L. Hanson, D. Shankweiler, F. W. Fischer (1983). Determinants of spelling ability in deaf and hearing adults: access to linguistic structure. *Cognition, 14*, 323–44.

"these strategies." D. Lillo-Martin, V. Hanson, and S. T. Smith (1989). Deaf readers' comprehension of complex syntactic structure. In D. S. Martin, ed., *Working Papers of the Second International Symposium on Cognition, Education and Deafness* (pp. 258–82). Washington, DC: Gallaudet University Press.

"English translations." V. Hanson and C. A. Padden (1989). Computers and Videodisc technology for bilingual ASL/English instruction of deaf children. In D. Nix and R. Spiro, eds., *Cognition, Education, and Multi-Media: Exploring Ideas in High Technology*. Hillsdale, NJ: Erlbaum.

180 "monolingual students." T. Skutnabb-Kangas (1988). Multilingualism and the education of minority children. In T. Skutnabb-Kangas and

J. Cummins, eds., *Minority Education: From Shame to Struggle* (pp. 9–44). Philadelphia: Multilingual Matters.

Page 181 "be integrated." I. Shor and P. Freire (1987). *A Pedagogy for Liberation*. South Hadley, MA: Bergin & Garvey.

182 "in Spanish." B. J. Mace-Matluck, W. A. Hoover, and R. C. Calfee (1984). *Teaching Reading to Bilingual Children*. Austin, TX: Southwest Educational Development Laboratory. Also see S. J. Campos and H. R. Keatinge (1988). The Carpinteria language minority student experience: from theory, to practice, to success. In T. Skutnabb-Kangas and J. Cummins. *Minority Education*. Philadelphia: Multilingual Matters, pp. 299–307.

"native language." M. Swain and S. Lapkin (1991). Additive bilingualism and French immersion education: the roles of language proficiency and literacy. In A. G. Reynolds, ed., *Bilingualism, Multiculturalism and Second Language Learning*. Hillsdale, NJ: Lawrence Erlbaum, pp. 203–16.

183 "Greek compositions." V. Kourbetis (1987). Deaf children of deaf parents and deaf children of hearing parents in Greece: a comparative study. Ph.D. dissertation, Boston University.

"secondary discourses." J. Gee (1986). Orality and literacy: from *The Savage Mind* to *Ways with Words*. *TESOL Quarterly*, *20*, 719–46; J. Gee (1990). *Social Linguistics and Literacies*. Philadelphia: Taylor and Francis.

184 "and poetry." S. Rutherford (1988). The culture of American Deaf people. *Sign Language Studies*, *59*, 129–47.

"some principles." R. E. Johnson, S. K. Liddell, and C. J. Erting (1989). Unlocking the curriculum: principles for achieving access in deaf education. *Gallaudet Research Institute Working Papers*.

191 "spring holidays." The description of the Gallaudet Revolution is an abridged version of "The week the world heard Gallaudet," *Gallaudet Alumni Newsletter*, *22*, 1988, 1–3, by Jack Gannon.

192 "academic underachievement." J. G. Carrier (1983). Masking the social in educational knowledge: the case of learning disability theory. *American Journal of Sociology*, *88(5)*, 949–74.

193 "rational decisions." S. Tomlinson (1982). *A Sociology of Special Education*. Boston: Routledge and Kegan Paul.

194 "several cities." *Coup d'Oeil*, Bureau 816, Ecole des Hautes Etudes en Sciences Sociales, 54 Boulevard Raspail, 75006 Paris, France. *Deux Langues Pour Une Education*, JUZES, 31540 St. Félix de Lauragais, France.

"the Sorbonne." A. Karakostas (1990). *Le pouvoir des signes*. Paris: Institut National des Jeunes Sourds; C. Cuxac. L'Education des sourds en France depuis l'abbé de l'Epée. Doctorat de Troisième Cycle, Université de Paris V, 1980. Reprint: *Le langage des sourds*. Paris: Payot, 1983; W. Moody (1983). *Introduction à l'histoire et à la grammaire de la langue des signes. Entre les mains des sourds*. Paris: International Visual Theater. The *Cahiers de l'histoire des sourds* is published by the Association Etienne de Fay, 46ter rue Ste. Catherine, 4500 Orléans. Also see J. Grémion (1990). *La planète des sourds*; Paris: Messinger.

195 "Great Britain." There is a trailblazing program at Durham University to prepare teachers of BSL. See A. C. Denmark (1990). British Sign Language tutor training course. In S. Prillwitz and T. Vollhaber, eds., *Sign Language Research and Application*. Hamburg: Signum, pp. 253–60.

"Malkowski." Ontario Ministry of Education (1989). *Review of Ontario Education Programs for Deaf and Hard-of-Hearing Students*. Toronto: Ministry of Education.

196 "in Germany." In S. Prillwitz and T. Vollhaber, eds. (1990). *Sign Language Research and Application*. Hamburg: Signum; P. Boyes-Braem (1991). Research cultures. *Signpost, 2(3)*, 2–4.

197 "educator writes." Cited in S. Davies (1991). *Bilingual Education of Deaf Children in Sweden and Denmark: Strategies for Transition and Implementation*. Washington, DC: Gallaudet Research Institute, p. 9. Also see I. Ahlgren (1990). Swedish conditions: sign language in deaf education (pp. 91–94). And: B. Bergman and L. Wallin (1990). Sign language research and the deaf community (pp. 187–214). In S. Prillwitz and T. Vollhaber, eds. (1990). *Sign Language Research and Application*. Hamburg: Signum.

198 "government mandate." S. Davies (1990). Two languages for deaf children in Sweden and Denmark. *International Rehabilitation Review, Ideas Portfolio, 11*. B. Hansen (1990). Trends in the progress towards bilingual education for deaf children in Denmark. In S. Prillwitz and T. Vollhaber, eds. *Sign Language Research and Application* (pp. 51–62). Hamburg: Signum.

199 "Spanish-speaking children." R. Porter (1990). *Forked Tongue: The Politics of Bilingual Education*. New York: Basic Books.

Part Seven. Bio-Power versus the Deaf Child

203 "social deviations." P. Rabinow, ed. (1984). *The Foucault Reader*. New York, Pantheon, p. 21.

205 "next child." Cochlear Corporation meeting in Boston, October 29, 1990. Scientists at the Cochlear Corporation list enrollment in an educational program with a strong oral/aural component as a criterion for patient selection: A. L. Beiter, S. J. Staller, and R. C. Dowell (1991). Evaluation and device programming in children. *Ear and Hearing*, Supplement, *12(4)*, 25S–33S.

"private therapists." E. H. Domico (1988). Managing a children's cochlear implant program. *Hearing Instruments, 39*. The implant team at the Manhattan Eye, Ear, and Throat Hospital reported in a promotional meeting sponsored in Boston on October 29, 1990, by the Cochlear Corporation that they work closely with the schools to emphasize oral skills, and seek adjustment of the IEP.

Page 205 "total communication." S. Staller of the Cochlear Corporation reported at the Third Symposium on Cochlear Implants in Children, held at Indiana University School of Medicine in January 1990, that among their selection criteria were an educational environment with a strong auditory component. When implanted children attending oral and total communication programs were matched for age at onset of deafness, there was no difference between the groups in performance on various speech perception measures. Staller et al. (1991) report that there was no difference between the speech perception scores of children in oral programs and those in total communication programs, once differences in age at onset of deafness in the two samples are controlled for. S. S. Staller, R. C. Dowell, A. L. Beiter, J. A. Brimacombe, and P. Arndt (1991). Perceptual abilities of children with the Nucleus 22-channel cochlear implant. *Ear and Hearing*, Supplement, *12(4)*, 34S–47S. A similar finding was obtained by M. J. Osberger, R. T. Miyamoto, S. Zimmerman-Phillips, J. L. Kemink, B. Stroer, J. B. Firszt, and M. A. Novak (1991). Independent evaluations of the speech perception abilities of children with the Nucleus 22-channel cochlear implant system. *Ear and Hearing*, Supplement, *12(4)*, 66S–80S.

206 "of time." R. I. Kohut, ed. (1988). Cochlear implants. *National Institutes of Health Consensus Development Conference Statement*, 7, 1–25, p. 16.

207 "medical problem." J. W. Evans (1989). Thoughts on the psychosocial implications of cochlear implantation in children. In E. Owens and D. Kessler, eds., *Cochlear Implants in Young Deaf Children* (pp. 307–14). Boston, MA: Little, Brown.

"States alone." A. House (1990). Cochlear implants in children; past and present perspectives. Address to the Third Symposium on Cochlear Implants in Children, Indiana University School of Medicine, Indianapolis, IN, January 1990.

208 "States alone." Food and Drug Administration, Center for Devices and Radiological Health (1990). Cochlear implant for children ages 2 through 17 years. Press release, June 28, 1990. Washington, DC: Department of Health and Human Services.

"hearing aid." R. I. Kohut, ed. (1988). Cochlear implants. *National Institutes of Health Consensus Development Conference Statement*, 7, 1–25, p. 4.

"to end." I. Illich (1976). *Medical Nemesis*. New York: Pantheon.

209 "of adults." P. Conrad and J. Schneider (1985). *Deviance and Medicalization*. New York: Merrill.

"private troubles." C. Wright Mills cited in S. Tomlinson (1982). *A Sociology of Special Education*. Boston: Routledge and Kegan Paul, p. 105.

"the school." "Many disabled people describe the feelings of 'belonging' to the medical profession who define us in terms of our diagnosis, 'she is a spastic,' e.g., who assess and define our rights to physical and financial assistance, who plan and manage our health care, whose signatures on bits of paper override our own judgment in even the most personal and fundamental areas of our lives." R. Rieser and M. Mason (1990). *Disability Equality in the Classroom: A Human Rights Issue*. London: ILEA, p. 14. Cited in J. Corbett (1990). Watching and listening: a pediatrician's career, 1944–1986. *Disability, Handicap and Society*, 5, 185–98, p. 185.

"of mind." P. Conrad and J. Schneider (1985). *Deviance and Medicalization*. New York: Merrill.

"that culture." B. J. Good and M.-J. Delvecchio Good (1982). Toward a meaning-centered analysis of popular illness categories: "fright illness" and "heart distress" in Iran. In A. J. Marsella and G. M. White, eds., *Cultural Conceptions of Mental Health and Therapy* (pp. 141–66). Dordrecht, Holland: Reidel.

"*Times Magazine*." B. Werth (1991). How short is too short? *New York Times Magazine*, June 16, 1991, 14–17, 28–29, 47.

210 "the individual." A. Caplan, H. T. Engelhardt, and J. J. McCartney, eds. (1981). *Concepts of Health and Disease* (pp. 119–29). Reading, MA: Addison-Wesley, p. xxv.

"different goals." P. Sedgwick (1981). Illness—Mental and otherwise. In A. Caplan, H. T. Engelhardt, and J. J. McCartney, eds., *Concepts of Health and Disease* (pp. 119–29). Reading, MA: Addison-Wesley, p. 123.

"or infirm." L. S. King (1981). What is disease? In A. Caplan, H. T. Engelhardt, and J. J. McCartney, eds., *Concepts of Health and Disease* (pp. 107–18). Reading, MA: Addision-Wesley, p. 111.

"specific illness." B. J. Good and M.-J. Delvecchio Good (1982). Toward a meaning-centered analysis of popular illness categories: "fright illness" and "heart distress" in Iran. In A. J. Marsella and G. M. White, eds., *Cultural Conceptions of Mental Health and Therapy* (pp. 141–66). Dordrecht, Holland: Reidel.

211 "in Denmark." N. E. Waxler (1981). The social labeling perspective on illness and medical practice. In L. Eisenberg and A. Kleinman, eds., *The Relevance of Social Science for Medicine* (pp. 283–306). Dordrecht, Holland: Reidel, p. 300.

"the treatments." H. T. Engelhardt (1981). The disease of masturbation: values and the concept of disease. In A. Caplan, H. T. Engelhardt, and J. J. McCartney, eds., *Concepts of Health and Disease* (pp. 267–80). Reading, MA: Addison-Wesley.

"social negotiations." N. E. Waxler (1981). The social labeling perspective on illness and medical practice. In L. Eisenberg and A. Kleinman, eds., *The Relevance of Social Science for Medicine* (pp. 283–306). Dordrecht, Holland: Reidel.

212 "or not." P. Ménière (1853). Quoted in A. Houdin, *De la surdi-mutité; examen critique et raisonné de la discussion soulevée à l'Académie Impériale de Médecine de Paris, séances des 19 et 26 avril 1853 sur cinq questions*. Paris: Lubé, 1855, p. 14.

"charged metal." Luigi Galvani (1737–1798), published in 1791.

"lymphatic excrement." A. Corone (1960). Contribution à l'histoire de la sonde d'Itard. *Histoire de la Médecine*, 10, 41–42.

Page 213 "without effect." J. M. G. Itard (1842). *Traité des maladies de l'oreille et de l'audition*, 2d ed.: Paris: Méquignon-Marvis fils, p. 342.

"dry up." P. Ménière (1853). *De la guérison de la surdi-mutité et de l'éducation des sourds-muets. Exposé de la discussion qui a eu lieu à l'Académie Impériale de Médecine, avec notes critiques*. Paris: Baillière, p. 47.

"about it." A. Esquiros (1847). Les Sourds-Muets. In *Paris au XIX siècle*, Vol. 2. Paris: Imprimerie Unis, pp. 391–492, p. 412.

"born parents." A. G. Bell (1920). Is race suicide possible? *Journal of Heredity*, *11*, 339–41.

214 "the desirables." A. G. Bell to David Fairchild, November 23, 1908. Bell papers, Library of Congress. Quoted in R. Winefield (1987). *Never the Twain Shall Meet*. Washington, DC: Gallaudet University Press, p. 83.

"the society." A. G. Bell (1883). *Memoir Upon the Formation of a Deaf Variety of the Human Race*. New Haven: National Academy of Sciences. A. G. Bell (1884). Fallacies concerning the deaf. *American Annals of the Deaf*, *29*, 32–69, p. 66. Reprint: Washington, DC: Gibson, 1884.

215 "hearing teachers." A. G. Bell (1883). *Memoir Upon the Formation of a Deaf Variety of the Human Race*. New Haven: National Academy of Sciences.

"the world?" Conference of Executives of American Schools for the Deaf (1884). *Proceedings*, p. 178.

"deaf education." S. Hegarty and P. Pocklington (1982). *Integration in Action*. Windsor: NFER-Nelson. Cited in T. Booth (1988). Challenging conceptions of integration. In L. Barton, ed., *The Politics of Special Educational Needs* (pp. 99–122). Philadelphia: Falmer Press, p. 120.

"educational programme." T. Cole (1986). *Residential Special Education*. Milton Keynes, Open University Press. Cited in T. Booth (1988). Challenging conceptions of integration. In L. Barton, ed., *The Politics of Special Educational Needs* (pp. 99–122). Philadelphia: Falmer Press, p. 120.

"not reproduce." R. H. Johnson (1918). The marriage of the deaf. *Jewish Deaf*, 5–6, p. 6.

"on Bell." Quoted in S. H. Mitchell (1971). The haunting influence of Alexander Graham Bell. *American Annals of the Deaf*, *116*, 349–56, p. 355.

"human stock." American Genetic Association, Eugenics Section (1912). . . . *American Sterilization Laws. Preliminary Report of the Committee of the Eugenics Section of the American Breeders Association to Study and to Report on the Best Practical Means for Cutting Off the Defective Germ Plasm in the Human Population*. London: Eugenics Educational Society, p. 3.

216 "degenerate persons." M. Haller (1963). *Eugenics: Hereditarian Attitudes in American Thought*. New Brunswick: Rutgers University Press, p. 133; D. May and D. Hughes (1987). Organizing services for people with mental handicap: The Californian experience. *Disability, Handicap and Society*, 2, 213–30, p. 215.

"eugenics movement." P. Conrad and J. Schneider (1985). *Deviance and Medicalization*. New York: Merrill, p. 12.

"hearing person." A. G. Bell (1891). Marriage. *Science, 17(424),* 160–163. Reprinted: *Silent World, 5(6),* 1891, 1,4; *Marriage: An Address to the Deaf,* 3rd ed. Washington, DC: Sanders, 1898.

217 "the surgery." J. Kveton (1991). The status of cochlear implantation in children. Surgery Subcommittee on Cochlear Implants, American Academy of Otolaryngology, Head and Neck Surgery. *Journal of Pediatrics, 118,* 1–7.

"Nucleus-22 device." N. Cohen, R. Hoffman, and M. Stroschein (1988). Medical or surgical complications related to the Nucleus multichannel cochlear implant. *Annals of Otology, Rhinology, and Laryngology,* Supplement, *97,* 8–13. Also see I. M. Windmill, S. A. Martinez, M. B. Nolph, and B. A. Eisenmenger (1990). Surgical and nonsurgical complications associated with cochlear prosthesis implantation. *The American Journal of Otology, 11,* 415–420.

"and complications." Food and Drug Administration (1990). *Summary of Safety and Effectiveness Data, Pre-Market Approval Application P890027.* June 27, 1990. Clark, Cohen, and Shepherd (1991) report a medical/surgical complication rate of 6.8 percent in 309 children. G. M. Clark, N. L. Cohen, and R. K. Shepherd (1991). Surgical and safety considerations of multichannel cochlear implants in children. *Ear and Hearing,* Supplement, *12(4),* 15S–24S.

"for life." A. House (1990). Cochlear implants in children: past and present perspectives. Address to the Third Symposium on Cochlear Implants in Children, Indiana University School of Medicine, Indianapolis, IN, January 1990.

"serious structural damage." G. E. Loeb (1989). Neural prosthetic strategies for young children. In E. Owens and D. Kessler, eds., *Cochlear Implants in Young Deaf Children* (137–52). Boston: Little, Brown, p. 142.

"no problem." Statements made at the Third Symposium on Cochlear Implants in Children, Indiana University School of Medicine, Indianapolis, IN, January 1990. Also see G. M. Clark, N. L. Cohen, and R. K. Shepherd (1991). Surgical and safety considerations of multichannel cochlear implants in children. *Ear and Hearing,* Supplement, *12(4),* 15S–24S.

218 "in the cochlea." J. B. Nadol, Y. S. Young, and R. J. Glynn (1989). Survival of spiral ganglion cells in profound sensorineural hearing loss: implications for cochlear implantation. *Annals of Otology, Rhinology and Laryngology, 98,* 411–16. Beiter, Staller, and Dowell (1991) state that "families should be counselled that the degree of auditory nerve viability is important to the amount of postoperative benefit realized with the [implant] device" but "preoperative predictors of the number of surviving cells are not available" (p. 28S). A. L. Beiter, S. J. Staller, and R. C. Dowell (1991). Evaluation and device programming in children. *Ear and Hearing,* Supplement, *12(4),* 25S–33S. Some patients with late-onset deafness of hereditary origin receive excellent benefit from a cochlear implant, however.

"growth occurs." A. House (1990). Cochlear implants in children:

past and present perspectives. Address to the Third Symposium on Cochlear Implants in Children, Indiana University School of Medicine, Indianapolis, IN, January 1990.

Page 219 "thumb's width." A. J. Hudspeth (1989). How the ear's works work. *Nature*, *341*, 397–404.

220 "from the implant." E. Owens (1989). Present status of adults with cochlear implants. In E. Owens and D. Kessler, eds., *Cochlear Implants in Young Deaf Children* (pp. 25–52). Boston: Little, Brown, p. 44.

"learning English." S. S. Staller, A. L. Beiter, J. A. Brimacombe, D. J. Mecklenburg, and P. Arndt (1991). Pediatric performance with the Nucleus 22-channel cochlear implant system. *American Journal of Otology*, Supplement, *12*, 126–36. In a later report, with typically ten more subjects on most open-set tests of speech perception, a third such test (Phonetically Balanced Kindergarten list, PBK) showed significantly improved scores after implantation and a year of training; these scores averaged 11.8 percent. Plots of individual data reveal that about half of the implanted children scored zero on these tests while using the implant, whereas the other half achieved scores ranging from a little above zero to 100 percent. Lip-reading scores were enhanced 20 percent and 12 percent on two different tests administered one year following implantation.

This article provides some information on the improvement in speech perception to be expected from longer-term implant use and training. Mean accuracy of sentence recognition ("CID Sentences") rose from 13 to 20 percent three years after implantation, but most early-deafened children still showed no ability to recognize sentences on this test after three years. The open-set test with mean score 11 percent cited above ("Spondee Recognition") rose to 20 percent three years after implantation. The increase in the third test in which there was significant improvement is not reported, but another open-set test (a linguistically and perceptually simple one, the "GASP") rose from 23 to 56 percent; however, the latter sample was a small subset of the original group. S. S. Staller, R. C. Dowell, A. L. Beiter, J. A. Brimacombe, and P. Arndt (1991). Perceptual abilities of children with the Nucleus 22-channel cochlear implant. *Ear and Hearing*, Supplement, *12(4)*, 34S–47S.

Osberger et al. (1991) examined twenty-eight children who had used the Nucleus 22-channel implant for an average of 1.7 years; the children varied in the age at which they had become deaf: some were born deaf and others deafened as late as ten years old. They scored an average of 6 percent correct on the PBK test and 15 percent correct on the common phrases test. A little more than half the children (61 percent) showed some open-set recognition; this more successful subset had mean scores of 11 and 24 percent correct on the two tests, respectively. Only six out of twenty-eight children scored better than zero on both tests. And "even those children who demonstrated open-set speech recognition in a quiet structured setting continue to experience communicative difficulty outside the clinic, especially in noisy classrooms" (p. 77S). Lip-reading scores were only slightly enhanced one year after implantation. M. J. Osberger, R. T. Miyamoto, S. Zimmerman-Phillips, J. L. Kemink, B. Stroer, J. B. Firszt, and M. A. Novak (1991). Independent evaluations of the speech perception abilities of children with the Nucleus 22-channel cochlear implant system. *Ear and Hearing*, Supplement, *12(4)*, 66S–80S. Tyler (1990) reports several measures of speech perception for five children ages six to ten using the Nucleus 22-channel implant who received training in lip-reading before implant and extensive auditory and verbal training (four to twenty months) after surgery. One child deaf since birth scored 6 percent on a test of open-set word recognition (the other child deaf since birth could not be tested with the standardized list). The remaining children scored 2, 10, and 46 percent correct. The child deafened latest, at age five, yielded the lowest score: 2 percent. The author concludes that the direct influence of the training is difficult to judge. It is clear that there is wide variability in outcomes as yet unaccounted for. R. Tyler (1990). Speech perception with the Nucleus cochlear implant in children trained with the auditory/verbal approach. *American Journal of Otology*, *11*, 99–107. Chute and colleagues (1990) in a study of six children, three with the single-channel and three with the Nucleus 22-channel implant, found performance that at best attained consistent word recognition (percent correct not reported). This occurred in two children. One child was deafened at age two, implanted two years later with a single-channel device, and tested five years later. The child is described as atypical and a "star performer." The other child became deaf at age six years three months and received a multichannel device ten years later. P. M. Chute, S. A. Hellman, S. C. Parisier, and S. H. Selesnick (1990). A matched-pairs comparison of single and multichannel cochlear implants in children. *Laryngoscope*, *100*, 25–28. Berliner and colleagues examined open-set speech recognition by children implanted with the House/3M device. Half of the children implanted at the House Ear Institute scored zero on the open-set task; the average score for the group of children, many of whom were postlingually deafened, was 17.3 percent correct. The average score of the thirty-four children implanted at the seven other surgical sites investigated was 10.1 percent. K. I. Berliner, R. A. Stovall, W. F. House, and H. E. Maddox (1990). Investigator differences in the cochlear implantation of children. *Otolaryngology, Head and Neck Surgery*, *102*, 683–89.

"even lower." Staller and colleagues report that on the GASP test of speech perception, congenitally deaf children with implants had an average score of 10 percent; "perilingually" deafened children, those deafened after birth but before age five, had an average score, when using their implant, of 25 percent; and postlingually deafened children an average score with prosthesis of 45 percent. S. S. Staller, A. L. Beiter, J. A. Brimacombe, D. J. Mecklenburg, and P. Arndt

(1991). Pediatric performance with the Nucleus 22-channel cochlear implant system. *American Journal of Otology*, Supplement, *12*, 126–36.

Page 220 "of ten." M. J. Osberger, A. M. Robbins, R. T. Miyamoto, S. W. Berry, W. A. Myres, K. S. Kessler, and M. L. Pope (1991). Speech perception abilities of children with cochlear implants, tactile aids, or hearing aids. *American Journal of Otology*, Supplement, *12*, 105–15. Also see R. T. Miyamoto, M. J. Osberger, A. M. Robbins, and W. A. Myres (1991). Comparison of speech perception abilities in deaf children with hearing aids or cochlear implants. *Otolaryngology, Head and Neck Surgery*, *104*, 42–46.

"rehabilitative services." R. T. Miyamoto, M. J. Osberger, A. M. Robbins, and W. A. Myres (1991). Comparison of speech perception abilities in deaf children with hearing aids or cochlear implants. *Otolaryngology, Head and Neck Surgery*, *104*, 42–46, p. 46.

"hearing-impaired." R. M. Horn, R. J. Nozza, and J. N. Dolitsky (1991). Audiological and medical considerations for children with cochlear implants. *American Annals of the Deaf*, *136*, 82–86, p. 85.

221 "trickle in." See reviews in E. Owens and D. K. Kessler (1989). *Cochlear Implants in Young Deaf Children*. Boston: Little, Brown; J. Kveton (1991). The status of cochlear implantation in children. Surgery Subcommittee on Cochlear Implants, American Academy of Otolaryngology, Head and Neck Surgery. *Journal of Pediatrics*, *118*, 1–7; *American Journal of Otology*, Supplement, *12*, 1991; *Ear and Hearing*, Supplement, *12*, 1991.

"poor indeed." One study of the speech perception of fifty children using the 3M/House single-channel implant, who became deaf at various ages, found the median number of common words correctly identified in a set of twelve was one; the average was two: K. I. Berliner, L. L. Tonokawa, L. M. Dye, and W. F. House (1989). Open set speech recognition in children with a single-channel cochlear implant. *Ear and Hearing*, *10*, 237–42. "The 3M/House single-channel device should be capable, at best, of converting a totally deaf child into the equivalent of a profoundly deaf child with a little residual hearing—that is, a child with a hearing loss in the 100 to 110 dB range and no useful hearing above 1000Hz": A. Boothroyd (1989). Hearing aids, cochlear implants and profoundly deaf children. In E. Owens and D. Kessler, eds., *Cochlear Implants in Young Deaf Children* (pp. 81–100). Boston: Little, Brown, p. 89.

"valid way." A. L. Beiter, S. J. Staller, and R. C. Dowell (1991). Evaluation and device programming in children. *Ear and Hearing*, Supplement, *12(4)*, 25S–33S, p. 28S.

222 "word recognition." S. S. Staller, A. L. Beiter, J. A. Brimacombe, D. J. Mecklenburg, and P. Arndt (1991). Pediatric performance with the Nucleus 22-channel cochlear implant system. *American Journal of Otology*, Supplement, *12*, 126–36.

"multiple-choice test." S. S. Staller, A. L. Beiter, J. A. Brimacombe, D. J. Mecklenburg, and P. Arndt (1991). Pediatric performance with the Nucleus 22-channel cochlear implant system. *American Journal of Otology*, Supplement, *12*, 126–36.

223 "born deaf." M. J. Osberger, S. L. Todd, S. W. Berry, A. M. Robbins, and R. T. Miyamoto (1991). Effect of age of onset of deafness on children's speech perception abilities with a cochlear implant. *Annals of Otology, Rhinology, and Laryngology, 100*, 883–88.

"cochlear implants." E. Owens (1989). Present status of adults with cochlear implants. In E. Owens and D. Kessler, eds., *Cochlear Implants in Young Deaf Children* (pp. 25–52). Boston: Little, Brown, p. 45.

"in school." T. Allen and M. Karchmer (1990). Communication in classrooms for deaf students: student, teacher, and program characteristics. In H. Bornstein, ed., *Manual Communication: Implications for Education*. Washington, DC: Gallaudet University Press, pp. 45–66.

"grade higher." T. E. Allen (1986). Patterns of academic achievement among hearing-impaired students: 1974 and 1983. In A. N. Schildroth and M. A. Karchmer, eds., *Deaf Children in America* (pp. 161–206). San Diego, CA: College-Hill, p. 165.

"speech production." A. E. Geers and J. S. Moog (1987). *Factors Predictive of the Development of Reading and Writing Skills in the Congenitally Deaf: Report of the Oral Sample. Final Report to NINCDS*. St. Louis, Mo: Central Institute for the Deaf, p. 34.

"intensive training." Geers in an address to the Third Symposium on Cochlear Implants in Children, Indiana University School of Medicine, Indianapolis, IN, January 1990, reported no advantage to language development in six children using the Nucleus implant.

"things worse." N. Tiber (1985). A psychological evaluation of cochlear implants in children. *Ear and Hearing, 6*, 48S–51S, p. 50S. There were improvements in scores on some IQ subtests, which the author attributes to a reduction in "hyperkinetic behavior" when using the implant on the second test administration. Practice effects cannot be ruled out, however, and parents did not report changes in child behavior and adjustment as a result of the implant.

224 "the brain." E. Newport (1990). Maturational constraints on language learning. *Cognitive Science, 14*, 11–28.

"six months." See the review in S. Curtiss (1989). Issues in language acquisition relevant to cochlear implants in young children. In E. Owens and D. Kessler, eds., *Cochlear Implants in Young Deaf Children* (pp. 293–306). Boston: Little, Brown. Also see K. Meadow-Orlans (1987). An analysis of the effectiveness of early intervention programs for hearing impaired children. In M. J. Guralnick and F. C. Bennett, eds., *The Effectiveness of Early Intervention for At Risk and Handicapped Children* (pp. 325–57). New York: Academic Press, p. 326.

"age three." K. Meadow-Orlans (1987). An analysis of the effectiveness of early intervention programs for hearing impaired children. In M. J. Guralnick and F. C. Bennett, eds., *The Effectiveness of Early Intervention for At Risk and Handicapped Children* (pp. 325–57). New York: Academic Press.

Page 224 "sensory milieu." D. Kessler and E. Owens (1989). Conclusions: current considerations and future directions. In E. Owens and D. Kessler, eds., *Cochlear Implants in Young Deaf Children* (pp. 315–30). Boston: Little, Brown, p. 325; S. Curtiss (1989). Issues in language acquisition relevant to cochlear implants in young children. In E. Owens and D. Kessler, eds., *Cochlear Implants in Young Deaf Children* (pp. 293–306). Boston: Little, Brown; H. J. Neville and D. Lawson (1987). Attention to central and peripheral visual space in a movement detection task. III. Separate effects of auditory deprivation and acquisition of a visual language. *Brain Research, 405,* 284–94.

"the station." Dr. Moise Goldstein called this possibility to my attention. See L. Petitto and P. F. Marentette (1991). Babbling in the manual mode: Evidence for the ontogeny of language. *Science, 251,* 1493–96. These authors contend that "babbling is thus the mechanism by which infants discover the map between the structure of language and the means for producing this structure," p. 1495; E. Newport and R. Meier (1986). Acquisition of American Sign Language. In D. I. Slobin, ed., *The Cross-Linguistic Study of Language Acquisition.* Hillsdale, NJ: Lawrence Erlbaum; E. Newport (1990). Maturational constraints on language learning. *Cognitive Science, 14,* 11–28.

225 "and intelligibility." M. J. Osberger (1989). Speech production in profoundly hearing-impaired children with reference to cochlear implants. In E. Owens and D. Kessler, eds., *Cochlear Implants in Young Deaf Children* (pp. 257–82). Boston: Little, Brown, p. 261.

"himself understood." M. J. Osberger, A. M. Robbins, S. W. Berry, S. L. Todd, L. J. Hesketh, and A. Sedey (1991). Analysis of spontaneous speech samples of children with a cochlear implant or tactile aid. *American Journal of Otology,* Supplement, *12,* 151–64. The preceding paper cites R. Stark and H. Levitt (1974). Prosodic feature reception and production in deaf children. *Journal of the Acoustical Society of America, 55,* S63(A), as showing that "production skills cannot be inferred from perception abilities."

"the implant." M. J. Osberger (1989). Speech production in profoundly hearing-impaired children with reference to cochlear implants. In E. Owens and D. Kessler, eds., *Cochlear Implants in Young Deaf Children* (pp. 257–82). Boston: Little, Brown.

"extensive training." S. Staller at the October 29, 1990, meeting convened by the Cochlear Corporation in Boston. Tobey and Hasenstab (1991) assessed the effects of implantation on the intelligibility of the speech of children who had participated in the Food and Drug Administration clinical trials. About half the children had become deaf from meningitis; many of these were presumably deafened after learning English, but the mean age of onset of deafness in the group as a whole was about a year and a half. Judges who were instructed to write down the key words in simple sentences ("The flag is red, white and blue") uttered by a sample of twenty-four children who had not yet received their implants averaged 28 percent correct; after a year of using the implant and training in speech and listening, the children were only slightly more intelligible: judges scored 36 percent correct on their key words. There was also no appreciable increase in the length of the children's spontaneous utterances after one year. E. A. Tobey and M. S. Hasenstab (1991). Effects of a Nucleus multichannel implant upon speech production in children. *Ear and Hearing,* Supplement, *12(4),* 48S–54S.

"hearing aids." M. J. Osberger (1989). Speech production in profoundly hearing-impaired children with reference to cochlear implants. In E. Owens and D. Kessler, eds., *Cochlear Implants in Young Deaf Children* (pp. 257–82). Boston: Little, Brown, p. 279. A similar conclusion is expressed in R. T. Miyamoto, M. J. Osberger, A. M. Robbins, and W. A. Myres (1991). Comparison of speech perception abilities in deaf children with hearing aids or cochlear implants. *Otolaryngology, Head and Neck Surgery, 104,* 42–46.

"be unintelligible." S. Wolk and A. N. Schildroth (1986). Deaf children and speech intelligibility: a national study. In A. N. Schildroth and M. A. Karchmer, eds., *Deaf Children in America* (pp. 139–60). San Diego, CA: College-Hill, p. 147.

"his life." M. J. Osberger, 1990, personal communication. In an address to the Research Laboratory of Electronics, M.I.T., December 1990, Dr. Osberger stated that even children who became deaf at a relatively late age and show large increases in speech perception with their prostheses continue to use ASL in academic situations and that all the children would use ASL for the rest of their lives.

226 "the implant." The child's name and the wording of the case history have been altered, so any resemblances to a particular child is coincidental.

"hearing parents." See, for example, D. Moores (1987). *Factors Predictive of Literacy in Deaf Adolescents with Deaf Parents. Final Report to NINCDS.* Washington, DC: Gallaudet University Press; A. Weisel and J. Reichstein (1988). Parental hearing status, reading comprehension skills, and social-emotional adjustment. In R. Ojala, ed., *Proceedings of the Tenth World Congress of the World Federation of the Deaf.* Helsinki: Finnish Association of the Deaf.

227 "(or eliminate) signing." N. Tye-Murray, ed. (1992). *Cochlear implants and children: A handbook for parents, teachers and speech and hearing professionals.* Washington, DC: A. G. Bell Assn., p. 51. The text further states: "Parents may observe their child using less sign language and relying more on speechreading and listening; encourage these behaviors" (p. 188).

"to be." E. Goffman (1963). *Stigma: Notes on the Management of Spoiled Identity.* Englewood Cliffs, NJ: Prentice-Hall, p. 87.

"of Deafness." J. W. Evans (1989). Thoughts on the psychosocial implications of cochlear implantation in children. In E. Owens and D. Kessler, eds., *Cochlear Implants in Young Deaf Children* (pp. 307–14). Boston: Little, Brown, p. 312.

228 "as schizophrenic." J. W. Small (1984). The crisis in adoption. *Journal of Social Psychiatry, 30,* 129–42.

Page 228 "and productivity." D. Ashmore (1990). Transcending the cultural conflicts between the deaf and hearing worlds: taming the stormy relationship. Unpublished ms., University of Tennessee, pp. 53–61.

229 "their teens." D. Kessler (1989). Present status of cochlear implants in children. In E. Owens and D. Kessler, eds., *Cochlear Implants in Young Deaf Children* (pp. 183–225). Boston: Little, Brown, p. 190. This "rash of adolescents who refuse to use the device" was reported at the Indiana meeting also. The Manhattan Eye, Ear and Throat Hospital team headed by Dr. Simon Parisier made a similar report in the Cochlear Corporation promotional meeting in Boston, October 29, 1990.

"cochlear implant." Manhattan Eye, Ear and Throat Hospital presentation at a meeting organized by the Cochlear Corporation in Boston, October 29, 1990.

"his skill." R. Mayberry and S. Fischer (1989). Looking through phonological shape to lexical meaning: the bottleneck of non-native sign language processing. *Memory and Cognition, 17*, 740–54.

"from birth." R. Mayberry (1990). Address to the Working Group on Concerns of the Deaf Community, National Institute on Deafness and Other Communicative Disorders.

"was deaf." J. W. Evans (1989). Thoughts on the psychosocial implications of cochlear implantation in children. In E. Owens and D. Kessler, eds., *Cochlear Implants in Young Deaf Children* (pp. 307–14). Boston: Little, Brown, p. 310.

"single-channel implant." A. L. Quittner, J. T. Steck, and R. L. Rouiller (1991). Cochlear implants in children: a study of parental stress and adjustment. *American Journal of Otology*, Supplement, *12*, 95–104.

230 "human narrative." O. Sacks (1990). Neurology and the soul. *New York Review of Books*. November 22, 1990, p. 45.

"the patient." A. Stewart, S. Greenfield, R. D. Hays, K. Wells, W. H. Rogers, S. D. Berry, E. McGlynn, and J. E. Ware (1989). Functional status and well-being of patients with chronic conditions: results from the medical outcomes study. *Journal of the American Medical Association*, 262, 907–13.

"life situation." E. Pellegrino and D. Thomasma (1988). *For the Patients' Good: The Restoration of Beneficence in Health Care*. New York: Oxford University Press, p. 78.

231 "statistical methods." Food and Drug Administration (1990). *Summary of Safety and Effectiveness Data, Pre-Market Approval Application P890027*. June 27, 1990.

"preschool years." M. J. Osberger, S. L. Todd, S. W. Berry, A. M. Robbins, and R. T. Miyamoto (1991). Effect of age of onset of deafness on children's speech perception abilities with a cochlear implant. *Annals of Otology, Rhinology, and Laryngology, 100*, 883–88.

"moral agents." P. Ramsey. *The Patient as Person*. New Haven: Yale University Press, 1970; P. Ramsey (1976). The enforcement of morals: Nontherapeutic research on children. *Hastings Center Report* 6 (August 1976), pp. 21–30; E. Pellegrino and D. Thomasma (1988). *For the*

Patients' Good: The Restoration of Beneficence in Health Care. New York: Oxford University Press.

232 "not encouraged." World Federation of the Deaf, Commission on Medicine, Audiology and Neuropsychiatry of the Tenth World Congress (1989). Recommendation 6, on cochlear implants. In R. Ojala, ed., *Proceedings of the Tenth World Congress of the World Federation of the Deaf*. Helsinki: Finnish Association of the Deaf.

"implant manufacturer." Letter from Dr. Jerome C. Goldstein, executive vice-president, American Academy of Otolaryngology—Head and Neck Surgery, to Mr. Charles Estes, executive director, National Association of the Deaf, dated February 13, 1991.

234 "and litigation." D. J. Rothman and S. R. Rothman (1980). The conflict over children's rights. *Hastings Center Reports, 10(3)*, 7–10.

"laws testify." C. Fried (1978). Children as subjects for medical experimentation. In J. van Eys, ed., *Research on Children* (pp. 107–15). Baltimore: University Park Press. J. Holt (1978). The right of children to informed consent. In J. van Eys, ed., *Research on Children* (pp. 5–16). Baltimore: University Park Press.

"an advocate." W. G. Bartholome (1978). Central themes in the debate over involvement of infants and children in biomedical research. In J. van Eys, ed., *Research on Children* (pp. 69–76). Baltimore: University Park Press. G. E. Pence (1980). Children's dissent to research: a minor matter? *IRB, 2*, 1–4.

"child advocate?" H. A. Cohen (1980). *Equal Rights for Children*. Totowa, NJ: Littlefield Adams. Howard Cohen makes the case that, on the grounds of social justice, we can have a single standard of rights for children and adults provided there are child agents—I have called them child advocates here—who give the child borrowed capacities he or she might otherwise lack.

235 "low enough." J. van Eys, ed. (1978). *Research on Children*. Baltimore: University Park Press.

"child is young." Staller et al. (1991) compared seventy implanted children who did better than chance at recognizing words with a like number who did not. There was no reliable difference between the groups in the number of years the children had been deaf before implantation. S. S. Staller, R. C. Dowell, A. L. Beiter, J. A. Brimacombe, and P. Arndt (1991). Perceptual abilities of children with the Nucleus 22-channel cochlear implant. *Ear and Hearing*, Supplement, *12(4)*, 34S–47S.

"would choose." R. A. McCormick (1976). Experimentation in children: sharing in sociality. *Hastings Center Report, 6(6)*, 41–46.

236 "the patient." E. Pellegrino and D. Thomasma (1988). *For the Patients' Good: The Restoration of Beneficence in Health Care*. New York: Oxford University Press, p. 113.

238 "it's a limitation." H. Fine and P. Fine, producers (March 1990). "60 Minutes." New York: Columbia Broadcasting System.

Index